METHODS IN MOLECULAR B

Series Editor
John M. Walker
School of Life Sciences
University of Hertfordshire
Hatfield, Hertfordshire, AL10 9AB, UK

For other titles published in this series, go to
www.springer.com/series/7651

METHODS IN MOLECULAR BIOLOGY™

Leukemia

Methods and Protocols

Edited by

Chi Wai Eric So

Professor and Chair in Leukaemia Biology, King's College London, London, UK

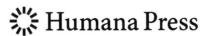 Humana Press

Editor
Chi Wai Eric So
Professor and Chair in Leukaemia Biology
King's College London
The University of London
London, UK
eric.so@icr.ac.uk

ISSN: 1064-3745   e-ISSN: 1940-6029
ISBN: 978-1-58829-989-5   e-ISBN: 978-1-59745-418-6
DOI: 10.1007/978-1-59745-418-6

Library of Congress Control Number: 2008941752

Cover illustration: Illustration by Pui Yi Tse.

Printed on acid-free paper

springer.com

Preface

Leukemia is a biologically and clinically diverse disease, and despite extraordinary advances in treatment over the past several decades, especially for childhood acute lymphoid leukemia, outcome remains poor for some subtypes and long-term therapy related side effects frequently associate with the treatment. There is considerable optimism however that the situation will improve.

Recent advances in molecular and cellular biology techniques have significantly improved our ability to detect, monitor, model and study the underlying molecular basis and aetiology of leukemia. The aim of this book "Leukemia" is to bring together a wide range of state-of-art laboratory methods and detailed protocols that are useful for both clinical and basic research scientists working on the disease. Leukemia contains chapters describing techniques for prenatal backtracking of leukemic clone, molecular diagnosis, detection of genome-wide genetic abnormalities and profiling, identification of unknown fusion genes, monitoring of minimal residual diseases, disease modelling using murine and human primary hematopoietic cells, studying of normal and malignant hematopoiesis, identification of interacting partners with leukemia associated oncoproteins, and global characterization of genome-wide epigenetic changes in leukemic cells. Leukemia should be of broad appeal to readers who are interested in molecular diagnosis, experimental Hematology, disease modelling and mechanistic studies of hematological malignancies.

Finally, I would like to express my greatest gratitude to all the authors for their useful and invaluable contributions, which constitute the most important elements of this book. Specific thanks are given to Mel Greaves for his constructive advice and support during the preparation of the book. Also I wish to thank Pui Yi Tse for assisting the editing, and professional graphic design. Clearly, we all share the same goal that this book will provide a useful reference to assist other investigators at different levels and aspects of leukemia research. Together, we will advance knowledge and have better understanding of the disease, which will ultimately improve anti-cancer therapy and quality of life for patients.

London, UK   *Chi Wai Eric So*

Contents

Contributors

SCOTT A. ARMSTRONG • *Department of Pediatric Oncology, Division of Hematology/Oncology, Children's Hospital, Dana Farber Cancer Institute, Harvard Medical School, Boston, MA, USA*

KERRY E. BARBER • *Cancer Sciences Division, University of Southampton, Southampton, UK*

DOMINIQUE BONNET • *Cancer Research UK London Research Institute, Haematopoietic Stem Cell Laboratory, London, UK*

SUE COLMAN • *Haemato-Oncology Section, The Institute of Cancer Research, London, UK*

ELAINE DZIERZAK • *Department of Cell Biology and Genetics, Erasmus University Medical Center, Rotterdam, The Netherlands*

CAROLYN A. FELIX • *Division of Oncology, Children's Hospital of Philadelphia, Philadelphia, PA, USA*

ZHAOHUI FENG • *Department of Pediatric Oncology, Division of Hematology/Oncology, Children's Hospital, Dana Farber Cancer Institute, Harvard Medical School, Boston, MA, USA*

MARIA EUGENIA FIGUEROA • *Developmental and Molecular Biology, Albert Einstein College of Medicine, Bronx, NY, USA*

MARIA-PAZ GARCIA-CUELLAR • *Department of Genetics, University Erlangen, Erlangen, Germany*

JOHN M. GREALLY • *Developmental and Molecular Biology, Albert Einstein College of Medicine, Bronx, NY, USA*

MEL GREAVES • *Haemato-Oncology Section, The Institute of Cancer Research, London, UK*

MANU GUPTA • *Cancer Research UK Medical Oncology Unit, Barts and the London School of Medicine and Dentistry, Queen Mary College, University of London, London, UK*

CHRISTINE J. HARRISON • *Cancer Sciences Division, University of Southampton, Southampton, UK*

JAY L. HESS • *Department of Pathology, University of Michigan Medical School, Ann Arbor, MI, USA*

MICHELLE KANG • *Laboratory for Molecular Epidemiology, University of California, San Francisco, CA, USA*

LYNDAL KEARNEY • *Haemato-Oncology Section, The Institute of Cancer Research, London, UK*

ZOË J. KONN • *Cancer Sciences Division, University of Southampton, Southampton, UK*

VALERIE KOUSKOFF • *Stem Cell Biology and Research, Paterson Institute for Cancer Research, University of Manchester, Manchester, UK*

ANDREI V. KRIVTSOV • *Department of Pediatric Oncology, Division of Hematology/ Oncology, Children's Hospital, Dana Farber Cancer Institute, Harvard Medical School, Boston, MA, USA*

GEORGES LACAUD • *Stem Cell Biology and Research, Paterson Institute for Cancer Research, University of Manchester, Manchester, UK*

CHRISTOPHE LANCRIN • *Stem Cell Biology and Research, Paterson Institute for Cancer Research, University of Manchester, Manchester, UK*

TERENCE R. LAPPIN • *Centre for Cancer Research and Cell Biology, Queen's University Belfast, Belfast, Ireland*

ROLF MARSCHALEK • *Institute of Pharmaceutical Biology, JWG-University of Frankfurt, Frankfurt, Germany*

GLENDA J. McGONIGLE • *Centre for Cancer Research and Cell Biology, Queen's University Belfast, Belfast, Ireland*

DENIZ MEDERER • *Department of Genetics, University Erlangen, Erlangen, Germany*

ARI M. MELNICK • *Developmental and Molecular Biology, Albert Einstein College of Medicine, Bronx, NY, USA*

CLAUS MEYER • *Institute of Pharmaceutical Biology, JWG-University of Frankfurt, Frankfurt, Germany*

THOMAS A. MILNE • *Laboratory of Biochemistry and Molecular Biology, The Rockefeller University, New York, NY, USA*

JAMES C. MULLOY • *Division of Experimental Hematology, Cincinnati Children's Hospital Medical Center, University of Cincinnati College of Medicine, Cincinnati, OH, USA*

KATRIN OTTERSBACH • *Department of Cell Biology and Genetics, Erasmus University Medical Center, Rotterdam, The Netherlands*

HELEN PARKER • *Leukaemia Research Cytogenetics Group, Cancer Sciences Division, University of Southampton, Southampton, UK*

STELLA PEARSON • *Stem Cell Biology and Research, Paterson Institute for Cancer Research, University of Manchester, Manchester, UK*

BLAINE W. ROBINSON • *Division of Oncology, Children's Hospital of Philadelphia, PA, USA*

HEIN SCHEPERS • *Department of Hematology, University Medical Center Groningen, University of Groningen, The Netherlands*

JAN JACOB SCHURINGA • *Department of Hematology, University Medical Center Groningen, University of Groningen, The Netherlands*

ROBERT K. SLANY • *Department of Genetics, University Erlangen, Erlangen, Germany*

CHI WAI ERIC SO • *The Institute of Cancer Research, and King's College London, London, UK*

PATRYCJA SROCZYNSKA • *Stem Cell Biology and Research, Paterson Institute for Cancer Research, University of Manchester, Manchester, UK*

JON C STREFFORD • *Leukaemia Research Cytogenetics Group, Cancer Sciences Division, University of Southampton, Southampton, UK*

ALEXANDER THOMPSON • *Centre for Cancer Research and Cell Biology, Queen's University Belfast, Belfast, Ireland*

VINCENT H.J. VAN DER VELDEN • *Department of Immunology, Erasmus MC, Erasmus University Medical Center, Rotterdam, The Netherlands*

JACQUES J.M. VAN DONGEN • *Department of Immunology, Erasmus MC, Erasmus University Medical Center, Rotterdam, The Netherlands*

YINGZI WANG • *Department of Pediatric Oncology, Division of Hematology/Oncology, Children's Hospital, Dana Farber Cancer Institute, Harvard Medical School, Boston, MA, USA*

JOSEPH WIEMELS • *Laboratory for Molecular Epidemiology, University of California, San Francisco, CA, USA*

SARAH L. WRIGHT • *Cancer Sciences Division, University of Southampton, Southampton, UK*

MARK WUNDERLICH • *Division of Experimental Hematology, Cincinnati Children's Hospital Medical Center, University of Cincinnati College of Medicine, Cincinnati, OH, USA*

JENNY YEUNG • *Haemato-Oncology Section, The Institute of Cancer Research, London, UK*

BRYAN D. YOUNG • *Cancer Research UK Medical Oncology Unit, Barts and the London School of Medicine and Dentistry, Queen Mary College, University of London, London, UK*

BERND ZEISIG • *Haemato-Oncology Section, The Institute of Cancer Research, London, UK*

KEJI ZHAO • *Laboratory of Molecular Immunology, National Heart, Lung and Blood Institute, National Institutes of Health, Bethesda, MD, USA*

Chapter 1

An Overview: From Discovery of Candidate Mutations to Disease Modeling and Transformation Mechanisms of Acute Leukemia

Chi Wai Eric So

Summary

Acute leukemia is an aggressive form of hematological malignancy, which is characterized and classified into different subtypes according to the morphology and immunophenotype of the leukemic blasts. However in the past decade, it became clear that it is the genetic makeup and probably the origin of leukemic stem cells, which determine the phenotype, aggressiveness, and prognosis of the disease. To further advance our knowledge, various molecular and cellular methodologies have been developed by clinical and basic researchers to not only identify and monitor these genetic changes in patients, but also model and dissect the underlying transformation mechanisms of the disease. In this chapter, I will summarize some of the key developments and latest technologies that have been instrumental to modern leukemia research.

Key words: Acute leukemia, Leukemic stem cells, Transcription factors, Epigenetics, Epigenome, Hematopoiesis, Self-renewal, Disease modeling

1. Introduction

Acute leukemia represents a group of complex and heterogeneous diseases, which are characterized by the accumulation of malfunctional and immature leukemic blasts in the bone marrow. Recurring chromosomal abnormalities found in over half of the patients are critical for classification of the disease, risk stratification, and design of treatment regiments. For example, 11q23 abnormalities involving *MLL* gene usually associates with poor prognosis, while t(15; 17) resulting in *PML-RARα* fusion

C.W.E. So (ed.), Leukemia, *Methods in Molecular Biology, vol. 538*
© Humana Press, a part of Springer Science + Business Media, LLC 2009
DOI: 10.1007/978-1-59745-418-6_1

is uniquely sensitive to the all-trans retinoic acid (ATRA) and arsenic trioxide (As$_2$O$_3$) treatment. Almost all the recurring primary abnormalities, with the exception of those affecting *ABL* gene, involve transcription factors, indicating a critical role of transcriptional deregulation in acute leukemogenesis *(1)*. The recent advances in the molecular and cellular biology techniques have greatly facilitated the functional characterization of candidate oncoproteins implicated in the pathogenic processes. An emerging common feature shared by these oncogenic transcription factors is their ability to enhance or even confer self-renewal to the targeted hematopoietic stem/progenitor cells, which allow accumulation of cooperative mutations for the development of full-blown leukemia *(2)*. Consistently, functional analyses using gene-targeted knockout approaches have also revealed their critical functions in generation and/or maintenance of hematopoietic stem cells (HSCs) for normal hematopoiesis *(3)*. Moreover, recent evidence from prenatal backtracking of the leukemic clone and disease modeling indicate that some of these recurring abnormalities, in particular, the formation of chimeric transcription factors, represent a very early and probably the initiating event in the leukemic stem cells (LSCs) that are critical for the induction and maintenance of the overt disease *(4)*. Further analyses of the leukemic cells from patients and animal models reveal transcriptional and epigenetic reprogramming mediated by oncogenic transcription factors, suggesting that aberrant recruitment of epigenetic regulator complexes may be a key and a potential therapeutic target for acute leukemia *(5)*. Although we start to get a grasp on the molecular and cellular basis of certain subtypes of leukemia, we are still at an early stage of the exploration and far from fully understanding the underlying mechanisms of the disease. Moreover, the collaborative mutations occurred in the leukemic cells and the genetic makeup of the leukemia, which does not carry notable genetic abnormalities, are still largely unknown. Thus further characterization and functional validation of candidate mutations identified by genomic approaches will inevitably be an important subject of intense research in the coming years.

2. Discovery and Characterization of Candidate Mutations

Conventional and molecular cytogenetics have been instrumental in identifying novel genetic mutations, and they remain as the major techniques for clinical diagnosis of specific subtypes of leukemia (*see* Chapter "Fluorescence In Situ Hybridization (FISH) as a Tool for the Detection of Significant Chromosomal Abnormalities in Childhood

Leukemia"). In combination with immunophenotyping, molecular cytogenetics also represents a powerful tool to identify the cell lineage in which the leukemia specific chromosome rearrangement occurs and has been used to identify putative preleukemic cells (*see* Chapter "Specialized Fluorescence In Situ Hybridization (FISH) Techniques for Leukemia Research"). In the case of chimeric fusions where only one of the partner genes is known, long-distance inversed polymerase chain reaction (LDI-PCR) (*see* Chapter "LDI-PCR: Identification of Known and Unknown Gene Fusions of the Human *MLL* Gene") and panhandle-PCR (*see* Chapter "Panhandle-PCR Approaches to Cloning *MLL* Genomic Breakpoint Junctions and Fusion Transcript Sequences") have been proved extremely useful for rapid identification of the fusion transcripts, which are critical for risk-stratification for disease treatment and monitoring of the minimal residual diseases (MRD) (*see* Chapter "MRD Detection in Acute Lymphoblastic Leukemia Patients Using Ig/TCR Gene Rearrangements as Targets for Real-Time Quantitative PCR"). With the explosion of array technology and bioinformatics, it is now possible to achieve high-resolution global assessment of genetic changes in the leukaemic cells. Array-based comparative genomic hybridization (aCGH) (*see* Chapter "Array-Based Comparative Genomic Hybridization as a Tool for Analyzing the Leukemia Genome") and single nucleotide polymorphisms (SNP) array (*see* Chapter "Application of SNP Genotype Arrays to Determine Somatic Changes in Cancer") are two major advances in the past decade that allow genome-wide detection of various submicroscopic somatic changes including loss, gain, and copy-neutral loss of heterozygosity (CN-LOH) that are frequently missed by cytogenetics and other conventional approaches. In addition to mutation discovery, it is equally important to identify the origin of the mutations and their functions in the leukemogenic processes. To unravel the clonal relationship and identify the origin of the disease in pediatric leukemia, prenatal backtracking has been one of the most powerful tools to trace back genetic events to early fetal origins using sensitive amplification methods (*see* Chapter "Backtracking of Leukemic Clones to Birth").

3. Functional Validation and Mechanistic Study on Candidate Mutations

To establish the pathological roles of candidate mutations identified in patients, it is essential to demonstrate their functions in disease progression. One of the most commonly used and successful methods for modeling leukemia is retroviral transduction and transformation assay (RTTA), in which purified populations of murine hematopoietic cells transduced with retroviruses-carrying candidate oncoproteins are transplanted into syngeneic mice for disease development (*see* Chapter "Retroviral/Lentiviral Transduction and Transformation Assay"). Using highly purified and distinctive populations of hematopoietic cells (*see* Chapter "Identification and Characterization of Hematopoietic Stem and Progenitor Cell Populations in Mouse Bone Marrow by Flow Cytometry") as the starting materials in RTTA in combination with expression array analysis, it allows characterization of the expression profile of the leukemic stem cells derived from distinctive cellular origins (*see* Chapter "Gene Expression Profiling of Leukaemia Stem Cells"), which are responsible for the initiation and probably maintenance of the disease. With the advances in developing immuno-compromised mouse models that can accept human xenografts, certain properties of leukemic stem cells can also be directly studied in human cell context via xenograft transplantation of purified leukemic cells into immunocompromised NOD/SCID mice (*see* Chapter "Humanized Model to Study Leukemic Stem Cells"). As a variant of murine RTTA (*see* Chapter "Retroviral/Lentiviral Transduction and Transformation Assay"), it is now possible to use human hematopoietic cells as the starting materials for transduction and transplantation assay into NOD/SCID mice, which may represent a step closer to humanized model (*see* Chapter "Model Systems for Examining Effects of Leukaemia Associated Oncogenes in Primary Human CD34+ Cells via Retroviral Transduction"). However, it is clear that only a subgroup of leukemic cells from patients can engraft and readout in NOD/SCID model. Ex vivo assays have thus been developed to assess the self-renewal property of leukemic cells by making use of well-established MS5 stromal cell culture (*see* Chapter "Ex Vivo Assays to Study Self-Renewal and Long-Term Expansion of Genetically Modified Primary Human Acute Myeloid Leukaemia Stem Cells"). In addition to malignant disease modeling, characterization of hematopoietic compartments by flow cytometry in genetically modified mice with targeted disruption of the candidate proteins can reveal their potential functions in normal hematopoiesis (*see* Chapter "Identification and Characterization of Hematopoietic Stem and Progenitor Cell Populations in Mouse Bone Marrow by Flow Cytometry"). Similar functional assessment can also be performed at even earlier developmental stages such as from embryonic stem cell (*see* Chapter "In Vitro Differentiation of ES Cells as a Model of Early Hematopoietic Development") and placental hematopoiesis (*see* Chapter "Analysis of the Mouse Placenta as a Hematopoietic Stem Cell Niche"). After characterization of the candidate mutations in normal and malignant hematopoiesis, it is essential to understand molecular functions of these mutations in order to design specific therapeutic strategy. Biochemical purification and yeast two-hybrid approaches (*see* Chapter "Identification of Protein Interaction Partners by the Yeast Two-Hybrid System") are two most common assays used for identification of interacting partners that are critical for transformation processes. Given the fact that transcriptional and epigenetic deregulation of important developmental genes such as *Hox* genes is central for acute leukemogenesis, assessment of global *Hox* expression (*see* Chapter "Complete Array of *HOX* Gene Expression by RQ-PCR") and genome-wide epigenetic changes in DNA (*see* Chapter "Genome-Wide Determination of DNA Methylation by *Hpa*II Tiny Fragment Enrichment by Ligation-Mediated PCR (HELP) for the Study of Acute Leukemias") and histone (*see* Chapter "Chromatin Immunoprecipitation (ChIP) for Analysis of Histone Modifications and Chromatin Associated Proteins") levels have and will continuously give important insights into the functions of candidate mutations and the composition of epigenome of the leukemic cells.

4. Conclusion

With the recent advances in cellular and molecular biology techniques, we are entering into a golden era where we can explore both the genome and epigenome of leukemia cells to identify and functionally validate critical events involved in the leukemogenic transformation. Having a better understanding of the biology of the disease, it will be possible to design and tailor specific approaches for detection, monitoring, and effective treatment regiments according to the cellular and molecular features of the diseases.

Acknowledgments

This work was supported by the Association for International Cancer Research (AICR), Cancer Research UK, the Kay Kendall Leukaemia Fund, Medical Research Council, Wellcome Trust, and Leukaemia Research Fund. Eric So is an AICR fellow and an EMBO young investigator.

References

1. Look AT. (1997). Oncogenic transcription factors in the human acute leukemias. *Science*;**278**(5340):1059–64.

2. Huntly BJ, Gilliland DG. (2005). Leukaemia stem cells and the evolution of cancer-stem-cell research. *Nat Rev Cancer*;**5**(4):311–21.

3. Pina C, Enver T. (2007). Differential contributions of haematopoietic stem cells to foetal and adult haematopoiesis: insights

from functional analysis of transcriptional regulators. *Oncogene*;**26**(47):6750–65.

4. Greaves MF, Wiemels J. (2003). Origins of chromosome translocations in childhood leukaemia. *Nat Rev Cancer*;**3**(9):639–49.

5. Rice KL, Hormaeche I, Licht JD. (2007). Epigenetic regulation of normal and malignant hematopoiesis. *Oncogene*;**26**(47):6697–714.

Chapter 2

Backtracking of Leukemic Clones to Birth

Joseph Wiemels, Michelle Kang, and Mel Greaves

Summary

Many of the acquired genetic changes that contribute to the molecular pathogenesis of leukemia are well characterized. The relative simplicity of the tumor genetics of the common subtypes of leukemia and the availability of archived material in the form of archived neonatal blood spots (ANB or Guthrie cards) has permitted the tracing of many genetic events to fetal origins using sensitive amplification methods. We here described methods for cloning translocations and other rearrangements for "backtracking" studies, and methods for sensitive detection of such rearrangements and a point mutation in ANB cards.

Key words: Leukemia, Translocation, Backtracking, Prenatal, KRAS2

1. Introduction

Childhood cancer, unlike most adult cancers, is a disease defined by relatively short latencies (or, time between the initiating mutation and clinically diagnosed tumor) which is at most the difference between the age of the child at diagnosis, and the embryonic origin of the organ or tissue from which the cancer arises. Given this short latency as well as the availability of archived stored material prior to the leukemia (i.e., ANB cards), it is possible to identify very early or initiating genetic events before birth. Leukemia, being a liquid tumor, is present in the general circulation without need for metastasis. Likewise, clinically silent preleukemic stem cells and their differentiated clonal progeny may also be present in circulation and therefore potentially detectable on a neonatal blood specimen at birth. This view is endorsed by the sharing of preleukemic clones by monozygotic twins via their common intraplacental vasculature (1). The knowledge that a particular

C.W.E. So (ed.), Leukemia, *Methods in Molecular Biology, vol. 538*
© Humana Press, a part of Springer Science + Business Media, LLC 2009
DOI: 10.1007/978-1-59745-418-6_2

mutation occurred before birth has several implications. First, it helps us understand the natural history, pathophysiology, and genetics of the most common cancer of childhood. Second, the information indicates the time period when key mutational events occur and can therefore help focus epidemiologic efforts to discover causes of leukemia. Third, a prenatal mutation is a potential target for early screening and intervention in leukemia. Finally, a positive result of the assay may have implications for the use of cord blood for transplantation purposes (2). While the assays we described in this section apply to ANB cards, they could also be used in studies of cord bloods. Cord blood has the advantage of containing RNA as a substrate for backtracking, but is much less available than ANB cards for research purposes and we confined our methods to ANB cards.

Genomic fusion gene sequences generated by chromosome translocations provide the ideal clonal marker for leukemia: (a) once formed they are stable, and (b) the unique nucleotide sequences present at fusion gene junctions provide good targets for PCR and can therefore be detected at high sensitivity coupled with high specificity. The essential caveats are that blood spots will only score positive if two conditions hold. One, that fusion gene function is a very early or initiating event in the particular leukemia being studied, and two, that the number of preleukemic progeny present in the blood at birth is sufficient to detect in a blood spot (at least one cell in ~30,000). A negative blood spot is uninterpretable. The detection of leukemia-specific genomic fusion sequences in Guthrie cards was first demonstrated for MLL-AF4 in infant ALL (3) and subsequently for the most common chromosome translocation of childhood B cell precursor ALL, TEL(ETV-6)/AML1(RUNX1) (4–6) and for other fusion genes, including those in childhood AML (7, 8). Fusion genes present in expanded cell populations of the "correct" lineage for the corresponding leukemia have also been demonstrated to exist at a relatively high frequency in unselected cord bloods via RT-PCR, RQ-PCR, and immuno-FISH methods (9). In cases where no unique fusion gene sequences are available, IGH or TCR clonotypic (rearranged) genomic sequences have been used as a surrogate marker of the leukemic clone (10–13). Although informative, these are not ideal or unambiguous markers as they are not always stable (i.e., continual rearrangements) and clone-specific rearrangements may exist in nontransformed cells. The most common genetic change in high hyperdiploid childhood acute leukemia is not currently amendable to high sensitivity molecular interrogation in blood spots. Nevertheless, retrospective analysis of archived cord blood (13) and twin studies (1) indicates that it too can be an early or initiating prenatal event in leukemogenesis.

Leukemia-specific point mutations have also been detected in ANB cards including most notably GATA1 mutations in patients with Down's syndrome and AMKL or neonatal transient myeloproliferative disease *(14)* and *NOTCH1* in T-ALL *(15)*. As microarray mapping of chromosome breakpoints becomes more available, more backtracking targets will be revealed. Here we considered the backtracking of chromosome abnormalities (translocations and deletions) and point mutations.

2. Materials

2.1. Patient Samples and DNA

1. Bone marrow cells from the leukemic patient (i.e., >40% blast cells). The patient sample should have full diagnostic information such as immunophenotype, karyotype, and any fluorescence in situ hybridization (FISH) data.
2. Matched ANB card for the same individual (*see* **Note 1**).
3. Ficoll solution for isolating mononuclear cells (Ficoll-Paque, Sigma-Aldrich) if bone marrow is fresh. (Frozen bone marrow can be used as well, but should not be subjected to mononuclear cell extraction.)
4. Appropriate reagents for DNA preparation: lysis buffer (10 mM Tris–HCL, pH 8.0, 100 mM EDTA, 0.5% SDS, 20 µg/ml RNAse A (added from a 10 mg/ml stock immediately before use), PCI (phenol, chloroform, isoamyl alcohol in a 25:24:1 ratio, Sigma-Aldrich), NH_4OAc (10 M), 100% ethanol, and 70% ethanol). Puregene Kit (Gentra/Qiagen) is a complete and excellent alternative and may be used in place of these reagents.
5. Large bore pipette tips (1 ml and 200 µl) or "cut tips" (conventional bore pipette tips with 5 mm cut off each tip to increase the bore).

2.2. PCR Reagents for Characterizing Leukemia DNA

1. Long distance polymerase. Elongase enzyme (Gibco BRL) is preferred for inverse PCR, but other LD polymerases are excellent for conventional long distance reactions (*see* **Note 2**).
2. If inverse PCR is indicated, 6- or 8-base restriction endonucleases should be chosen carefully, as appropriate for the PCR design (*see* **Subheading 3.3, step 2** and **Fig. 1b**).
3. QIAquick® gel extraction kit (Qiagen) for clean-up of ligation reaction for inverse PCR.
4. Isopropanol for use with the gel extraction kit.
5. 3 M sodium acetate (pH 5.0) and ethanol for use during ethanol precipitations of DNA.

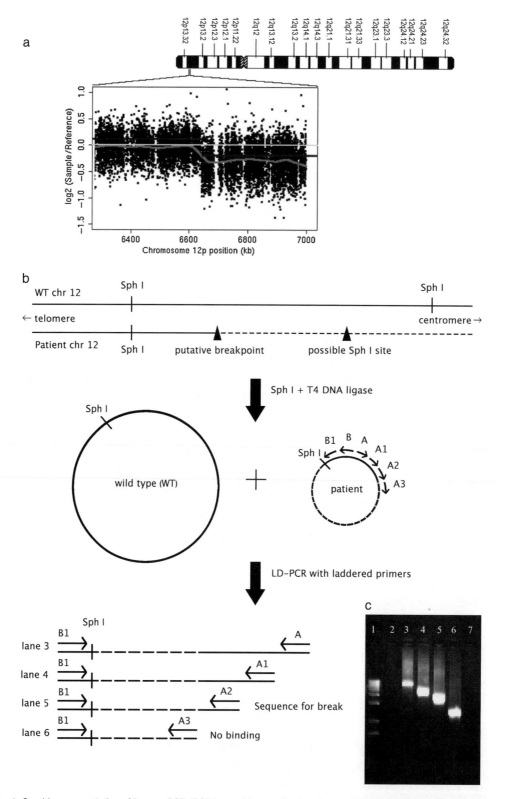

Fig. 1. Graphic representation of inverse PCR. IPCR is used to amplify an unknown sequence of DNA. (a) Map of a portion of chromosome 12 indicating base pair position and array comparative genomic hybridization data (Nimblegen array). The break in the arm of chromosome 12 can be seen as a drop in log$_2$ ratio at the right end of the figure. Directly in the center the drop in the log$_2$ ratio is shown as a disjoint in "change point" statistical analysis. (b) IPCR procedure.

6. Mineral Oil (Sigma, nuclease free) to prevent evaporation during long distance PCR.

7. Conventional short distance *Taq* polymerase required for confirming breakpoints (Roche, Applied Biosystems, others).

8. Deoxynucleotidyl transferases (dNTPs, set of four, dATP, dTTP, dCTP, dGTP), 10 mM stock of each (when combined in one solution), from manufacturers such as Applied Biosystems, Roche, etc.

9. High-quality oligonucleotides for long distance polymerization, available from multiple suppliers. In our experience, HPLC purification is not necessary and HPSF purification (MWG Biotech) is sufficient and excellent. Store as 100 µM stock at –80°C, and 10 µM aliquots at –20°C for usage within 6 months.

2.3. PCR Reagents for Characterizing ANB Cards Using Conventional PCR

1. AmpDirect buffers (Shimadzu, and Rockland Immunochemicals): a product that inhibits the deleterious effects of blood proteins and heme on PCR amplification (necessary only for cards stored at room temperature, *see* **Note 3**).

2. Blood card DNA purification kit (Qiagen QIAamp Micro DNA prep) necessary only for ANB cards stored at –20°C or colder.

3. Poly(A)+ RNA carrier RNA to increase DNA recovery during isolation (from manufacturers such as Sigma-Aldrich or Promega).

4. 10 mM Tris–HCl, pH 8.5 for DNA elution. Also sold under the name Buffer EB (Qiagen).

2.4. Reagents for Backtracking KRAS2 Point Mutations

1. REMS-PCR Buffer (*see* **Note 4**): 50 mM Tris–Cl, 100 mM NaCl, 4 mM MgCl$_2$, and 1 mM DTT in water. Adjust to pH 8.3 at 25°C.

2. Three required primer sets: (a) diagnostic primer set: 5BKIT [5′-TATAAACTTGTGGTAGTTGGACCT-3′], 3K2 [5′-CGTCCACAAAATGATTCTGA-3′]; (b) restriction enzyme control primers: 5BK36 [5′-CTAGAACAGTAGACACAAA CCA-3′], 3K3 [5′-GATTTTGCAGAAAACAGATC-3′]; (c) 5BK38 [5′-GTACACATGAAGCCATCGTATA-3′] and 3K39

Fig. 1. (continued) Known sequence (solid line) adjacent to unknown sequence (dashed line) is used to choose and design restriction endonucleases (*Sph*I in this case) and primers, which will cut and amplify unknown sequence, respectively. The DNA is digested by the *Sph*I, followed by a ligation to circularize the DNA. Since the wild type sequence *Sph*I site is 20 Kb distal, an *Sph*I site would be predicted to occur earlier on the mutated sequence. LD-PCR amplifies the region of unknown sequence. Products can by analyzed with electrophoresis. (**c**) 1% agarose gel of laddered products. Lane 1, 1 Kb ladder; *lane 2*, blank; *lane 3–7*, laddered PCR products on patient DNA, *lane 7*, primer A4 does not bind to the DNA because it is inside the unknown sequence region.

Table 1
TaqMan + REMS-PCR primers

Primer name	Amplicon length	Primer purpose	Primer sequence
5BKIT	82 bp	Diagnostic	5'- TATAAACTTGTGGTAGTTGGACCT -3'
3K2	82 bp	Diagnostic	5'- CGTCCACAAAATGATTCTGA -3'
5BK36[a]	130 bp	RE Control	5'- CTAGAACAGTAGACACAAACCA -3'
3K37[a]	130 bp	RE control	5'- GATTTTGCAGAAAACAGATC -3'
5BK38[a]	215 bp	PCR Control	5'- GTACACATGAAGCCATCGTATA -3'
3K39[a]	215 bp	PCR control	5'- CCACTTGTACTAGTATGCCTTAAG -3'
KRAS2-probe	n/a	n/a	5'- CAAAATGATTCTGAATTAGCTGTATCG -3'

[a]The RE control and PCR control primer sets are not analyzed through TaqMan. The probe is only specific for the diagnostic amplicon. RE Control, restriction enzyme control

[5'-CCACTTGTACTAGTATGCCTTAAG-3'] (from manufacturers such as MWG Biotech, Invitrogen, along with others) (*see* **Table 1**). HPSF purification (MWG Biotech) gives satisfactory results.

3. *Bst*NI restriction enzyme (from manufacturers such as New England Biolabs or Roche).

4. AmpliTaq® DNA Polymerase required for PCR amplification (Applied Biosystems).

5. TaqStart™ antibody and diluent to preserve enzyme activity (Clontech Laboratories).

6. dNTP mix (as above).

7. ROX Reference Dye as a passive dye reference for TaqMan + REMS-PCR (Roche Applied Science).

8. TaqMan probe, [5'-FAM – CAAAATGATTCTGAATT-AGCTGTATCG – TAM -3'] that has been HPLC purified (MWG Biotech).

3. Methods

A choice of backtracking target is determined by the research question – a variety of molecular alterations found in leukemia cells may be "backtracked" to birth on ANB cards. Most translocations in childhood leukemias have defined, albeit not small, breakpoint cluster regions that are amenable to sequencing with long distance or long distance-inverse PCR. Rearrangements with less well-defined regions such as interchromosomal deletions require additional techniques, such as FISH and/or array-based CGH to localize the breakpoints. A second class of targets are those defined by single base pair mutations (e.g., *RAS, BRAF, cKIT*), these are much easier to ascertain in leukemia cells through standard mutation detection techniques but more difficult to develop specific assays due to the likelihood of false positives. *IG* variable regions can be backtracked similar to translocations and their identification and sequencing are much easier *(16)*.

The typical research question in such studies is determining a binary answer – yes or no – regarding the presence of a mutation at birth, and assays are designed to run at a maximal level of sensitivity. Sensitivity here means being able to identify as little as a single target in 10^4 cells, which represents a portion of a card which will not have more than 100,000 cells total (1–1.5 cm² card). By far the largest technical issue is maximal sensitivity balanced with minimization of false positives. Other questions, such as the relationship between numbers of mutations at birth and risk of leukemia or age of onset, have not been adequately addressed and will require some refinement of the techniques reported here.

Because backtracking assays are designed to be sensitive, all good laboratory practices concerning PCR should be in place. A separate set of pipettemen for loading gels is a must. Positive displacement pipettes should be considered for PCR set up. PCR set up, patient DNA, and ANB cards should all be well-separated in the laboratory, preferably in separate rooms. Special care should be taken when setting up secondary reactions so that PCR products and patient DNA do not contaminate the ANB card reactions.

3.1. Preparation of DNA

For translocations and deletions, high molecular weight DNA is required. For backtracking small rearrangements, such as *IGH* rearrangements or point mutations, any size DNA is sufficient (*see* **Note 5**). If bone marrow is fresh, then mononuclear cells should be purified. This will remove neutrophils and result in a purer blast cell preparation. DNA from frozen bone marrow is also adequate. If using cryopreserved mononuclear cells, wash cells once and proceed to **Subheading 3.1.2**. Repeated freeze-thawing of bone marrow and DNA should be avoided.

3.1.1. Isolation of Mononuclear Cells

1. Fresh bone marrow. Dilute bone marrow $3 \times$ in RPMI-1640, and carefully layer on top of a 1/3 volume Ficoll. Spin tubes at $400 \times g$ for 30 min (with the brake off), and remove the mononuclear cell layer (a cloudy layer above the Ficoll) with a transfer pipette. Add the cells to 10 ml PBS, spin at $200 \times g$, and discard the supernatant.

2. Frozen bone marrow. Dilute frozen marrow 1:1 in PBS (phosphate buffered saline) which will aid in red cell lysis. Spin mixture at $3,500 \times g$, and pour off (but save, just in case!) the red

supernatant. The pellet contains a mass of sticky lysed cells. If there is no pellet, then degraded DNA may be isolated from the supernatant.

3.1.2. High Molecular Weight DNA (See Note 6)

Use large bore or cut tips throughout.

1. Vortex the pelleted fresh cells or frozen cell at low speed to disperse the pellet. Add 500 µl lysis buffer (*see* **Subheading 2.1, item 4**) to ~2×10^6 cells in the pellet, and mix with wide bore pipette. If you are isolating DNA from the supernatant (*see* **Subheading 3.1.1.2**), use equal volumes of $2 \times$ concentrate of lysis buffer and proceed to the next step, adjusting volumes as appropriate (for instance, use 1 ml PCI if lysis solution is 1 ml).

2. Add 500 µl PCI, rock tube for 30 min. Do not vortex. Spin at $10,000 \times g$ for 10 min.

3. Remove aqueous supernatant carefully to a new tube, not disturbing the PCI layer, and discard PCI. Add 1:10 volume 10 M NH_4OAc; rock tube to mix, and add $2 \times$ volume ethanol. Rock the tube to mix ethanol and precipitate the DNA.

4. Remove the ethanol mixture with a pipetteman, being careful not to remove the precipitated DNA, which should appear white and wispy. This can be done without centrifugation, but DNA can be centrifuged at $500 \times g$ if desired prior to removing the ethanol mixture. Wash the precipitate one time with 500 µl 70% ethanol, and then remove all traces of ethanol with a pipetteman and a kimwipe. Add 200 µl of TE and let DNA dissolve for 24 h before use. Finally, pipette the DNA through a wide bore or cut tip to dissolve completely, and quantify DNA.

3.1.3. Low Molecular Weight DNA and Small Numbers of Leukemia Cells

Many manufacturers produce DNA purification kits that use columns and beads that tend to shear DNA via physical and hydrodynamic forces. These column methods are good for isolating high-quality DNA of any quantity, but the DNA will be lower average molecular weight. Qiagen Micro and Mini kits are recommended for this purpose. The DNA that results is ideal for PCR-based assays to ascertain *IGH* and *TCR* rearrangements and point mutations at leukemia oncogenes.

3.2. Cloning a Chromosomal Rearrangement When Both Breakpoints Can Be Estimated from High Density Arrays, Fiber-FISH, or Other Assays of Intermediate Precision (1–50-Kb Resolution)

Chromosomal rearrangements such as translocations and deletions result in a single breakpoint, but two strands of DNA must break for this to form. For chromosomal translocations where both partner locations are established via FISH or karyotype, a long distance PCR (LD-PCR) design can be used to locate the breakpoint (protocol in the current section). In the case of a deletion identified by FISH (a broken probe) (Chapter "Fluorescence In Situ Hybridization (FISH) as a Tool for the Detection of Significant Chromosomal Abnormalities in Childhood Leukemia," "Specialized Fluorescence In Situ Hybridization (FISH) Techniques for Leukemia Research") or array-CGH (Chapter "LDI-PCR: Identification of Known and Unknown Gene Fusions of the Human MLL Gene"), with no apparent partner, a one-sided method is required to identify the breakpoint: inverse PCR (IPCR, *see* **Subheading 3.3**) (also Chapter "Application of SNP Genotype Arrays to Determine Somatic Changes in Cancer" of this book).

1. Estimate the location of breakpoints on either side using known exon/intron boundaries, or other techniques such as high-resolution array-based comparative genomic hybridization (aCGH).

2. Design PCR primers at 5–10 Kb intervals to the left and right hand sides, respectively, of the predicted breakpoint. The 5′–3′ direction of the primers should be directed towards the putative breakpoint. Primers should be 25–35 bp in length, have T_m of 68°C, and be composed of unique sequence in the human genome, without runs of four or more mononucleotides. T_m should be "salt adjusted" to a typical PCR buffer of 50 mM Na$^+$ (*see* **Note 7**). If the regions are estimated to be larger than 10 kb or are not well-defined, then multiple primers will be needed, and spaced at 5–10 Kb intervals.

3. Perform long distance PCR is as recommended by the manufacturer of the polymerase (*see* **Note 2**). Set up a master mix (*see* **Table 2**). Add 100 ng of DNA template to the reaction. If DNA is limiting for the patient and multiple primer pairs are required (due to ill-defined breakpoints) then primer sets may be combined, as many as three forward and three reverse in one reaction. An example of this

Table 2
Long distance PCR master mix

Component	Volume (μl)	Final concentration
Water	to 50	–
5 × Buffer A	3	60 mM Tris–SO$_4$ (pH 9.1),
5 × Buffer B	7	18 mM (NH$_4$)$_2$SO$_4$, 1.3 mM MgSO$_4$
10 mM dNTP mix	1	200 μM each dNTP
Forward primer, 10 μM	2	400 nM
Reverse primer, 10 μM	2	400 nM
Template DNA	5–10[a]	≥100 ng
Elongase® Enzyme Mix	0.75	–

[a]The volume of DNA template is subject to change depending on the concentration of the DNA. Add at least 100 ng to each reaction for LD-PCR; less is okay for inverse PCR

Table 3
Elongase® reaction cycling program for LD-PCR

Preamplificationt	Thermal cycling (40 cycles)		Postcycling	
Initial denaturation	Denaturation	Annealing + extension	Extension	Hold
94°C for 30 s	94°C for 30 s	68°C for 20 min	68°C for 7 min	4°C

is shown in **ref.**5. Run reaction with the standard LD-PCR cycling program (*see* **Table 3**). Visualize 5–10 µl of the sample by electrophoresis.

4. Evaluate PCR products. LD-PCR has a tendency to produce false bands from mishybridization more often than conventional short PCR. PCR bands should be cut out of the gel and purified using Qiagen gel purification kit, and sequenced using the same primers used for the PCR. If both primers produce bona-fide sequence consistent with the predetermined breakpoint location, the band can be pursued as a "bona-fide" PCR band.

5. Design a set of PCR primers internal to one primer at 1 Kb intervals toward the putative breakpoint. Test these new primers with the single reverse primer, using PCR product from **step 4**, to gauge where the breakpoint would be located. This "laddering procedure" (*see* **Fig. 1b** and also **Subheading 3.3**, **step 8**) helps to localize the breakpoint. Sequence the smallest product produced.

3.3. Cloning a Chromosomal Rearrangement with a Single Gene Sequence: Inverse PCR

1. Perform preliminary examination of chromosomal rearrangements with fluorescence in situ hybridization (FISH), karyotype, or array-based comparative genomic hybridization for deletions (with manufacturers such as Nimblegen, *see* **Fig. 1a**) to identify breakpoint locations. Use IPCR to sequence the rearrangement when only one side of the breakpoint can be defined well (i.e., within 10–50 Kb of the breakpoint). If both sides can be defined, then use LD-PCR (*see* **Subheading 3.2**).

2. Design IPCR assay: Examine the 60 Kb region surrounding the putative break in the chromosome (30 Kb upstream and downstream, respectively) (*see* **Fig. 1a** and **Note 8**). Create a restriction map of this region based on the known sequence. Find a restriction endonuclease that will cut at least 7 Kb before the break (on the retained sequence) and at least 15 Kb after the break (on the other side of the putative breakpoint location) (*see* **Note 9**). Design two primers adjacent to the

restriction site prior to the chromosomal break, and several that will ladder in toward the putative break point (*see* **Fig. 1b**). These primers should be 25–30 nucleotides in length, with a T_m of 68°C (*see* **Note 10**), and be spaced at 500 bp intervals.

3. After the assay is designed, digest 500 ng of high molecular weight DNA (*see* **Note 11**) with the 10 U of the chosen restriction endonuclease for 2 h at 37°C in the appropriate buffer.

4. PCI extract the digest to denature the endonuclease, followed by an ethanol precipitation of the DNA with 0.1 volume of 3 M sodium acetate and 2.5 volumes of ethanol.

5. Add 449 µl of water to the precipitated DNA. Pipette up and down gently to reconstitute the sample. Add 50 µl of T4 DNA ligase reaction buffer. Circularize the digested product using 1 µl (~5 Weiss units) of T4 DNA ligase (400,000 U/ml) in a total reaction volume of 500 µl. Mix carefully by pipetting up and down and incubate at 16°C for 16 h. The diluted conditions of this reaction ensure intramolecular rather than intermolecular ligations.

6. Use the QIAquick® gel extraction kit (Qiagen) after ligation to extract the DNA. Transfer the ligation reaction to a 15-ml centrifuge tube. Add 1.5 ml of Buffer QG to the ligation reaction and mix. Add 500 µl of isopropanol and mix. Place the QIAquick spin column in a 2-ml collection tube. Add 500 µl of the sample to the column and centrifuge for 1 min at 14,000 RCF (which is 13,000 rpm in an Eppendorf 5415C rotor). Discard the flow-through and place column back in the collection tube. Repeat this step twice to apply the rest of the sample to the column (*see* **Note 12**). Add 500 µl of Buffer QG to the column and centrifuge for 1 min at 14,000 RCF. Discard the flow-through and replace the column. Wash the column with 750 µl of Buffer PE and centrifuge 1 min at 14,000 RCF. Discard the flow-through and centrifuge for 1 min at 14,000 RCF to get rid of residual ethanol. Place the column in a clean, labeled microcentrifuge tube. Add 30 µl of Buffer EB to the center of the membrane. Let the column stand for 1 min and then centrifuge for 1 min at 14,000 RCF. To preserve the DNA, add EDTA to a final concentration of 1 mM to the eluted DNA.

7. Perform a primary LD-PCR reaction using Elongase® enzyme mix. Set up a master mix (*see* **Table 2**). Add 2 µl of the DNA template to the reaction (at most, 30 ng). Use the primers that are furthest away from the restriction site and the putative break. Run the reaction with the LD-PCR cycling program (*see* **Table 3**). Visualize the 5–10 µl of the sample by electrophoresis (1% agarose gel).

8. Perform a secondary reaction using the primer set just inside the previously used set, i.e., ladder inward (*see* **Fig. 1b**). In this reaction, use only 0.5 µl of primary DNA template as a maximum. Primary product may be diluted 1:20 to reduce aberrant amphibication. Continue to test different primers, moving closer to the breakpoint. Once you have passed the break, no band will appear on the gel because there will be no binding site for annealing (*see* **Note 13**).

9. Sequence the PCR product, using the last primer that produced a band on the ladder. This sequencing reaction should identify the exact DNA sequence of the breakpoint.

3.4. Backtracking Chromosomal Rearrangements for ANB Card Stored at Room Temperature

DNA is often bound to the paper if stored at room temperature for a length of time, making extraction difficult or impossible. For this reason the card itself is used in the PCR reaction without extraction. If the ANB card was stored frozen, use **Subheading 3.5**.

1. Design a nested PCR assay that crosses the breakpoint with four PCR primers (a nested reaction). The external primer pair should not exceed 250 bp and the internal primer pair should not exceed 150 bp (*see* **Note 7**).

2. Test the external primer pair in a PCR reaction using a 1:10 dilution series of patient DNA to establish the sensitivity of the primer pair. 100 ng/µl patient DNA diluted down to 1 pg (five dilutions) in a solution of 100 ng/µl normal DNA will establish sensitivity to one cell (~6 pg DNA). The PCR should include controls such as blanks and other DNA samples from healthy individuals and leukemia patients to establish specificity of the primer pair. Run PCR using conventional *Taq* polymerase and buffers (short distance PCR, **Table 4**).

3. Place 0.5 µl of the original PCR reaction as a template into a second PCR reaction which has the internal primer pair, and run for 35 cycles. Load first and second round PCR products on a 2% agarose gel only after the second round PCR (to help avoid contamination). If a sensitivity of 10 pg of patient DNA is achieved, ANB cards can be tested. If not, reevaluate the PCR primer design and order more primers if appropriate.

Table 4
Taq DNA polymerase reaction cycling program for short distance PCR

Preamplification	Thermal cycling 25–35 cycles			Postcycling	
Initial denaturation	Denaturation	Annealing	Extension	Final extension	Hold
94°C for 4 min	94°C for 45 s	55°C for 30 s	72°C for 90 s	72°C for 7 min	4°C

4. After establishing sensitivity, the dilution series can be run along with ANB cards. Set up an Ampdirect PCR. Create a master mix with 10 µl of both Ampdirect A and Amp Addition-1, 1 µl dNTPs (10 mM each), 0.5 µM each primer (external), and 1.25 units *Taq* DNA polymerase, and water, for 50 µl per reaction.

5. For a card 1 cm in diameter, cut a 1/8 portion of card using a fresh sterile scalpel. If cards are 1.5 cm in diameter, use a 1/16 portion. Up to four ANB card portions can be run at once, and should be interspersed with control Guthrie cards from nondiseased people or "mock" cards created in the laboratory from healthy blood and aged at room temperature for at least a month.

6. Place the card segments directly into the PCR reactions. Run primary reaction, and then a secondary reaction using 1 µl of the primary PCR as a template, using conventional short distance PCR reagents and cycle parameters as shown in **Table 4** for both reactions.

3.5. Backtracking a Chromosomal Rearrangement for an ANB Card Stored at −20°C Or Colder

DNA is readily extractable from cards stored frozen in a government or hospital repository. Since the assays are much cleaner with DNA as a substrate, investigators should attempt this extraction procedure before moving to Ampdirect methods (**Subheading 3.4**).

1. Isolate ANB card DNA using the QIAamp DNA micro kit (Qiagen). Using a sterile scalpel, cut out 1/8 of a 1-cm diameter ANB card and place into a 1.5-ml microcentrifuge tube.

2. Add 180 µl Buffer ATL. Add 20 µl proteinase K mixture (supplied with the kit) and mix thoroughly by vortexing. Be sure that the card is completely submerged in the buffer. Place the tube in a thermomixer or heated orbital incubator, and incubate for 1 h at 56°C with shaking at 900 rpm (*see* **Note 14**).

3. Centrifuge the 1.5-ml tube to remove residual liquid from the lid. Add 1 µg of carrier RNA (*see* **Note 15**). Add 200 µl Buffer AL and then mix by vortexing for 10 s (*see* **Note 16**). Incubate 1.5-ml tube at 70°C with shaking at 900 rpm for 10 min (*see* **Note 17**).

4. Centrifuge the tubes. Transfer the lysate to the QIAamp MiniElute Column. Avoid wetting the rim of the column. Centrifuge at $6,000 \times g$ for 1 min. Discard flow-through and place column in a clean 2-ml collection tube (*see* **Note 18**).

5. Add 500 µl Buffer AW1 without wetting rim and centrifuge 1 min at $6,000 \times g$. Place column in a clean collection tube and discard flow-through.

6. Add 500 μl Buffer AW2 without wetting the rim and centrifuge 1 min at 6,000 × g. Discard flow-through and place in a clean collection tube.

7. Centrifuge at 20,000 × g for 3 min. Place the column in a clean, labeled 1.5-ml microcentrifuge tube. Apply 15 μl of Buffer AE and 15 μl of Buffer EB to the center of the membrane (*see* **Note 19**). Incubate at room temperature for 2 min. Centrifuge for 1 min at 20,000 × g.

8. Quantify the DNA isolated from the ANB card (*see* **Note 20**).

9. The samples are then ready to be backtracked for chromosomal rearrangements or point mutations. Follow all steps in **Subheading 3.4** above for chromosomal rearrangements, but substitute conventional PCR buffers for Ampdirect buffers. For *KRAS2* mutations, follow **Subheading 3.6**.

3.6. Cloning Other Rearrangements, Including IGH Sequences and Point Mutations: Example of KRAS2

IGH sequences can be cloned using primer sets maximized to capture all possible *IGH* rearrangements. Both complete and incomplete (i.e., *D-J*) rearrangements can be utilized, and illegitimate rearrangements at *TCR* loci have also proven to be good clonal markers. Standardized methodology for *IGH* and *TCR* sequencing have been developed by the clinical community for use as minimal residual disease markers *(16)*. Other mutated genes with potential for backtracking in leukemia include *RAS*, *BRAF*, *FLT3*, *cKIT*, *NOTCH*, etc. Methodology to characterize specific mutations is particular to each gene, and we have only covered *KRAS2* for which we demonstrated backtracking. *KRAS2* mutations occur in about 10% of pediatric leukemias (ALL and AML) and an appropriate number of diagnostic leukemias should be acquired and screened with this in mind. We have briefly described the method of screening with denaturing high-pressure liquid chromatography (DHPLC), but many other methods have been described, including oligonucleotide hybridization, SSCP, and direct sequencing.

1. PCR amplify 10 ng patient bone marrow DNA (>40% blast cells) with the following PCR primers (5′-CAGAGAGT-GAACATCATGGAC-3′, and 5′-GGACCCTGACATACTC-CCAAG-3′) with a high fidelity polymerase (optimase polymerase, transgenomics; regular *Taq* polymerase error rate is high and will ensure artifactual mutation detection by this method!)

2. Denature samples at 100°C, renature on ice, and run samples on WAVE DHPLC system (Varian Inc.) at a 55.5°C column temperature. Sequence those PCR products that display a wavelike pattern different than control, nonmutant PCR products. *KRAS2* mutations at codon 12 may be backtracked by the methods described in the next section.

3.7. Backtracking a Point Mutation: KRAS2

Two techniques are used simultaneously to backtrack point mutations in exon 12 of *KRAS2*: (1) REMS-PCR and (2) Taq-Man. Combination of these assays allows for increased sensitivity, enabling point mutation detection at a high sensitivity (1:10,000 mutant:normal targets). Either method alone is appropriate if a lower sensitivity is desired (1:1,000). These methods may be modified to fit other targets.

1. Prior to backtracking the point mutation on the ANB card DNA, it is important to test the sensitivity of the primers on patient DNA. Make a tenfold dilution series from 100 ng to 1 pg of patient DNA into wild-type DNA, maintaining 100 ng of total DNA, which represents about 15,000 cells (an ANB card contains 30–60,000 cells).

2. Prepare the master mix for the combined TaqMan and REMS-PCR reactions (*see* **Tables 1** and **5**). Each reaction should be performed in triplicate or quadruplicate to ensure validity of the results. Mix the AmpliTaq® DNA polymerase and the TaqStart™ antibody at a 1:5 molar ratio in the provided TaqStart™ antibody diluent. Incubate the mixture at room temperature for 15 min before adding it to the master mix. The restriction endonuclease control is run without any added restriction endonuclease. Perform real-time analysis of the DNA of the dilution series (*see* **Table 6**) using the absolute quantification setting of a quantitative PCR machine such as the Applied Biosystems 7900HT (*see* **Fig. 2**).

3. After the reaction is complete analyze it by electrophoresis using a 5% Nusieve® GTG agarose gel. While the probe is solely able to detect the amplification of the diagnostic amplicon, electrophoresis allows for visualization of the two control products. To ensure the sensitivity of the assay, this dilution curve should be run each time an ANB card is tested. The resultant bands will give: (a) a 215 bp region of exon 4b of *KRAS2*, amplified by the PCR control primers; (b) an 82 bp region, amplified by diagnositic primers; (c) a 130 bp region of exon 3 of *KRAS2*, amplified by restriction endonuclease primers (*see* **Fig. 3**).

4. Upon satisfactory amplification, the ANB card DNA can be tested in the same manner as the patient DNA dilution series, using the patient dilution series as a control each time the assay is performed.

Backtracking currently is limited to DNA targets since RNA is unstable for long periods on a neonatal blood spot. Furthermore, RNA sequences derived from fusion genes are not clone patient specific. Future backtracking efforts may focus on proteins in neonatal blood spots, as well as frozen (viable) cord blood cells which are an excellent source for high throughput efforts (*9, 17*).

Table 5
TaqMan + REMS-PCR master mix

Component	Volume (μl)	Final concentration
Water	to 20	–
5 × Reaction buffer	4	1×
10 mM dNTP mix	0.1	50 μM each dNTP
5BKIT, 10 μM	2	1 μM
3K2, 10 μM	2	1 μM
5BK36, 1 μM	0.8	40 nM
3K37, 1 μM	0.8	40 nM
5BK38, 1 μM	0.8	40 nM
3K39, 1 μM	0.8	40 nM
ROX Ref dye, 10 μM	0.6	300 nM
TaqMan probe, 10 μM	0.5	250 nM
BstNI[a], 10,000 U/ml	2	20 U
Template DNA	2[b]	≥100 ng
AmpliTaq® DNA Polymerase, 5 U/μl[c]	0.6	3 U

[a]Restriction endonuclease control contains no BstNI
[b]Volume will vary with DNA concentration
[c]Mix with TaqStart™ antibody at a molar ratio of 1:5. Incubate at room temperature for 15 min before addition to mix. Total volume of AmpliTaq® DNA Polymerase: TaqStart® Antibody will be 0.95 μl

Table 6
TaqMan + REMS-PCR reaction cycling parameters

	Thermal cycling			
Preamplification	10 cycles		50 cycles	
Initial denaturation	Annealing + extension	Denaturation	Annealing + extension	Denaturation
94°C for 2 min	58°C for 2 min	92°C for 20 s	58°C for 1 min	92°C for 20 s

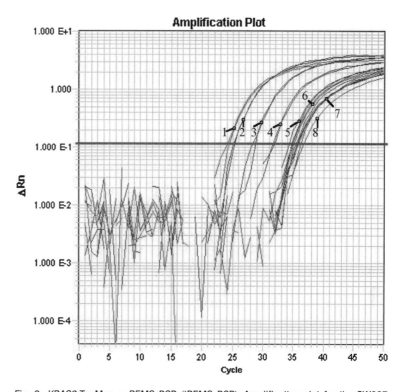

Fig. 2. *KRAS2* TaqMan + REMS-PCR (tREMS-PCR). Amplification plot for the SW837 dilution series (i.e., PCR products from *Fig.* 3). Each line represents the amplication of differing concentrations of mutant DNA diluted in REH. All reactions were conducted in duplicate and contained 50 ng of DNA, 1 μM of each diagnostic primer, and 250 nM of probe. SW837 was diluted in REH (wild type). Decreasing amounts of mutant template result in increased cycle thresholds. *1*, SW837 with no BstNI tREMS-PCR product; *2*, SW837 tREMS-PCR product DNA; *3*, SW837 tenfold dilution in REH REMS-PCR product DNA; *4*, SW837 100-fold dilution in REH REMS-PCR product DNA; *5*, SW837 1,000-fold dilution in REH REMS-PCR product; *6*, SW837 10,000-fold dilution in REH REMS-PCR product DNA; *7*, REH REMS-PCR product DNA; *8*, blank.

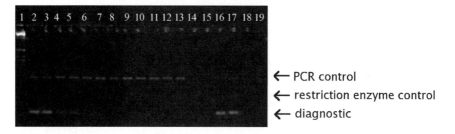

← PCR control

← restriction enzyme control

← diagnostic

Fig. 3. KRAS TaqMan + REMS-PCR. Dilution series of SW837 DNA amplification, showing the sensitivity of assay. SW837 contains a *KRAS2* mutation at the first nucleotide in codon 12 (G > T). 5% NuSieve GTG agarose gel. *Lanes 1*, 1 Kb DNA ladder; *lane 2 & 3*, SW837; *lane 4 & 5*, SW837 diluted tenfold into REH; *lane 6 & 7*, SW837 diluted 100-fold into REH; *lane 8 & 9*, SW837 diluted 1,000-fold into REH; *lane 10 & 11*, SW837 diluted 10,000-fold into REH; *lane 12 & 13* REH; *lane 14 & 15*, blank; *lane 16 & 17*, SW837 with no BstNI. Each reaction had 70 ng of total DNA. SW837, mutant. REH, wild type. Diagnostic primers, 5BKIT and 3K2, amplify an 82-bp region of exon 1 of the *KRAS2* gene. PCR control primers, 5BK38 and 3K39, amplify a 215-bp region of exon 4b of the *KRAS2* gene. Restriction endonuclease control primers, 5BK36 and 3K37, amplify a 130-bp region of exon 3 of the *KRAS2* gene.

4. Notes

1. One significant consideration not addressed in this monograph is the ethical and logistic considerations for obtaining and using ANB cards. Locating matched neonatal blood spots requires the use of extensive identification information such as hospital of birth, parent's names, and birthdates. A human research ethics board that is organized under the Helsinki Doctrine should approve all research using leukemia samples and ANB cards.

2. Elongase enzyme has a reduced propensity to yield aberrant products in a second, or nested, round of PCR. All other polymerases that we have tested have seemingly greater activity to produce products other than those intended, and should be avoided for nested PCR. Elongase polymerase is not the 'best' long-distance polymerase, since it does not yield extremely long products (>15 Kb) or products of high intensity. The greater activity of other polymerases besides Elongase (sold by Stratagene, Roche, Takara) work well for single-round PCR when there is less chance of side products.

3. It is very difficult to extract DNA from ANB cards stored at ambient temperatures, and AmpDirect buffers eliminate the need for extraction. For cards stored frozen, blood card extraction protocol (Qiagen micro Genomic DNA kit) works well. Storage conditions for ANB cards vary widely however depending on location of the child's birth.

4. Store REMS-PCR buffer at –20°C in aliquots. We preferred to make a 5 × stock, stored in 1 ml aliquots.

5. Extraction of DNA is one of the most ubiquitous protocols; however, we have mentioned two extraction protocols here, since high molecular weight DNA is critical for the long distance methods here, and many modern DNA extraction protocols are geared for short distance PCR. For both protocols mentioned, the user should avoid vortexing and rough handling.

6. These methods are appropriate when large numbers of leukemia cells are available (>10^6 cells). The Puregene kit (Gentra, sold by Qiagen) has an equivalent lysis buffer and avoids the use of toxic reagents. The Puregene method can be used with small amounts of DNA when glycogen is added to the DNA prior to purification to assist in the DNA precipitation step (see manufacturer's recommendations).

7. Short-range PCR primers should have annealing temperature in the range of 60°C. An excellent resource for designing

primers is Primer 3.0 (http://frodo.wi.mit.edu/). The pair should not produce a PCR product when tested, on UCSC in silico PCR website (http://genome.ucsc.edu/cgi-bin/hgPcr).

8. Do not place primers in genomic repeat regions. These regions are easily identified on the UCSC Genome Browser, which is the best source for human DNA sequence (http://genome.ucsc.edu/). Sequence output formats allow the annotation of repeat regions.

9. Use of six-cutter restriction enzymes is preferred due to the frequency of restriction sites spread across the genome. We found that designing a reaction with at least two enzymes is necessary. Some enzymes will not give satisfactory results due to the investigator being "blind" to the presence of a restriction site on the hidden side of the break.

10. The oligonucleotides require a higher T_m because this will be a LD-PCR reaction. Additionally, when designing primers, take into consideration repeats, runs, palindromes, dimer formation, and hairpin loops. GC content should be at least 35%. An excellent web-based resource for primer design, including T_m calculations, a BLAST link, and primer secondary structure calculations is: http://www.basic.northwestern.edu/biotools/oligocalc.html. When designing the primers that ladder in toward the putative break site, begin 2–5 Kb away from the break, spacing each subsequent primer 1–2 Kb apart.

11. It is possible to use less DNA for the digest, down to 50 ng. However, results may vary depending on quality of the DNA.

12. A vacuum manifold may be used in substitution for a centrifuge for the steps up until Buffer PE. The vacuum manifold may save some time because it allows the quick application of the sample to the column. After washing the sample with Buffer PE, transfer the column to a 2-ml collection tube and centrifuge 1 min at 14,000 RCF. Continue on with the elution instructions above (*see* **Subheading 3.3**; **step 6**).

13. The design of more oligonucleotides for long distance PCR will be necessary to hit the break point. The products should get increasingly smaller as you approach the break point. Beware of contamination issues because these are nested reactions.

14. We have found that shaking at a lower frequency (400 rpm) is adequate. Use of a water bath or heat block requires vortexing of the tube for 10 s every 10 min. This will improve lysis. Increased incubation time will not affect sample quality.

15. Buffer AL and AW1 contain guanidinium chloride. Do not add bleach or acidic solutions to sample waste.

16. The Qiagen kit includes carrier RNA (unknown concentration) that can be added to Buffer AL prior to use. The carrier RNA increases DNA binding to the column. However, we add a known quantity of carrier RNA, 1 μg per each isolation. Adjusting the amount of carrier RNA can increase DNA yield from the ANB cards.

17. Again, vortexing is required if using a water bath or heat block for 10 s every 3 min.

18. The 2-ml collection tubes can be reused between wash steps to cut down on plastic use. Discard flow-through and reuse tube.

19. Though EDTA slows degradation of stored DNA, it can inhibit amplification. We use Buffer EB, which lacks EDTA, to reduce the 0.5 mM EDTA of Buffer AE.

20. While there is no gold standard for DNA quantification and various methods can produce significantly differing results, use of one method within an assay will ensure consistency. We use the FL_x800 Microplate Fluorescence Reader (Bio-Tek), which makes use the Quant-iT® PicoGreen® dsDNA reagent (Invitrogen) to measure DNA concentration. The amount of DNA in the preceding REMS-PCR reaction is vital to the success of the assay. Anything lower than 50 ng of DNA is pushing the lower limit of the assay.

Acknowledgements

This work was supported by the National Institutes of Health (R01CA89032), the Leukemia and Lymphoma Society of America, and the Leukaemia Research Fund of the UK. JLW is a scholar of the Leukemia and Lymphoma Society of America.

References

1. Greaves, M. F., Maia, A. T., Wiemels, J. L., and Ford, A. M. (2003) Leukemia in twins: lessons in natural history, *Blood* **102**, 2321–33.

2. Greaves, M. F. (2006) Cord blood donor cell leukemia in recipients, *Leukemia* **20**, 1633–34.

3. Gale, K. B., Ford, A. M., Repp, R., Borkhardt, A., Keller, C., Eden, O. B., and Greaves, M. F. (1997) Backtracking leukemia to birth: identification of clonotypic gene fusion sequences in neonatal blood spots, *Proceedings of the National Academy of Sciences of the United States of America* **94**, 13950–4.

4. Hjalgrim, L. L., Madsen, H. O., Melbye, M., Jorgensen, P., Christiansen, M., Andersen, M. T., Pallisgaard, N., Hokland, P., Clausen, N., Ryder, L. P., Schmiegelow, K., and Hjalgrim, H. (2002) Presence of clone-specific markers at birth in children with acute lymphoblastic leukaemia, *British Journal of Cancer* **87**, 994–99.

5. McHale, C. M., Wiemels, J. L., Zhang, L., Ma, X., Buffler, P. A., Guo, W., Loh, M. L., and Smith, M. T. (2003) Prenatal origin of TEL-AML1-positive acute lymphoblastic leukemia in children born in California, *Genes Chromosomes Cancer* **37**, 36–43.

6. Wiemels, J. L., Cazzaniga, G., Daniotti, M., Eden, O. B., Addison, G. M., Masera, G., Saha, V., Biondi, A., and Greaves, M. F. (1999) Prenatal origin of acute lymphoblastic leukaemia in children, *Lancet* **354**, 1499–503.

7. McHale, C. M., Wiemels, J. L., Zhang, L., Ma, X., Buffler, P. A., Feusner, J., Matthay, K., Dahl, G., and Smith, M. T. (2003) Prenatal origin of childhood acute myeloid leukemias harboring chromosomal rearrangements t(15;17) and inv(16), *Blood* **101**, 4640–1.

8. Wiemels, J. L., Xiao, Z., Buffler, P. A., Maia, A. T., Ma, X., Dicks, B. M., Smith, M. T., Zhang, L., Feusner, J., Wiencke, J., Pritchard-Jones, K., Kempski, H., and Greaves, M. (2002) In utero origin of t(8;21) AML1-ETO translocations in childhood acute myeloid leukemia, *Blood* **99**, 3801–5.

9. Mori, H., Colman, S. M., Xiao, Z., Ford, A. M., Healy, L. E., Donaldson, C., Hows, J. M., Navarrete, C., and Greaves, M. (2002) Chromosome translocations and covert leukemic clones are generated during normal fetal development, *Proceedings of the National Academy of Sciences of the United States of America* **99**, 8242–7.

10. Taub, J. W., Konrad, M. A., Ge, Y., Naber, J. M., Scott, J. S., Matherly, L. H., and Ravindranath, Y. (2002) High frequency of leukemic clones in newborn screening blood samples of children with B-precursor acute lymphoblastic leukemia, *Blood* **99**, 2992–6.

11. Yagi, T., Hibi, S., Tabata, Y., Kuriyama, K., Teramura, T., Hashida, T., Shimizu, Y., Takimoto, T., Todo, S., Sawada, T., and Imashuku, S. (2000) Detection of clonotypic IGH and TCR rearrangements in the neonatal blood spots of infants and children with B-cell precursor acute lymphoblastic leukemia, *Blood* **96**, 264–8.

12. Fischer, S., Mann, G., Konrad, M., Metzler, M., Ebetsberger, G., Jones, N., Nadel, B., Bodamer, O., Haas, O. A., Schmitt, K., and Panzer-Grumayer, E. R. (2007) Screening for leukemia- and clone-specific markers at birth in children with T cell precursor ALL suggests a predominantly postnatal origin, *Blood* **110**, 3036–8.

13. Maia, A. T., Tussiwand, R., Cazzaniga, G., Rebulla, P., Colman, S., Biondi, A., and Greaves, M. (2004) Identification of preleukemic precursors of hyperdiploid acute lymphoblastic leukemia in cord blood, *Genes Chromosomes Cancer* **40**, 38–43.

14. Ahmed, M., Sternberg, A., Hall, G., Thomas, A., Smith, O., OÕMarcaigh, A., Wynn, R., Stevens, R., Addison, M., King, D., Stewart, B., Gibson, B., Roberts, I., and Vyas, P. (2004) Natural history of GATA1 mutations in Down syndrome, *Blood* **103**, 2480–89.

15. Eguchi-Ishimae, M., Eguchi, M., Kempski, H., and Greaves, M.F. (2008) NOTCH1 mutation can be an early, prenatal genetic event in T-ALL, *Blood* **111**, 376–8.

16. van Dongen, J. J., Langerak, A. W., Bruggemann, M., Evans, P. A., Hummel, M., Lavender, F. L., Delabesse, E., Davi, F., Schuuring, E., Garcia-Sanz, R., van Krieken, J. H., Droese, J., Gonzalez, D., Bastard, C., White, H. E., Spaargaren, M., Gonzalez, M., Parreira, A., Smith, J. L., Morgan, G. J., Kneba, M., and Macintyre, E. A. (2003) Design and standardization of PCR primers and protocols for detection of clonal immunoglobulin and T-cell receptor gene recombinations in suspect lymphoproliferations: report of the BIOMED-2 Concerted Action BMH-CT98-3936, *Leukemia* **17**, 2257–317.

17. Olsen, M., Madsen, H. O., Hjalgrim, H., Ford, A., and Schmiegelow, K. (2006) Stability of cord blood RNA measured by house keeping transcripts: relevance for large-scale studies of childhood leukaemia, *Leukemia* **20**, 2214–7.

Chapter 3

Fluorescence In Situ Hybridization (FISH) as a Tool for the Detection of Significant Chromosomal Abnormalities in Childhood Leukaemia

Zoë J. Konn, Sarah L. Wright, Kerry E. Barber, and Christine J. Harrison

Summary

Cytogenetics is integral to the diagnosis of childhood leukaemia, particularly in relation to the risk stratification of patients for treatment. Fluorescence in situ hybridization (FISH) has become an important complementary technique, expanding chromosomal analysis into the molecular arena. It has greatly improved the accuracy and applicability of cytogenetics and led to the discovery of novel chromosomal changes of prognostic significance. Many probes are now commercially available, providing robust and reliable detection of chromosomal abnormalities. Since the cloning of the human genome, it is now possible to access detailed genomic information and develop FISH probes for virtually any known DNA sequence. The range of procedures necessary for the successful application of FISH in the accurate detection of significant chromosomal abnormalities in childhood acute leukaemia is described here.

Key words: FISH probes, Cytogenetics, Bone marrow, Chromosomal abnormalities

1. Introduction

Cytogenetics plays a pivotal role in the diagnosis of childhood leukaemia, by exploiting the association between certain chromosomal abnormalities and the different disease subtypes. The independent prognostic association of specific chromosomal changes has been known for some time. For example, the chromosomal rearrangements involving core binding factor genes: the translocation, t(8;21)(q22;q22), and the inversion of

C.W.E. So (ed.), Leukemia, *Methods in Molecular Biology, vol. 538*
© Humana Press, a part of Springer Science + Business Media, LLC 2009
DOI: 10.1007/978-1-59745-418-6_3

chromosome 16, inv(16)(p13q22), are associated with a favourable outcome in acute myeloid leukaemia (AML) *(1)*. In childhood acute lymphoblastic leukaemia (ALL), high hyperdiploidy (51–65 chromosomes) is linked to a good outcome whilst the translocation, t(9;22)(q34;q11.2), which gives rise to the Philadelphia chromosome, is a high-risk abnormality in both children and adults *(2)*. Such chromosomal changes are now used in the risk stratification of patients for treatment, thus, their precise identification is vital. FISH and other molecular techniques were developed throughout the 1990s. These procedures led to the discovery of the genes involved in these rearrangements, for example, the fusion of the *BCR* and *ABL* genes resulted from the t(9;22)(q34;q11.2). In addition, new recurring chromosomal abnormalities were identified. Of note was the finding of the cryptic translocation, t(12;21)(p13;q22), giving rise to the *ETV6-RUNX1* fusion. It was observed in ~25% childhood ALL and was associated with a good outcome *(3)*. FISH has now become integrated into routine laboratory practice to ensure the accurate identification of these significant chromosomal abnormalities. At the same time, FISH screening has increased their detection rate among patients in whom cytogenetic analysis either failed or revealed a normal karyotype.

FISH uses fluorescently labelled probes specific for genes or whole chromosomes. It is based on the ability of a single-stranded DNA probe to anneal to its complementary sequence in a target genome. Many probes are now commercially available, offering reliable detection of the range of significant chromosomal abnormalities. It is possible to access detailed genomic information and develop FISH probes for virtually any known DNA sequence. These probes are made by standard procedures for DNA extraction and labelling. There are three main types of FISH probes: (i) repetitive sequences, which hybridize to repetitive alpha (or beta) satellite sequences present in the centromeres of all human chromosomes. These can be used to identify the origin of chromosomes in metaphase and enumerate specific chromosomes in interphase cells, providing a rapid and accurate method to ascertain chromosome copy number; (ii) locus-specific, usually focused on genes, which are used to identify rearrangements, deletions, and gains in both interphase and metaphase cells; (iii) whole chromosome paints, chromosome-specific probe libraries prepared from flow-sorted chromosomes. They are applied to metaphase chromosomes to determine the origin of structural abnormalities.

This chapter describes, in detail, those procedures necessary for the successful application of FISH in the detection of the important chromosomal abnormalities in childhood acute leukaemia.

2. Materials

It is assumed that the following protocols will be carried out in a laboratory provided with standard equipment, including an autoclave, bench-top centrifuge, micro-centrifuge, water bath, thermometer, pH meter, and balance, as well as a range of pipettes, microtubes, glass slides, an assortment of plastics and glassware. The main reagents required are listed below. A suggested supplier and catalogue number have been given for the less common items. Good laboratory practice should be followed at all times.

2.1. Culturing and Slide Preparation

1. RPMI 1640 culture medium, supplemented with 25% fetal calf serum and 1% antibiotics (penicillin/streptomycin). Supplemented medium should be stored at 4°C.

2. Red cell lysis reagent (Zap-OGLOBIN® II Lytic Reagent, Beckman Coulter, CA). Once opened, store at 4°C.

3. Colchicine solution (Colcemid, Sigma, Dorset). Once opened, store at 4°C.

4. Potassium Chloride (KCl) hypotonic solution 0.075 M (5.56 g/L). Dissolve in sterile water. Store at room temperature.

5. Virkon disinfectant (3% solution). Keep at room temperature. Discard after use or if colour changes.

6. Fixative: Analar methanol: Analar glacial acetic acid ratio 3:1. Make fresh each day. All procedures involving fixative should be carried out in a fume extraction hood.

7. 70% acetic acid. Store at room temperature.

2.2. Growing and Preparing FISH Probes

1. Clone stabs requested from an appropriate source (*see* **Subheading 3.3.1**).

2. Agar plates inoculated with the appropriate antibiotic, LB agar (1 L): 10 g Tryptone, 5 g yeast extract, 10 g $NaCl_2$, 15 g Agar. Make up to 1 L with distilled water. Autoclave immediately, allow to cool to less than 50°C, add appropriate antibiotics, pour into sterile petri dishes. Store at 4°C for up to 1 month.

3. LB broth (1 L): 10 g Tryptone, 5 g yeast extract, 10 g $NaCL_2$, make up to 1 L with distilled water and autoclave immediately. Store at room temperature.

4. Spectrum red/green dUTP: Spectrum red dUTP (Abbott Diagnostics, IL, catalogue number 06J94-020), spectrum green dUTP (Abbott Diagnostics, catalogue number 06J94–010), 50 nmol spectrum red (or green) dUTP. Reconstitute in 50 µL distilled water, aliquot 10 µL into five microtubes. Add a further 40 µL distilled water at the time of use to give a 0.2°mM solution. Store at –20°C.

5. 0.5°M EDTA pH 8.0 (1 L):186.1 g ethylenediamine-tetraacetic acid (EDTA), ~20 g sodium hydroxide (NaOH), make up to ~800 mL with distilled water, adjust to pH 8.0 with NaOH. Note EDTA will only dissolve at pH 8.0. Make up to 1 L with distilled water. Store at room temperature.

6. 1 M Tris–HCL pH 7.4 (1 L): 121.1 g Tris-base, add distilled water, adjust to pH 7.4 with HCl. Store at room temperature.

7. TE buffer pH 7.4 (1 L): 10 mL of 1 M Tris–HCL, pH 7.4, 2 mL of 0.5 M EDTA, pH 8.0, make up to 1 L with distilled water. Store at room temperature.

8. Glycerol.

9. Plasmid purification kit (mini-kit, Qiagen, West Sussex, catalogue number 12123 or midi-kit catalogue number 12143).

10. Isopropanol.

11. 70% ethanol.

12. Nick translation kit (Abbott Diagnostics, catalogue number 07J00–001).

13. Sephadex G-50 columns (Amersham, Buckinghamshire, catalogue number 27-5330–02). Store at room temperature.

14. Human COT-1 DNA (Invitrogen, Paisley, catalogue number15279-011). Store at –20°C.

15. 3 M Sodium acetate. Store at room temperature.

16. Hybridization buffer. Available from all manufacturers of commercial FISH probes (e.g., Abbott Diagnostics, catalogue number 32–804826). Store at –20°C.

17. Ice-cold ethanol. Store at –20°C.

2.3. FISH

1. FISH probes (commercial or home-grown).

2. 10-mm circular coverslips: These are required if multiple FISH tests are to be set up on one slide (VWR, Leicestershire, catalogue number 631–0170).

3. 13-mm circular coverslips: These are more useful when applying probes to metaphases, as they cover a larger area.

4. 24 × 50 mm² coverslips for final slide mounting.

5. Slide mounting medium: Vectorshield (Peterborough) containing 4′,6-diamidino-2-phenylindole (DAPI) (Vector Laboratories, catalogue number H-1200).

6. Rubber cement/solution: Rubber solution for bicycle tyre puncture repair works well. This is available from a number of suppliers (our preference is Halfords).

7. Parafilm: Cut into pieces slightly smaller than the slide area.

8. Block: Dried milk powder solution (~0.1 g in 15 mL of distilled water). Store at 4°C.

9. Phosphate buffered saline (PBS): Prepare according to manufacturer's instructions. Store at room temperature.

10. Detection reagents for indirectly-labelled probes: Avidin-Fluorescein for biotin labelled probes (Roche, East Sussex, catalogue number 1 975 595) and Anti-Digoxigenin-rhodamine Fab fragments for digoxigenin labelled probes (Roche, catalogue number 1 207 750). Reconstitute the reagents as directed, and then store Avidin-Fluorescein in 2 μL aliquots and Anti-Digoxigenin-Rhodamine Fab fragments in 10 μL aliquots. Store long-term at –20°C. Working solution: Make up to 2 mL with PBS and store at 4°C for up to 1 month. Protect from light.

11. 2× SSC (1 L): 100 mL of 20× SSC, 900 mL of distilled water. Store at room temperature.

12. Wash 1 (1 L): 20 mL of 20× SSC, 980 mL of distilled water, 3 mL of Np40 or Tween 20 detergent. Store at room temperature.

13. Wash 2 (1 L): 100 mL of 20× SSC, 900 mL of distilled water, 1 mL of Np40 or Tween 20. Store at room temperature.

14. Wash 3 (1 L): 200 mL of 20× SSC, 800 mL of distilled water, 1 mL of Np40 or Tween 20. Store at room temperature.

15. Nail varnish to seal the slide edges after analysis for long-term storage.

2.4. Analysis

1. A microscope equipped for epifluorescence. The minimum filter set required for standard three colour FISH are DAPI (counterstain) and appropriate filters for the red and green florochromes (**Subheading 3.8.1**).

---

3. Methods

3.1. Setting Up Bone Marrow/Blood Cultures for Cytogenetic Analysis and FISH

Bone marrow and/or blood samples are often received by post or courier. They should be processed as soon as possible to increase the chance of achieving a successful result. Until the sample is fixed, it should be handled in a class II safety cabinet.

3.1.1. Bone Marrow

1. Spin the sample for 5 min at $200 \times g$ in a bench-top centrifuge (*see* **Note 1**).

2. Remove and discard supernatant into 3% Virkon solution (*see* **Note 2**). Do not pour.

3. Re-suspend the cell pellet in supplemented RPMI culture medium to a sufficient volume to allow 0.5 mL per culture. The number and type of culture is dependent on the disease type and number of cells available (*see* **Note 3**).

4. Inoculate a culture tube containing 4.5 mL of supplemented RPMI with 0.5 mL of re-suspended bone marrow. Ensure that the culture is well mixed and incubate at 37°C.

Alternatively, a total cell count may be performed in order to assess the cell numbers for the optimum density in culture. If the cells are too dense they may become contact inhibited, while if they are too sparse division may be arrested.

1. Add 50 μL of bone marrow suspension into a small sterile container, for example, an Eppendorf tube.

2. Add 50 μL of red cell lysis reagent and shake gently to mix.

3. Count the cells using a haemocytometer. Multiply the cell number by 2 (dilution factor) and then by 10^4 to obtain the number of cells/mL in the original sample.

4. Spin the sample for 5 min at 200 × g in a bench-top centrifuge.

5. Remove and discard the supernatant into 3% Virkon solution (*see* **Note 2**). Do not pour.

6. Re-suspend the bone marrow cells in an appropriate volume of supplemented medium in a culture tube to allow the accurate addition of 5×10^6 cells per culture (1×10^6/mL). Ensure that the culture is well mixed and incubate at 37°C (*see* **Note 3**).

3.1.2. Peripheral Blood

Occasionally a peripheral blood sample is received, for example, when the marrow tap was dry or the blood sample contained a high number of circulating leukaemic blasts.

1. The white cell count (WCC) must be known ($\times 10^9$/L).

2. From the WCC the number of cells/mL may be calculated.

3. Inoculate the supplemented culture media with sufficient blood to give 5×10^6 white cells per culture. Ensure that the culture is well mixed and incubate at 37°C (*see* **Note 3**).

3.2. Harvesting and Slide Making

3.2.1. Harvesting

The cell suspension obtained after harvesting is used to make slide preparations for both cytogenetic analysis and FISH.

1. Add 50 μL of the mitotic spindle poison, colchicine, to each culture to be harvested.

2. After the appropriate time in colchicine (*see* **Note 4**), spin the sample for 5 min at 200 × g in a bench-top centrifuge.

3. Remove and discard the supernatant into 3% Virkon solution (*see* **Note 2**). Do not pour.

4. Re-suspend the cell pellet by gently flicking the tube and add sufficient 0.075 M KCl hypotonic solution to the culture tube to fill (~10 mL). KCl may be pre-warmed to 37°C (*see* **Note 5**).

5. Re-spin the tube immediately for 5 min at 200 × *g* (*see* **Note 6**).

6. Remove and discard the supernatant into 3% Virkon solution (*see* **Note 2**). Do not pour.

7. Re-suspend the pellet by gentle flicking.

8. Keeping the pellet mobile using a vortex (*see* **Note 7**), add fixative (3:1 methanol:acetic acid) drop-wise for the first mL, then generously to 5 mL. Stop the vortex and top up with more fixative (to ~10 mL) (*see* **Note 8**).

9. Leave the fixed cells at –20°C for a minimum of 1 h or preferably overnight (*see* **Note 9**).

3.2.2. Post-Harvest Fixative Changes

1. Spin the sample for 10 min at 200 × *g* in a bench-top centrifuge (*see* **Note 10**).

2. Remove and discard the supernatant, do not pour.

3. Re-suspend the pellet and top up to ~10 mL with fresh fixative.

4. Repeat **steps 1–3**.

5. Spin again, as **step 1**.

6. Remove and discard the supernatant, do not pour.

7. Re-suspend the pellet by flicking gently. The cell suspension is now ready for slide making (*see* **Note 11**).

8. For longer term storage transfer the cells to a small screw-topped Eppendorf tube with the pellet re-suspended in ~1 mL of fixative. Store at –20°C.

3.2.3. Making Slide Preparations for FISH

3.2.3.1. Slides for Interphase FISH

1. Make the slides for only one patient at a time.

2. Clearly label the slide with appropriate identification, such as name, test, and unique laboratory number.

3. Dilute the re-suspended pellet with fresh fixative until it appears slightly cloudy (*see* **Note 12**).

4. Using a p20 Gilson pipette, drop 2 μL of cell suspension onto the slide.

5. While the spot is drying, mark the outside edges with a diamond pen (*see* **Note 13**).

6. If multiple testing is to be carried out on one slide, a template may be useful (*see* **Fig. 1**) (*see* **Note 14**).

7. Examine the slide under low power on a phase-contrast microscope. For best results, nuclei should appear grey (not phase bright) and flat, with no residual cytoplasm. Cells should be

spread with minimal touching between nuclei but at a sufficiently high density to allow easy scoring on high power (*see*
Fig. 2) (*see* **Note 15**).

8. Slides should be kept for a minimum of 20 min on a hot plate
at ≥60°C.

9. Usually, slides made in this way require no further pre-treatment.

**3.2.3.2. Slides for
Metaphase FISH**

1. Make the slides for only one patient at a time.

2. Clearly label the slide with appropriate identification, such as
name, test and unique laboratory number.

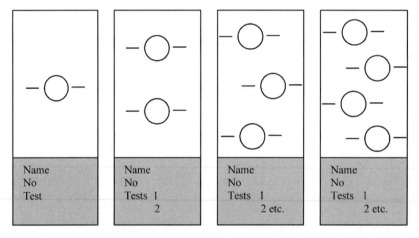

Fig. 1. Slide template. Proposed slide template for undertaking multiple interphase FISH tests on a single slide.

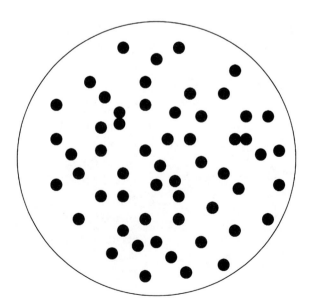

Fig. 2. Illustration of the appropriate density nuclei
for interphase FISH. Low power (10×) representation of the optimum cell density for interphase
FISH scoring.

3. Dilute the re-suspended pellet with fresh fixative until it appears slightly cloudy (*see* **Note 12**). Under dilution of a cell suspension may lead to poorly spread metaphases; over dilution and subsequent over spreading may lead to chromosome loss. If necessary, experiment to find the optimum dilution.

4. Using a p20 Gilson pipette, drop 2 μL of cell suspension onto the slide.

5. While the spot is drying mark the outside edges with a diamond pen (*see* **Note 13**).

6. Examine the metaphase quality under a low power lens (10×) on a phase-contrast microscope.

7. Consider the variations described in **Note 15**, to assist the spreading of chromosomes.

8. Slides should be aged for a minimum of 20 min on a hot plate at ≥60°C.

9. Often, slides require no further pre-treatment for successful metaphase FISH.

3.3. Growing and Preparing FISH probes

Please note that the following protocols are given for research purposes; if the probes are required for diagnostic testing then additional quality control procedures may be required.

3.3.1. Identifying Appropriate Probe Design

The following probe designs and applications apply to both home-grown and commercially available, ready labelled probes.

Dual Colour

Dual Colour Breakapart

These probes are designed to visualize disruption at a specific chromosomal breakpoint. Spectrum red (R) and Spectrum green (G) labelled probes are designed to hybridise to either side of a known breakpoint cluster, or to span a gene of interest. When the probe is hybridised to normal cells, the red and green signals are juxtaposed and appear as a yellow fusion (F) signal. A 0R0G2F signal pattern is produced in interphase, representing the intact locus on two normal homologous chromosomes. If a break occurs in the chromosome at this locus, the red and green signals become separated and appear as single signals. The resulting signal pattern is a "split" of one fusion signal into the component red and green parts (1R1G1F). This type of probe is particularly useful when the partner gene in a rearrangement is unknown, or when the target gene has multiple partners, for example, the *MLL* locus on chromosome 11q23 has more than 40 different partner genes.

Single Fusion

The single fusion probe is used for identification of specific gene rearrangements. It operates in the opposite sense to the breakapart probe. The red and green probes hybridise individually to specific genes of interest. The normal signal pattern is two red and two green signals (2R2G0F). When one red and one green signal become juxtaposed as the result of the gene fusion, they become aligned and appear as a yellow fusion signal on the derived chromosome 2, with the signal pattern 1R1G1F (*see* **Fig. 3a**).

Extra Signal and Dual Fusion

The same principle applies to extra signal and dual fusion probes. In extra signal probes, one of the probes extends beyond the breakpoint region of interest (the red signal on the normal chromosome in **Fig. 3b**). When the region is disrupted as a result of the gene fusion, part of the probe will remain in the original location on derived chromosome 1, forming the "extra signal" whilst the other part moves to derived chromosome 2, where it forms a fusion as described for the single fusion probe. The standard abnormal signal pattern for this type of probe will be 2R1G1F (red extra signal) or 1R2G1F (green extra signal).

In dual fusion probes both probes are extended beyond the breakpoint of both chromosomes. Thus, when the translocation occurs, two fusions are formed, one on each derived chromosome (**Fig. 3c**). The standard abnormal signal pattern in this situation is 1R1G2F.

The benefit of extra signal and dual fusion probes is that they reduce the incidence of false-positive cells as these signal patterns rarely arise by chance. These probes also provide additional information. For example, screening for the *BCR-ABL* rearrangement with the BCR-ABL dual fusion probe allows the detection of a deletion at the breakpoint of the derived chromosome 9 *(4)*.

Single Colour

If the genomic region of interest is small (50–200 kb), it may be covered by a single clone, which may be labelled with either Spectrum red or Spectrum green. If this region is involved in a

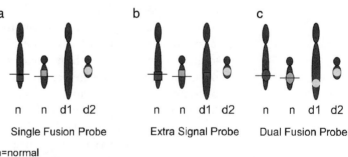

a   b   c

n   n   d1 d2   n   n   d1 d2   n   n   d1 d2

Single Fusion Probe   Extra Signal Probe   Dual Fusion Probe

n=normal
d1=derived chromosome 1
d2=derived chromosome 2

Fig. 3. Diagrammatic representation of (**a**) single fusion, (**b**) extra signal, and (**c**) dual fusion probes. Different sizes and positioning of probes on normal chromosomes produces a range of signal patterns for the same cytogenetic rearrangement. Probes which span a chromosomal breakpoint will produce a split signal between both derivative chromosomes. Normal chromosomes (n) show a single *red* or *green* signal, the derived chromosomes 1 and 2 (d1 and d2) show the patterns expected for each probe type. (*see* Color Plates)

chromosomal rearrangement, the probe will become split into two. Unlike the breakapart probe, which produces red and green portions (*see* **Subheading 3.5.1**), the splitting probe produces two signals in the same colour. Hence, a normal cell will have two signals and a "split" cell will have three. When an unknown cell is analysed, single colour probes cannot distinguish between a gain in copy number of the region and a "split."

Problems relating to the gain of a signal vs. splitting may be overcome by use of an internal control. Another probe is added to the hybridisation, usually a centromeric or locus-specific probe for the same chromosome, labelled in the opposite colour. A centromeric probe will provide information on chromosome copy number, confirming the presence of a split clone, while an additional locus-specific probe will indicate the efficiency of the hybridisation.

Painting Probes

Whole Chromosome Paints

These probes are derived from flow-sorted chromosomes. The DNA sequences from the chromosome of interest are labelled. Repetitive sequences are suppressed to prevent cross-hybridisation with similar sequences of other chromosomes. On hybridisation, only regions from the chromosome of interest will fluoresce. This allows identification of accurate location of specific regions of DNA within metaphase chromosomes. Paints are used to identify the origin of chromosomes involved in rearrangements. They are particularly useful in the identification of unknown partner chromosomes or regions.

Chromosome Arm Paints

These function in the same way as whole chromosome paints, but are specific for the short or long arms only. They are useful for refined analysis of a chromosome of interest.

3.3.2. Acquiring Clones

1. Identify the clones for BAC, PAC, and/or fosmids corresponding to the chromosomal region of interest using an appropriate website: ensembl: http://www.ensembl.org/index.html, UCSC http://genome.ucsc.edu/cgi-bin/hgGateway, NCBI: http://www.ncbi.nlm.nih.gov/(*see* **Note 16**).The clones are transported as agar stabs or glycerol stocks (*see* **Note 17**). Although it is advisable to use them immediately, stabs may be stored for up to 3 months at 4°C without any detrimental effects. Glycerol stocks can be stored indefinitely at –20 or –80°C

3.3.3. Streaking Plates (Day 1)

1. Set the incubator to 37°C.
2. Turn on the bunsen burner to a hot flame.
3. Sterilise the inoculating loops in the flame (or use disposable sterile inoculating loops).
4. Allow the loop to cool briefly before inserting into the tube containing the clone. Touch only the tip of the agar/glycerol stock.

5. Streak the clone onto an agar plate inoculated with the appropriate antibiotic (**Fig. 4**) (*see* **Note 18**). Replace lid.

6. Invert the plate and incubate upside–down in the incubator at 37°C overnight (~16 h) (*see* **Note 19**).

3.3.4. Inoculating Broth (Day 2)

1. Check the plates for growth of colonies.

2. Set the shaking incubator to 37°C at 200–250 rpm.

3. Turn the bunsen burner to a hot flame.

4. Pour 4–5 mL of LB broth (if using a plasmid purification mini-kit) into a 15-mL screw-top tube (*see* **Note 20**).

5. Sterilise the inoculating loops in the flame (or use disposable sterile inoculating loops).

6. Allow the loop to cool briefly.

7. Pick a single colony from the plate.

8. Briefly stir the colony into the LB broth.

9. Loosely tighten the screw cap onto the tube and secure with masking tape to ensure that the lid remains in position whilst shaking.

10. Place the tube into the shaking incubator at 37°C at ~200–250 rpm overnight (~16 h).

3.3.5. Making a Glycerol Stock and Extracting DNA (Day 3)

Glycerol Stock

1. Remove 850 μL of the bacteria-containing broth and place it into a screw-top microtube.

2. Add 150 μL of glycerol into the microtube.

3. Flick the tube to mix.

4. Store at –80°C (*see* **Note 21**).

DNA Extraction

1. Extract the DNA from the remaining bacteria-containing broth using a suitable plasmid purification kit. Follow the kit instructions.

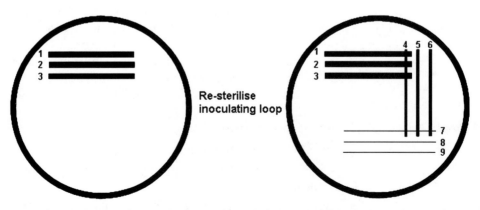

Fig. 4. Streaking plates. Streak each plate in the illustrated numerical order, re-sterilising the inoculating loop after streak 3. Single colonies are most likely to be found on streak 9.

At the final stage:

2. Re-suspend the extracted DNA in 40 μL (Mini) or 200 μL (Midi) of sterile distilled water, but not in TE buffer (*see* **Note 22**).

3. Leave at room temperature for 2 h to fully dissolve.

4. Optional step: A small amount of extracted DNA may be run on a 1% agrose gel to confirm the presence of DNA.

5. Store at –20°C until required for labelling (*see* **Note 23**).

3.3.6. Labelling (Day 4)

Using the Nick translation kit, choose to label the probes either with Spectrum red or Spectrum green dUTP.

1. Set the water bath to 16°C (*see* **Note 24**).

2. Thaw the kit reagents except for the enzyme, which should remain in the freezer until required.

3. Work on ice (*see* **Note 25**). Make up two tubes:

   a) A master mix of 0.1 mM of dNTP: 22 μL of 0.3 mM dATP, 0.3 mM of dCTP, and 0.3 mM of dGTP (provided with the kit, sufficient for six reactions).

   b) 0.1 mM of dTTP: 11 μL of 0.3 mM of dTTP (provided with the kit), and 22 μL of nuclease-free water (provided with kit).

4. Label a microtube for each probe being made.

5. Add: 2.5 μL of 0.2 mM Spectrum red (or green) dUTP, 5 μL of 0.1 mM dTTP, 10 μL of 0.1 mM dNTP, 5 μL of 10× nick translation buffer (supplied with the kit), and 17.5 μL of DNA.

6. Flick the tube to mix.

7. Remove the nick translation enzyme from the freezer and place on ice. It will thaw very quickly. Add 10 μL of enzyme to each reaction tube. Return the remaining enzyme to the freezer immediately.

8. Flick the tube to mix.

9. Pulse spin to concentrate the solution in the bottom of the tube.

10. Place the tube into the water bath at 16°C for 3¼ h.

11. Stop the reaction by adding 3 μL of 0.5 M EDTA (pH 8).

3.3.7. Probe Clean-Up

Using Sephadex G-50 columns follow the instructions provided or follow the protocol given below:

1. Flick the column to re-suspend the granules.

2. Snap-off the bottom section.

3. Place it into a clean microtube.

4. Unscrew the cap for ¼ turn.

5. Spin the tube for 1 min at 2,000 × *g* at 4°C in a micro-centrifuge.

6. Discard the supernatant.

7. Add 50 μL of TE buffer onto the granules in the column.

8. Spin for 1 min at 2,000 × *g* at 4°C in a micro-centrifuge.

9. Discard the waste collection tube and place the Sephadex column into a clean microtube to collect the labelled DNA.

10. Place the labelled DNA into the middle of the Sephadex column.

11. Spin for 2 min at 2,000 × *g* at 4°C.

12. As the labelled DNA is now eluted into the microtube, discard the Sephadex column (*see* **Note 26**).

13. Optional step: A small amount may be run on a 1.5% agrose gel to determine the size of the labelled DNA.

3.3.8. Probe Precipitation

1. To the labelled DNA (probe) add: 10 μL of Cot-1 DNA, 5 μL of 3 M sodium acetate, and 125 μL of ice cold 100% ethanol (*see* **Note 27**).

2. Vortex the mixture briefly.

3. Incubate at –20°C for 1–2 h.

4. Place into the micro-centrifuge, noting tube orientation (*see* **Note 28**).

5. Spin for 30 min at maximum speed at 4°C.

6. Remove and discard all the supernatant using a pipette, being careful not to dislodge the pellet (*see* **Note 29**).

7. Dry the pellet at room temperature with the lid of the tube removed for ~1 h.

8. Add 6 μL of distilled water and 14 μL of hybridization buffer.

9. Vortex to mix.

10. Store the probe at –20°C until required (*see* **Note 30**).

3.3.9. Probe Validation

The chromosomal location of the probes should be verified by hybridization to metaphases from a normal control. This may be facilitated by the co-hybridization of a centromeric probe, specific for the relevant chromosome (*see* **Note 31**). Cut-off scores for each new probe should be determined as described in **Subheading 3.8.3**.

3.3.10. Overcoming Problems

Cross-hybridisation and high background levels can usually be reduced and often eliminated by increasing the stringency of the washes. This may be achieved by increasing the temperature of Wash 1, reducing the SSC concentration of Wash 1, and leaving the slide in Wash 1 for a longer time or a combination of the three. If the cross-hybridisation signals are intense, this usually indicates a high degree of sequence homology, for example, when the clone is located close to the centromere or in a region of heterochromatin. This type may be impossible to eliminate and needs to be taken into consideration when interpreting results. Alternatively, varying the denaturation temperature by a degree or two and/or increasing or decreasing the denaturation time may be of assistance. Sometimes the FISH procedure fails to produce signals for no apparent reason; in these circumstances the hybridization should be repeated before re-labelling the DNA is considered.

3.4. In Situ Hybridisation, Post-Hybridisation and Visualization of Probes

The basic protocol used in our laboratory is a simple one, with only slight variations in the denaturing temperature and time dependent on the probe. The first time a probe is used, the manufacturer's protocol should be followed for optimum results. Often, if the probes are robust and the slide preparation is good, many of the manufacturer's recommendations for pre-treatment may subsequently be omitted without discernable reduction in signal visibility or hybridization efficiency.

3.4.1. Probe Dilutions and Mixes

Commercial Probes

These probes should always be diluted according to manufacturers' instructions. However, it is possible to obtain a result from a smaller area of the slide, using a correspondingly smaller quantity of probe at the same probe: buffer ratio. Most probes are used at a working dilution of 1/10 probe in buffer mix. The total volume of probe mix used is dependent upon the size of the coverslip. For example, 3 µL is sufficient for a 13-mm coverslip. Multiples of the volume of the probe may be prepared at one time if more than one slide is to be hybridised with the same probe mixture.

Home-Grown

The protocol for in-house probe growing and labelling (**Subheading 3.3**) produces a final working probe volume re-suspended in hybridization buffer. The probe can be applied to the slide individually or in a mixture with other probes.

3.4.2. Denaturing

For commercial probes, the manufacturers' protocols should be employed the first time a probe is used. For home-grown probes (**Subheading 3.3**), this standard protocol should apply.

1. Remove the probes from the freezer 5 min before use and leave at room temperature to thaw (*see* **Note 32**).

2. Label a microtube with each probe name or mixture of probes to be applied.

3. Pulse probes (in buffer) briefly in a micro-centrifuge to mix and collect all liquid together at the bottom of the tube.

4. Aliquot the appropriate amount of probe, taking care to avoid cross contamination.

5. Flick the tube to mix, or vortex briefly. Pulse the probe mix in a micro-centrifuge as **step 3** above.

6. Apply the appropriate volume of probe mix for the coverslip size.

7. Invert the region of the slide to be hybridised onto the coverslip, aligning the coverslip with the diamond marks and the spot of cell suspension. Surface tension will adhere the coverslip to the slide when it is turned over to coverslip-side-up.

8. Allow the probe mix to spread underneath to the edges of the coverslip. This will usually require applying gentle pressure (*see* **Note 33**).

9. Seal the edges of the coverslip with rubber cement.

10. Place the slide in a hybridisation machine (*see* **Note 34**), set to the appropriate programme (see specific manufacturers instructions or use 72°C for 2 min to denature the probe and target followed by overnight hybridisation at 37°C) (*see* **Note 35**).

3.4.3. Post-Hybridisation Washes

This protocol uses the same washes and times for all types of probe.

1. Switch on the water bath to 72°C and immediately place it into a coplin jar containing stringent Wash 1 (*see* **Notes 36 and 37**). Do not overfill the jar as the addition of slides will displace the liquid.

2. Fill two more coplin jars: One with 2× SSC and one with Wash 2. Leave at room temperature.

3. When the water bath and the solution in the coplin jar have reached the required temperature, remove the slides one at a time from the hybridization chamber. Using forceps, carefully remove the rubber cement.

4. Slide the coverslips off into a sharps disposal bin and place the slide in 2× SSC (*see* **Note 38**). If the coverslips do not detach easily, place the slide into 2× SSC, where they will eventually soak off or become loose enough to detach in ~10 min (*see* **Note 39**).

5. Repeat **steps 1–4** until all of the slides are in 2× SSC or until the coplin jar is full (*see* **Note 40**).

6. Transfer the slides quickly to Wash 1 for 2 min. Ensure that the slides are in separate slots of the coplin jar. Start the timer after the last slide has been added. This is a stringent wash, therefore accurate timing is important.

7. Remove the slides from Wash 1 in the same order as they were put in to keep timings as similar as possible for each slide. Transfer to Wash 2 for 30 s to 2 min. This wash reduces non-specific binding of probe and prevents the slide from drying out whilst preparing for the next stage.

3.4.4. Detection of Indirectly Labelled Probes

If a probe is directly labelled proceed to **Subheading 3.4.5**

1. Remove the slides from Wash 2 and drain off excess fluid from the tissue. Place the slides face up and add an excess (~100 μL) of block (*see* **Note 41**).

2. Cover with a temporary "coverslip" (*see* **Note 42**) and incubate at room temperature in a humid chamber (to prevent slide from drying out) for 15 min.

3. Carefully remove the coverslip and discard. Drain any excess block from the slide and apply an excess of detection reagent. Cover with a coverslip (as **step 2** above) and incubate at room temperature in a humid chamber for 10 min (*see* **Note 43**).

4. Carefully remove the coverslip and place the slides in Wash 3 for 1–2 min. This wash removes any unbound detection reagent.

5. Mount the slides as described below.

3.4.5. Mounting of Slides

1. Place the appropriate number of 24 × 50-mm² coverslips on absorbent paper. Add 7 μL of slide mounting medium to each one.

2. Taking each slide in turn, drain off the excess liquid. Wipe the back of the slide on the paper, taking care to wipe the correct side!

3. Invert the slide onto the coverslip to come into contact with the slide mounting medium. Surface tension will adhere the coverslip to the slide. Press firmly but carefully on the back of the slide whilst it is face down on the paper. This will allow excess fluid to be absorbed.

4. Turn the slide over and push out the air bubbles (*see* **Note 33**).

5. Re-blot the slide.

6. Store the slide at 4°C in the dark until required.

7. For long-term storage, the edges of the coverslip should be sealed with nail varnish. This prevents the slides drying out. Store in slide boxes at 4°C.

3.5. Breakpoint Mapping and Identification of Partner Genes

Breakpoint mapping identifies the breakpoint involved in a chromosomal rearrangement. Although chromosome banding and/or painting may indicate the chromosome arm or region involved, it may be novel or distant from one with a known probe associated with it. Starting from a known region or probe, clones to cover the region of interest should be selected. Practically, it is easier to handle not more than ten clones at any one time. Initially widely spaced clones, several Mb apart, should be used to narrow down a large region. Metaphases are required to map the breakpoints of balanced rearrangements to locate the positions of probes on the derived chromosomes. Once the relevant region has been narrowed down to ~1 Mb, the separation of clones designed as breakapart probes will be informative in interphase.

Breakpoint mapping may be performed in interphase nuclei if the rearrangement is unbalanced. For example, a der(7)t(7;10)(q22;24) will show monosomy for the region distal to 7q22. Thus, probes representative of this region will show a single copy in interphase.

1. Order the clones corresponding to evenly-spaced intervals across the region of interest.

2. Grow and label the probes as described in **Subheading 3.3**.

3. Apply the probes sequentially (*see* **Subheading 3.7**) to abnormal metaphases in order to identify the derived chromosome to which they hybridise.

4. Continue in this way until the region is narrowed down and the breakpoint is identified to be within two neighbouring clones (*see* **Fig. 5**). Interpretation becomes more precise if the breakpoint arises in a single clone, resulting in a split (*see* **Subheading 3.5.3**).

5. Once the breakpoint has been identified as closely as possible by FISH, the genes in the region may be assessed using online resources. Ideally, the breakpoint will be further characterised using additional molecular techniques, such as RT-PCR or long distance inverse-PCR.

3.6. Sequential Metaphase FISH

This approach is highly effective for the characterisation of chromosomal abnormalities. By re-hybridisation of the same metaphase several times with different probes, direct comparisons can be made. This allows the identification of partner chromosomes in balanced and unbalanced rearrangements, leading to definition of the regions or genes involved (*see* **Fig. 6**).

1. Prepare metaphase spreads onto slides (*see* **Subheading 3.2.3**).

2. Hybridise the initial probe(s) (*see* **Subheading 3.4**).

3. Scan the slide using a low magnification lens and a DAPI filter to locate metaphases. Carefully record their location using an England Finder or Vernier scale.

4. Capture images of suitable metaphases using the appropriate filters.

5. Remove the probe by:
    (a) Wiping the oil off the cover slip.
    (b) Placing the slide in 2× SSC for 1 h (*see* **Note 44**).
    (c) Washing the slide for 20 min in Wash 2 (*see* **Note 45**).
    (d) Air drying the slide (*see* **Note 46**).

6. Hybridise the second probe(s) as **step 2** (*see* **Note 47**).

7. Relocate and recapture images of the metaphases.

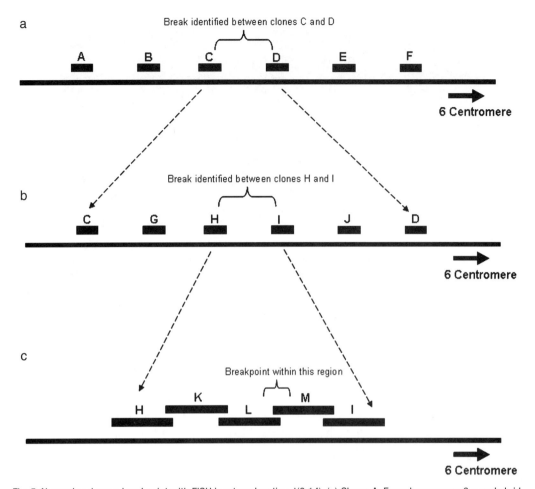

Fig. 5. Narrowing down a breakpoint with FISH in a translocation, t(6;14). (**a**) Clones A–F on chromosome 6 were hybrid-ised initially. The breakpoint was identified to be located between clones C and D with clones D–F remaining on the derived chromosome 6, der(6), and clones A–C moving to the der(14). (**b**) New clones G–J (between clones C and D) were hybridised. The breakpoint was identified to be between clones H and I. (**c**) Overlapping clones K, L, and M were hybridised. Clone L was found to relocate to the der(14), but clone M remained on the der(6). The breakpoint was identi-fied to be within clones L and M.

8. Analyse the images by comparing relative probe positions from the sequential hybridisations to fully characterise the abnormalities of interest. With some imaging software it may be possible to superimpose the images. Care should be taken in interpretation of results as residual signals may remain from a previous hybridisation.

3.7. Analysis and Interpretation of Results

3.7.1. Microscope Set Up

The microscope used for analysis of the FISH slides will need to be equipped for epifluorescence. The minimum filter set required for standard three colour FISH are DAPI (counterstain) and appropriate filters for the red and green florochromes. The green filter is most commonly FITC (which also allows visualisation of

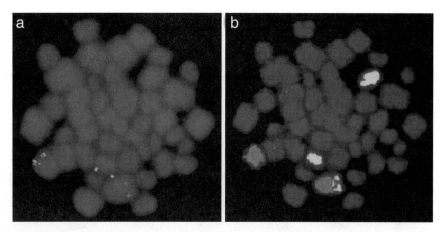

Fig. 6. Sequential metaphase FISH to identify a chromosomal partner. (**a**) A breakapart locus-specific probe to *TLX3* shows a split signal pattern. The intact fusion hybridises to 5q35, the red signal remains on the derived chromosome 5, der(5), and the green signal has translocated to an unknown partner chromosome. (**b**) After washing and re-hybridising with whole chromosome paint 5 (*red*) and 7 (*green*), the partner chromosome is identified as chromosome 7. Further FISH may be carried out to identify the partner gene involved, using published data on known genes, or by breakpoint mapping (*see* **Subheading 3.7**). (*see* Color Plates)

Fluorescein) but the choice of red filter is dependent on whether the red fluorochrome is TRITC, Rhodamine, or Texas red. A dual filter (which allows visualization of both red and green florochromes at the same time) is the one most frequently used for interphase analysis. Most imaging software packages allow for easy switching between filters. Alternatively, the filters may be switched into position manually. Images may be captured if the appropriate camera and software are in use.

3.7.2. Interphase FISH Analysis

It is recommended that results, especially if they are to be used for diagnostic purposes, should be generated from the combined interpretation of two independent analysts. For a standard interphase FISH test on an acute leukaemia sample, 100 successful nuclei should be scored by each analyst, providing a total of ≥200 cells. If a sample is very sparse, a result from ≥100 cells may be acceptable with both analysts scoring at least 50 cells.

It is vital that the analyst has knowledge of the probe used and the expected signal patterns. Consider these questions before analysing a case:

(i) Is the probe single or dual colour?

(ii) Is it designed to detect a gain, loss or gene fusion?

(iii) Is it a breakapart or a fusion probe?

(iv) What chromosome(s) or region(s) do the probes hybridise to?

(v) What is the normal signal pattern for this probe?

(vi) What is the standard abnormal signal pattern for this probe?

(vii) Is there any indication from a cytogenetic or molecular result (if available) to expect an unusual signal pattern?

(viii) All analysts should score the slides "blind," without knowledge of the other analyst's results.

1. Select the correct area of cells to be analysed on a low power lens (10 or 16×) using the DAPI filter.

2. Switch to a high power lens (100×) and refocus the slide.

3. Use the dual filter to locate signals in the nuclei (*see* **Note 48**).

4. Determine the signal pattern and record it for each nucleus in turn. Avoid damaged nuclei and clumps of cells with indistinct boundaries.

5. Analyse 100 cells. A second analyst should analyse a further 100 cells from a different region of the area covered by the probe.

3.7.3. Calculation of Cut-Off Values

There is a possibility of accidental juxtaposition of red and green signals in a normal cell, which may be interpreted as a positive result in a normal case. To take such chance findings into account in the interpretation of results and to determine the false-positive level, a cut-off score should be calculated for every probe used. Five samples from normal individuals should be evaluated. The sample type should be the same as the samples to be tested (bone marrow for leukaemia patients) and 200 nuclei should be scored by each analyst on all five cases. The false-positive rate for each and the mean false-positive rate for all five cases should be calculated. The cut-off level is the mean false-positive rate plus 3 standard deviations. This is expressed as a percentage and may differ between analysts. To maintain maximum accuracy, cut-off values should be revaluated periodically.

3.7.4. Interpretation of Interphase FISH Results

Any population in the patient sample of a higher level than the cut-off value should be considered as positive. Although very low level positive results, close to the cut-off value, are rare in diagnostic acute leukaemia samples, they may occur from time to time. The results should be scrutinised and if possible the sample tested with an alternative probe or an appropriate molecular test.

The results from the two analysts should be in close agreement in terms of the cell populations present in the sample and their relative sizes, as interpreted from the FISH signal patterns and the number of cells with each pattern. If the results disagree, then a third independent analysis is required. The two sets of results which most closely agree after the third analysis should be used to provide the definitive result. Sometimes discrepant results may arise from poor probe hybridisation. In these circumstances the test should be repeated or an alternative informative probe is used.

4. Notes

1. Samples are usually received in transport medium containing RPMI, preservative-free heparin and a small amount of foetal calf serum, to support the bone marrow cells during transit. The sample is centrifuged and the cells are transferred to fresh complete medium to encourage growth.

2. 3% Virkon is used as an appropriate strength disinfectant against infectious bacteria (e.g., tuberculosis).

3. Blast cells from patients with acute leukaemia must be cultured over short time periods as they die rapidly in vitro.

4. The time in colchicine varies according to laboratory practice, ranging from 15 min to 2 h. Sometimes overnight incubation is carried out, although this results in highly condensed chromosomes.

5. Pre-warming the KCl solution prevents cold shock to the leukaemic cells.

6. Cells may be incubated in KCl at 37°C before spinning to promote metaphase spreading when slide making. This depends on the sample type, which may be determined empirically.

7. If a sample is contaminated with red blood cells, vortexing during fixation is particularly important to prevent clumping of white cells. If the red blood cells have been removed prior to cell culture the white cells become more fragile. Thus, keeping the pellet mobile by flicking gently with one finger as the fixative is added reduces the chance of the cells rupturing during the fixation process.

8. At this first fixation step the suspension will appear brown due to the presence of lysed red blood cells.

9. Acetic acid softens the cell membrane; therefore overnight fixation improves the spreading of the chromosomes, as the cell membranes rupture more easily upon contact with the glass slide.

10. At this stage, the cell pellet has become more fragile and the cells require longer centrifugation to minimise cell loss.

11. Slide making may be carried out immediately or postponed, if so the cell suspension should be topped up with fresh fixative to prevent evaporation, and stored at –20°C.

12. The concentration of the cells in suspension depends on the purpose for the slide being made. It is possible to achieve good results from a very small aliquot of cell suspension: ~2 μL is usually adequate for most interphase and metaphase FISH. In contrast, cell suspensions used to make slides for

conventional cytogenetic analysis need to be more dilute and larger quantities are required.

13. Marking the limits of the cell suspension "spot" helps to relocate the cells while the probe is being applied and later to read the result.

14. Up to four tests may be easily performed on a single slide. Thus the diamond pen markings are important to relocate the areas.

15. (a) Slide making is a sensitive procedure, susceptible to subtle variations in temperature, air current, and humidity. In general, warmer, moist, and still conditions produce the best slides. Conditions are less critical for slides made for interphase FISH as many probes are sufficiently robust to hybridise well to sub-optimal slides. A number of steps may be added to improve slide quality and assist the spreading of cells.

   (i) The slide should be cleaned before use (wipe with a tissue soaked in a small amount of fixative).

   (ii) Breathe on the slide to add a layer of condensation immediately prior to dropping the cell suspension.

   (iii) Drop the cell suspension in a single motion.

   (iv) Rotate the slide once after dropping the cells.

   (v) Add a second drop of fixative to the slide as the edges of the spot begin to dry: at the time that the Newton's rings become visible.

   (vi) Add 3–4 drops of 70% acetic acid in methanol at the time that the Newton's rings become visible. Cover the spot and allow the acetic acid to remain on the slide and evaporate slowly. Leave for ~2–3 min, rotating the slide occasionally to ensure contact is maintained with the spot. Drain excess acetic acid from the slide onto a tissue and air dry.

   (vii) Keep the slide motionless whilst drying to avoid unnecessary air currents.

   (viii) Dry the slide slowly on a damp paper towel (to create a humid atmosphere).

   (ix) Dry the slide by warming on the back of the hand.

   (b) Cells from different disease types behave differently during the preparation of metaphases:

AML samples
Generally, AML cells spread more easily than those from ALL samples, which makes them prone to over-spreading. A single, additional drop of fixative, added when the Newton's rings form on the slide, is usually the best additional step to use. The use of

70% acetic acid in methanol (*see* **Note 15a** (vi)) is not advisable for AML samples as it may induce over spreading, leading to loss of nuclei from the slide.

ALL samples

It is more difficult to obtain good quality metaphases from ALL samples. The addition of one or more drops of fixative onto the slide whilst it is drying may improve spreading (*see* **Note 15a** (v)). Alternatively, the addition 70% acetic acid in methanol may be effective (*see* **Note 15a** (vi)).

16. It should be verified that the chosen clones are positioned to the same chromosomal location by more than one website. If there is a discrepancy between sites it is advisable to choose an alternative clone. Note that not all sites list the same clones. Specific clone requirements will depend on the project being undertaken. If the probe is being created for the detection of a translocation it is advisable to choose two clones and to label them with different fluorochromes (*see* **Subheading 3.5.1**). Clones may be purchased from companies such as Invitrogen (Invitrogen Ltd), BACPAC Resources Center (BACPAC Resources, CA) and Geneservice (Geneservice Ltd, Cambridge).

17. Delivery time for stabs may be up to 6 weeks.

18. It must be ascertained that the plate is free from contamination before use (especially if it has been stored for more than 2 weeks). A fresh plate should be used for each clone. Each plate must be labelled with the date and clone name. Information supplied with the clone will identify the antibiotic to be used. The bacteria tend to be densely packed within the agar stabs, so it is important to re-flame the inoculating loops to ensure that only single colonies are grown without cross contamination.

19. It is important to incubate (and store) the plates upsidedown in order to prevent condensation dripping onto the colonies, which may lead to cross contamination. Plates may be stacked one on top of the other in the incubator. They may be stored upside-down at 4°C for several weeks. Taping stacks of plates together with masking tape reduces the risk of them being knocked over and contaminated.

20. A plasmid mini-kit will provide sufficient material for ~20 FISH tests. If a larger volume is required a midi- or maxi- kit should to be used. Larger volumes need to be grown in a larger container, either a conical or bacteria flask (ridged conical flask). The broth should not occupy more than one third of the total vessel volume to allow appropriate aeration of the culture.

21. Glycerol stocks may be stored for many years at –80°C. They may be used to re-grow clones as required.

22. TE buffer may interfere with downstream applications (subsequent experiments) of the DNA.

23. Avoid repeated rounds of freeze thawing as this will damage the DNA.

24. Use a standard water bath placed in a 4°C cold room to maintain 16°C. Alternatively a thermocycler or cooling water bath may be used.

25. It is important that all reagents are maintained on ice to prevent the temperature of the reaction mixture being above 16°C. Temperatures above this can cause inefficient dye incorporation into the DNA.

26. Although probes may be stored at –20°C prior to the probe precipitation step, this is not advisable as it may lead to an increase in background signals when the probe is hybridised.

27. It is advisable to store a 50 mL tube of 100% ethanol permanently at –20°C.

28. It is important to note the orientation of the tube in the centrifuge as the DNA is unlikely to be visible after spinning.

29. It is important to remove all supernatant to facilitate complete drying of the pellet.

30. Probes may be stored for several years at –20°C. Probe efficiency may be reduced after about 2 years.

31. It is critical to validate the chromosomal location of probes, as their genomic positioning by the public databases may sometimes be incorrect or, occasionally, clones may have become cross contaminated. This validation will also confirm the efficiency of the probe, identify any cross hybridization and determine the level of background staining before the probe is used on valuable research material.

32. Directly labelled probes should be protected from light to prevent bleaching of the fluorochromes.

33. Air bubbles must be removed as they prevent efficient probe hybridisation/probe visualisation. Use a pipette tip, blunt pencil or the barrel of a Gilson pipette to apply gentle pressure to the coverslip from the middle outwards.

34. Alternatively, denaturation may be carried out by placing the slide onto a hotplate at 72°C for 2 min followed by hybridisation in a humid chamber (either a box floating in a water bath or a box containing damp paper towels in an oven) at 37°C overnight.

35. Hybridisation of the slide for longer than 16 h (overnight) at 37°C may increase the levels of background staining.

36. Coplin jars break easily when exposed to sudden changes in temperature.

37. The detergent in Wash 1 removes background staining from the slides.

38. The coverslip may adhere to the rubber cement while it is being removed. This is not a problem as the lump of rubber cement which gathers on the end of the forceps may be used as a handy non-slip tool to assist in the sliding of the coverslip to the edge of the slide for easy removal into the sharps bin.

39. Care must be taken to appropriate disposal of coverslips which have detached into the Coplin jar containing 2× SSC.

40. Add not more than five slides to each Coplin jar. The addition of each slide will cool down the solution and it is important that the temperature is maintained at 72°C.

41. Block is a weak solution made from dried milk powder (available from any supermarket) and is used to prevent non-specific binding of the fluorochromes during the detection stage.

42. Pieces of "Parafilm" is cut to size to make excellent temporary "coverslips."

43. The time in block or detection reagent is not critical, although it should be no longer than 2 h.

44. The coverslip should detach from the slide whilst in this solution. If not, agitate the slide at intervals and continue soaking until it does so. The coverslip may be gently slid off once loose, although care must be taken not to damage the metaphases.

45. Some probes are not easily removed, so it may be necessary to increase the time in Wash 2 or to introduce an additional 2 min incubation in Wash 1 at 72°C, after the 2× SSC step.

46. Sometimes salt crystals will appear on the slide. However, these do not appear to affect subsequent hybridisations.

47. Consider the probe locations and, if possible, alternate the red and green labelling of these probes which are likely to hybridise adjacent to one another in order to facilitate the interpretation of results. Since paints tend to be more difficult to remove than locus-specific probes, it is advisable to apply the locus-specific probes prior to the paints. Our experience has shown that it is possible to apply at least five rounds of FISH sequentially onto the same metaphase, although 13 rounds have been achieved *(5)*. Note that repeated hybridisation leads to increasing degradation of the chromatin and reduced DAPI staining, making relocation of the metaphases increasingly difficult.

48. Signals may not be located within a single plane of focus, and therefore when the nuclei are scanned it is important to focus up and down through the nuclei.

References

1. Grimwade D, Walker H, Oliver F, Wheatley K, Harrison CJ, Harrison G, et al. (1998). The importance of diagnostic cytogenetics on outcome in AML: Analysis of 1,612 patients entered into the MRC AML 10 trial. *Blood* **92**(7):2322–33.

2. Harrison CJ, Foroni L. (2002). Cytogenetics and molecular genetics of acute lymphoblastic leukemia. *Rev Clin Exp Hematol*;**6**(2):91–113.

3. Romana SP, Poirel H, Leconiat M, Flexor MA, Mauchauffe M, Jonveaux P, et al. (1995). High frequency of t(12;21) in childhood B-lineage acute lymphoblastic leukemia. *Blood*;**86**:4263–9.

4. Robinson HM, Martineau M, Harris RL, Barber KE, Jalali GR, Moorman AV, et al. (2005). Derivative chromosome 9 deletions are a significant feature of childhood Philadelphia chromosome positive acute lymphoblastic leukaemia. *Leukemia*;**19**(4):564–71.

5. Pinson MP, Martineau M, Jabbar MS, Kilby AM, Walker H, Harrison CJ. (2000). Sequential FISH reveals an abnormal karyotype involving 14 chromosomes in a child with acute lymphoblastic leukemia. *Leukemia*;**14**(9):1705–7.

Chapter 4

Specialized Fluorescence In Situ Hybridization (FISH) Techniques for Leukaemia Research

Lyndal Kearney and Sue Colman

Summary

Fluorescence in situ hybridization (FISH) provides one of the few ways of analysing the genotype of individual cells, an important consideration for mixed cell populations such as those found in leukaemia. A more sophisticated variation combines fluorescence immunophenotyping and FISH for specific leukaemia-associated chromosome rearrangements. Combined immunophenotyping and FISH is a powerful tool to identify the cell lineage in which the leukaemia-specific chromosome rearrangement occurs and has been used to identify putative pre-leukaemic cells in normal cord blood. Another valuable FISH-based research technique is multi-fluor FISH (M-FISH). This multicolour approach is effectively a molecular karyotype of individual cells and has a range of applications, from chromosome breakage studies and characterising mouse models of leukaemia, to providing a perfect complementary approach to the emerging genomic microarray technologies.

Key words: Fluorescence immunophenotyping, FISH, M-FISH

1. Introduction

The development of techniques based on fluorescence in situ hybridization (FISH) has been a major advance in cytogenetic analysis. With the widespread availability of high-quality commercial FISH probes for leukaemia-associated chromosome abnormalities, these techniques are now incorporated into the diagnostic cytogenetics profile alongside conventional karyotyping. This chapter will concentrate on two specialized FISH-based techniques that we have found particularly useful in childhood leukaemia research. The first of these, combined immunophenotyping

C.W.E. So (ed.), Leukemia, *Methods in Molecular Biology, vol. 538*
© Humana Press, a part of Springer Science + Business Media, LLC 2009
DOI: 10.1007/978-1-59745-418-6_4

and FISH, allows the simultaneous visualization of fluorescence immunophenotype and FISH for specific leukaemia-associated chromosome abnormalities (**Fig. 1a, b** *(1)*. Our previous screening of a large series of unselected cord bloods by RT-PCR revealed that approximately 1% of normal cord blood samples harboured clones with the *TEL-AML1* fusion *(1)*. This is approximately 100 times higher than the incidence of leukaemia and indicates that the fusion itself is insufficient for the development of leukaemia. In this study, the *TEL-AML1* fusion gene was present in the CD19+ (pan B lineage), but not the CD13/33+ (pan myeloid) or CD3+ (pan T cell) fraction, providing evidence that these are pre-leukaemic cells containing the initiating genetic event for the development of leukaemia. More recently, we investigated a pair of monochorionic twins, one of whom was diagnosed with pre-B cell acute lymphoblastic leukaemia (ALL) at age 2 *(2)*. Combined immunophenotyping and FISH of her leukaemic blasts revealed the *TEL-AML1* gene fusion with additional loss of the normal *TEL* allele. In the peripheral blood lymphocytes of her healthy co-twin, we identified a low frequency (~1%) of CD19+ cells with the *TEL-AML1* fusion. However, these cells contained the normal *TEL* allele, consistent with pre-leukaemia status (**Fig. 1b**) *(2)*.

The second method included here is multi-fluor (also called multicolour) FISH (M-FISH) (**Fig. 1c**) *(3)*. M-FISH and the related variants spectral karyotyping (SKY) *(4)* and combined binary and ratio labelling (COBRA) *(5)* has been one of the great successes of molecular cytogenetics in the past decade. Designed to provide a "molecular" karyotype, this technique has spawned many variations with chromosome arm-specific *(3, 6)*, region-specific *(7, 8)*, centromeric *(9)*, and subtelomeric probe sets *(10, 11)*. Although the main application has been to elucidate complex karyotypes, the technique lends itself to a diverse range of biological questions, notably the 3D analysis of nuclear structure and function *(12)*, and the analysis of mouse models of leukaemia using murine M-FISH paints *(13)*. We have demonstrated that M-FISH perfectly complements the new genomic microarray technologies (array CGH), which are designed to detect regions of gain or loss *(14)*.

2. Materials

2.1. Combined Immunophenotyping and FISH

1. Lamb's immuno slide staining trays (Raymond A. Lamb Ltd., Eastbourne, UK).
2. DakoCytomation delimiting pen S2002 (DakoCytomation, Ely, Cambridgeshire, UK).

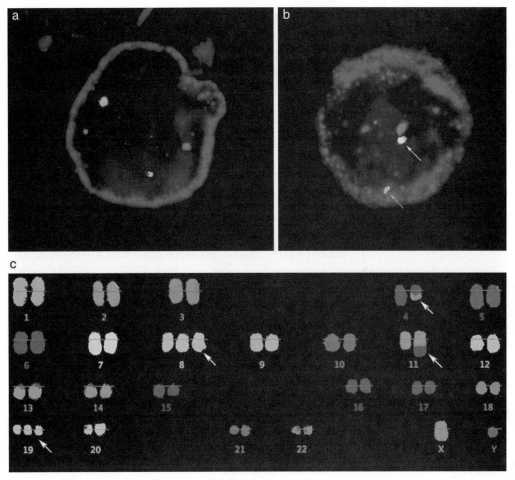

Fig. 1. Examples of combined immunophenotyping and FISH and M-FISH. (**a**) Combined fluorescence immunopheno-typing of a normal cord blood cell stained for CD33 (AMCA-blue fluorescence) and FISH with centromeric probes for chromosomes 7 (SpectrumOrange, red fluorescence) and 12 (SpectrumGreen, green fluorescence). (**b**) Combined fluorescence immunophenotyping of a putative pre-leukaemic cell stained for CD19 (AMCA, *blue*) and FISH for the *TEL-AML1* fusion gene. The yellow fluorescence denotes the fusion gene (indicated here by a *yellow arrow*); the small red signal the residual piece of the *AML1* gene resulting from the translocation and the large red signal the second (normal) copy of the *AML1* gene. Note that the second copy of the *TEL* gene (the allele not involved in the translocation) is present (green signal, indicated by a *green arrow*). (**c**) M-FISH karyotype of the MV4:11 leukaemia-derived cell line containing the t(4;11)(q21;q23), which results in the *MLL-AF4* fusion gene. Other abnormalities identified here are an additional copy of chromosome 8 and 19. Each of the abnormalities is indicated by an *arrow*. (*see* Color Plates)

3. Vulcanising rubber solution (www.weldtite.co.uk).

4. Vectashield mountant (Vector Laboratories, Peterborough, UK).

5. Phosphate buffered saline (PBSa): Dissolve the following in 800 mL of H_2O: 10 g NaCl, 0.25 g KCl, 1.437 g KH_2PO_4, 0.25 g Na_2HPO_4. Adjust pH to 7.2 with HCl. Make up to 1 L with distilled water.

6. 10× Phosphate (PN) buffer: 57.7 mL 1 M Na_2HPO_4, 42.3 mL 1 M NaH_2PO_4. Dilute 1 in 10 with water for use.

7. Primary antibody: Mouse monoclonal anti-human antigen of interest (e.g. CD19 clone HD37, DakoCytomation).

8. Secondary antibody: Goat F(ab')$_2$ anti-mouse IgG biotin labelled (Cambridge BioScience Ltd., Cambridge, UK).

9. Avidin D AMCA (Vector Laboratories, Peterborough, UK).

10. 20× SSC (3 M NaCl, 0.3 M trisodium citrate, pH 5.2): 175.3 g NaCl, 88.2 g trisodium citrate in 800 mL of H$_2$O. Adjust pH to 5.2 with HCl. Make up to 1 L with water.

11. Denaturation buffer (70% formamide, 2× SSC, pH 7.0): 35 mL Fluka formamide, 5 mL 20× SSC at pH 5.2, 10 mL dH$_2$O. Check the pH with pH paper.

12. 20× SSC (3 M NaCl, 0.3 M trisodium citrate, pH 7.0): 175.3 g NaCl, 88.2 g trisodium citrate in 800 mL of H$_2$O. Adjust pH to 7.0 with HCl. Make up to 1 L with water.

13. 2× SSC/0.1% (v/v) NP-40: 100 mL 20× SSC (pH5.2), 850 mL H$_2$O, 1 mL NP-40. Mix thoroughly until NP-40 is dissolved. Make up to 1 L with water.

14. 0.4× SSC/0.3% (v/v) NP-40: 20 mL 20× SSC (pH 5.2), 950 mL H$_2$O, 3 mL NP-40. Mix thoroughly before making up to a final volume of 1 L.

2.2. Multicolour FISH (M-FISH)

2.2.1. Pre-treatment of Chromosomal DNA on Slides

1. Phosphate buffered saline (PBSa): Dissolve the following in 800 mL of H$_2$O: 10 g NaCl, 0.25 g KCl, 1.437 g KH$_2$PO$_4$, 0.25 g Na$_2$HPO$_4$. Adjust pH to 7.2 with HCl. Make up to 1 L with distilled water.

2. PBS/50 mM MgCl$_2$: 50 mL of 1 M MgCl$_2$, 950 mL of 1× PBS.

3. 1% Formaldehyde in PBS/50 mM MgCl$_2$: 2.7 mL formaldehyde (40% w/v) in 100 mL PBS/MgCl$_2$. Make up freshly each time.

4. Pepsin stock (10 mg/ mL): Mix 10 mg pepsin (Sigma P-6887) with 1 mL of water, pre-warmed to 37°C. Aliquot and store at –20°C until ready to use.

5. 30 µg/ mL pepsin: Add 150 µL of pepsin stock to 50 mL of 0.01N HCl (pre-warmed to 37°C). Make up freshly each time

2.2.2. Hybridization and Washes

1. Vysis SpectraVysion M-FISH whole chromosome painting kit (Abbott Molecular).

2. Denaturation solution (70% formamide, 2× SSC, pH 7.0): 35 mL ultrapure formamide (Fluka, Sigma-Aldrich), 5 mL 20× SSC (pH 5.2), 10 mL dH$_2$O, 25 µL 0.25 M EDTA. Measure the pH with pH paper to verify if it is pH 7.0–8.0.

3. Formamide wash solution (50% formamide, 2× SSC, pH 7.0): 75 mL ultrapure formamide (Fluka, Sigma-Aldrich),

15 mL 20× SSC at pH 5.2, 60 mL distilled H_2O. Check the pH using pH paper

4. 20× SSC (3 M NaCl, 0.3 M trisodium citrate, pH 5.2): 175.3 g NaCl, 88.2 g sodium citrate in 800 mL of H2O. Adjust pH to 5.2 with HCl. Make up to 1 L with water.

5. 20× SSC (pH 7.0): 175.3 g NaCl, 88.2 g trisodium citrate in 800 mL of H_2O. Adjust pH to 7.0 with HCl. Make up to 1 L with water.

6. 1× SSC: 50 mL 20× SSC, 950 mL H_2O.

7. 2× SSC, pH 7.0: 100 mL 20× SSC, 900 mL H_2O.

8. 4× SSCT (4× SSC with 0.05% (v/v) Tween 20): 200 mL 20× SSC, 800 mL H_2O, 0.5 mL Tween 20. Mix thoroughly.

9. Vectashield with DAPI: 1 μL of 1 mg/ mL DAPI stock in 1 mL of Vectashield mountant (Vector Laboratories).

2.2.3. M-FISH Image Capture and Analysis

1. Epifluorescence microscope fitted with narrow bandpass filters for the component fluorochromes in the paint set. For the Vysis SpectraVysion probes, filters for SpectrumGreen, SpectrumAqua, SpectrumGold, SpectrumRed and SpectrumFRed, as well as the DAPI counterstain, are required.

2. CCD camera: We use a Photometrics Sensys cooled CCD camera with a Kodak KAF 1400 chip (Photometrics, Tucson, USA)

3. M-FISH Software: We use Digital Scientific SmartCapture and M-FISH software (Digital Scientific, Cambridge UK).

3. Methods

3.1. Combined Fluorescence Immunophenotyping and FISH

This technique allows the simultaneous assessment of cell surface markers and FISH signals for specific genetic abnormalities. In the following protocol, fluorescence immunophenotyping is performed first, followed by FISH, without any additional fixation steps in between the two. Although directly labelled antibodies can be used for immunophenotyping, we find that it is preferable to use a sandwich technique to increase the intensity of the fluorescence, as this is decreased by the subsequent FISH procedures. The FISH method given here is for a commercial dual colour fusion gene probe set. However, in general, FISH can be carried out using any FISH protocol, always omitting any preceding protease/pepsin steps, as this would remove the immunofluorescence sandwich.

3.1.1. Preparation of Cells

The quality of cellular preparations is even more important for combined immunophenotype and FISH procedure than it is for FISH alone. Where possible, we prefer to use cytospin slides of the cell of interest, although the technique has been successfully used on bone marrow or peripheral blood smears, tumour imprints, and even paraffin embedded bone marrow trephines *(15)*. Cytospins can be prepared on mononuclear cells after Lymphoprep gradient centrifugation, or on cell subsets enriched by magnetic bead sorting or fluorescence activated cell sorting (FACS). For cytospin preparations of FACS cell subsets, it is necessary to have at least 10,000, and preferably 20,000–30,000 cells, in order to obtain 200 cells for FISH scoring. It is important that the cells are well spaced (not too dense or too sparse), as this helps to reduce non-specific antibody staining, and makes scoring of the FISH signals easier. Freshly prepared slides should be air dried at room temperature for several hours. They can then be processed immediately, or wrapped individually in foil and stored at –80°C until required. Remove individual slides from the freezer for use, to avoid thawing the remaining slides in the batch.

3.1.2. Fluorescence Detection of Cell Surface Markers (1)

1. The slides are removed from –80°C and brought to room temperature before removing from foil (to prevent condensation damage to cells).

2. The slides are fixed in acetone for 7 min at room temperature.

3. The slides are allowed to air dry for 10 min before being rehydrated in PBSa for 10 min.
   All the following procedures are carried out in a humidified chamber (*see* **Note 1**):

4. The area of the slide containing the cells of interest is marked either using a diamond pen, or a delimiting pen (*see* **Note 2**).

5. 25 µL normal human serum (1:10) is placed on the area containing the cells for 10 min at room temperature to block non-specific protein binding sites.

6. Excess blocking solution is removed by gently tipping the slide and draining onto a paper towel.

7. 25 µL of primary antibody (mouse monoclonal anti-human antibody against the antigen of interest) (*see* **Note 3**) is applied to the marked area of the slide and incubated for 45 min at room temperature.

8. The slides are washed in PBSa (in waterbath with agitation) for 15 min (3 × 5 min).

9. 25 µL of secondary antibody (biotinylated goat F(ab')$_2$ anti-mouse IgG, Southern Biotechnology Associates, Birmingham AL, USA) (1:20) is applied and incubated for 45 min at room temperature (*see* **Note 4**).

10. The slides are washed in three changes of PBSa for 5-min each (with agitation).

11. 20 µL of Avidin D AMCA (1:25) is applied to the marked area of the slide and incubated for 45 min at room temperature.

12. The slides are washed in three changes of PBS for 5-min each (with agitation).

13. At this stage slides can be stored in phosphate buffer (in coplin jars in the fridge) for several weeks before proceeding with the FISH. The success of the immunostaining can be monitored by mounting the slides in phosphate buffer (avoid glycerol as this may cause hybridization artefacts).

An alternative fluorescence detection protocol is given in **Note 5**.

3.1.3. FISH

1. The FISH probe is prepared in an appropriate volume of hybridization buffer according to the manufacturer's instructions.

2. The probe DNA is denatured in a waterbath at 73°C for 5 min. Place in a waterbath at 45°C until ready to apply to slide.

3. The chromosomal DNA on slides is denatured in denaturation buffer at 73°C (in waterbath under a fume hood) for 5 min (*see* **Notes 6** and **7**).

4. The slides are dehydrated through an ethanol series (70%, 90%, absolute) for 3-min each. Just before the probe is ready to apply, the slides are air dried.

5. The denatured probe (10 μL) is applied onto the marked area of the slide, covered with a 22 × 22 mm² coverslip and sealed with vulcanising rubber solution (www.weldtite.co.uk).

6. The rubber solution is allowed to dry briefly and the slide is placed in a humidified chamber at 37°C overnight (*see* **Note 8**).

7. The next day, the rubber solution is removed using forceps and the slide placed in 2× SSC to release the coverslip. The coverslip is tipped off into a sharps bin.

8. The slides are washed in 0.4× SSC/0.3% NP-40 at 73°C for 2 min.

9. The slides are transferred to 2× SSC/0.1% NP-40 at room temperature for 5 min.

Alternative post-hybridization washes are given in **Note 9**.

10. The slides are drained of excess fluid and then mounted in Vectashield mountant without DAPI counterstain.

11. The slides are viewed under epifluorescence using the appropriate filters: DAPI or DEAC for AMCA immunostaining, FITC and Texas Red/Rhodamine for the FISH signals.

12. The appropriate area of the slide is selected under a low power objective (16× or 20×) using the DAPI filter.

13. Once the cells are located, the 100× oil lens is used to view the fluorescence immunophenotype and FISH signals.

14. The cells are scanned using the DAPI filter to locate cells positive for the antigen of interest, and then reviewed on the red and green filters for the FISH signals.

15. A dual colour filter can be used to locate the cells and the signals in the nucleus, but it is important to review the signals through the single FITC and Rhodamine/Texas Red filters.

16. At least 100 cells (for rare populations at least 1,000) are analysed and the FISH signal pattern recorded for each. Clumps of cells and damaged nuclei should be avoided.

17. Tips for troubleshooting FISH are given in **Note 10**.

18. Cut-off levels are established for each probe by recording the signal pattern on at least three normal slides of a cell type similar to the test cells. A useful cut-off for false-positivity is the mean + 2 standard deviations.

3.2. Multicolour FISH (M-FISH)

In 1996, two groups reported successful 24-colour karyotyping, termed multi-fluor FISH (M-FISH) *(3)* and spectral karyotyping (SKY) *(4)* respectively. Both approaches made use of the new cyanine dyes and a combinatorial labeling approach using five fluorochromes. Using this strategy, the total number of colours achievable (N) is given by the equation $N = 2^n-1$, where n = number of spectrally separate fluorochromes. Whereas, SKY uses a dedicated imaging system that incorporates Fourier transform spectrometry to analyze the spectral signature at each pixel of the image *(4)*, M-FISH uses a conventional epifluorescence microscope equipped with specific narrow bandpass fluorescence filter sets. The critical features of M-FISH are: (a) the accurate alignment of the individual fluorochrome planes; (b) a reduction (or elimination) of chromatic crosstalk; and (c) quantitation of the intensity of each fluorochrome *(16)*. These features have been met by modern epifluorescence microscopes that incorporate up to eight narrow bandpass filters and M-FISH software that computes the combinatorial labelling algorithm and allows separation and identification of all chromosomes, generating a colour karyotype in which each chromosome is given a characteristic pseudocolour.

The generation of combinatorially labelled probes for M-FISH is a complex procedure, requiring access to purified flow sorted or microdissected chromosomes and skill in labelling and fluorescence imaging. Commercial versions of M-FISH whole chromosome painting sets are now available which obviate the need to undertake such procedures. Some of these are tied to the particular company's instrumentation. We use the Vysis Spectra-Vysion M-FISH whole chromosome painting kit that can be used with any M-FISH imaging software. The SpectraVysion system uses five proprietary fluorochromes, Spectrum Aqua, Spectrum-Green, SpectrumGold, SpectrumRed and SpectrumFRed. The following protocol is based on the manufacturer's recommendations, but uses simultaneous denaturation of probe and chromosomal DNA and a modified post-hybridization wash series.

3.2.1. Pre-Treatment of Slides

1. The slides are treated with 100 µL of RNase (100 µg/ mL) under a 24 × 50 mm^2 coverslip and incubated in a humid chamber at 37°C for 30min-1 h.

2. The slides are washed twice (3-min each) in 2× SSC at room temperature (with agitation).

3. The slides are incubated in 30 µg/ mL of pepsin at 37°C for 2–5 min (depending on the amount of cytoplasm present).

4. The slides are washed twice (5-min each) in 1× PBS, with agitation.

5. The slides are incubated in PBS/50 mM MgCl$_2$ for 5 min at room temperature.

6. The slides are fixed in 1% formaldehyde in PBS/50 mM MgCl$_2$ for 10 min at room temperature.

7. The slides are washed in PBS for 5 min at room temperature (with agitation).

8. The slides are dehydrated through an alcohol series and allowed to air dry. At this stage they can be stored desiccated at 4°C for up to 1 month before use.

3.2.2. Hybridization

1. The area to be hybridized is marked either using a diamond pen underneath the area, or in soft pencil on the edge of the slide.

2. 10 µL of SpectraVysion probe is applied to the appropriate area of the slide, covered with a 22 × 22 mm^2 coverslip and sealed with rubber solution to ensure that there are no bubbles in the hybridization area. This can be done on a hotplate at 37°C to allow the solution to fill the area more easily.

3. The sealed slide is placed on a hotplate at 72°C (+/–1°C) under a fume hood for 2–5 min. The optimum denaturation time needs to be determined for each batch of slides by carrying out a time course. Use single whole chromosome paints for this to avoid wasting expensive reagent. However, if the slides require significantly less than, or more than 5 min, separate denaturation of slides and probe should be performed (*see* **Note 11**).

4. The slide is placed in a humid chamber at 37°C and allowed to hybridize for 24–48 h.

3.2.3. Post-Hybridization Washes

1. The rubber solution is removed using forceps and the slide placed in 2× SSC for 5 min to loosen the coverslip. The coverslip is then gently removed.

2. The slides are immersed in 1× SSC at 65°C for 5 min (prewarm the solution for at least 30 min beforehand).

3. The slides are transferred to 4× SSCT at room temperature for 5 min. (*see* **Note 9** for alternative formamide washes).

4. The excess liquid is drained from the slide before dehydrating the slides in 70, 90, and 100% ethanol.

5. The slides are mounted in Vectashield with DAPI and covered with a 24×50 mm^2 coverslip.

3.2.4. M-FISH Imaging and Analysis

Accurate imaging and analysis of M-FISH is critical to obtain meaningful results. In choosing an epifluorescence microscope for M-FISH it is imperative to select the appropriate filter sets for the discrimination of the chosen fluorochromes. This requires the optimal combination of excitation, emission, and dichroic beamsplitter filters. This can be achieved using a combination of filter wheel (containing excitation filters only) and specific filter blocks in the microscope, or a filter turret with individual narrow bandpass filter blocks (each block comprised of the excitation, emission, and dichroic filters). The lamp must be properly centred as it is essential to have even illumination for M-FISH imaging. It was originally recommended to use two different light sources: a 75 W xenon arc lamp (superior for the cyanine dyes) and a 100 W mercury lamp (superior for the blue end of the spectrum), and a switching mechanism to alternate between the two sources. However, we find that a single 100 W mercury lamp is suitable for all of the commonly used fluorochromes. For image capture we use a Sensys cooled CCD camera with a Kodak KAF 1400 chip. The following recommendations are specific for the fluorochromes used in the SpectraVysion system:

1. The hybridized area is located under low power using the Spectrum Gold or Spectrum Red filter set. Exposure to the ultaviolet DAPI excitation light at this stage should be avoided as it will cause degradation of all fluorochromes.

2. The fluorochrome planes are captured in the following order: Spectrum Gold first, followed by Spectrum FRed, then Spectrum Aqua, Spectrum Red, Spectrum Green can be captured in any order, and finally DAPI.

3. Proceed with an appropriate M-FISH software programme. We use Digital Scientific M-FISH software that applies intensity threshold levels for each fluorochrome. Chromosomes are segmented and separated, then karyotyped using a look-up table for colour classification before assigning a pseudocolour. The karyotype can then be edited manually by the operator using the inverted DAPI (banded) image.

4. At this stage it is useful to view the individual fluorochrome channels in the karyotype format. It is also important to be aware that spurious chromosome assignments can be given due to the overlap of fluorochromes at translocation borders. It is always wise to check the findings of multicolour karyotyping using single or dual colour FISH.

Other troubleshooting tips are given in **Note 12**.

4. Notes

1. We use a purpose made perspex box with a lid and an integral staining rack to hold the slides. A small amount of water or PBSa is placed in the bottom to humidify the atmosphere. Alternatively, Lamb's immuno slide staining trays can be used.

2. Wiping around the marked area of the slide will prevent the solution from spreading over the rest of the slide.

3. For each antibody layer, it is necessary to perform an antibody titration to determine optimum dilution. Antibodies are diluted in PBSa.

4. Cell subsets positively enriched by FACS or MACS will have primary antibody on the cell surface: In this case, begin at this step (anti-mouse layer).

5. Alternative fluorescence detection *(17, 18)*: The following fluorochrome conjugated secondary and tertiary antibody layers can be used (all from Jackson ImmunoResearch) in place of the biotin and avidin conjugated antibodies (all diluted 1:20 with PN buffer). Slides are incubated in each for 30 min at room temperature:

    (i)   AMCA-rabbit anti-mouse IgG.

    (ii) AMCA- goat anti-rabbit IgG.

6. Use a fume hood both for making up all formamide solutions and for incubation in hot formamide. Always check the temperature of the formamide in the coplin jar, not of the waterbath.

7. Alternative hybridization using simultaneous denaturation of probe and chromosomal DNA on a hotplate (substitute for **steps 2–6** in **Subheading 3.1.4**):

    (i)   Place 10 mL of probe in hybridization buffer on the cell-containing area of the slide and cover with a 22 × 22 mm² coverslip. Seal with rubber solution.

    (ii) Place on a hotplate at 73°C and heat for 2–5 min. The denaturation time for each batch of slides will need to be established using a time course.

    (iii) Incubate slides at 37°C and allow to hybridize overnight.

8. We use a humid chamber consisting of a plastic microscope slide storage box with a lid (floated in a waterbath). In this case it is not necessary to put any moisture in the chamber. However, if hybridizing in a dry oven, put some moist tissue at the bottom and suspend the slides above this on a rack. Alternatively, use Lamb's immuno slide staining trays placed in a waterbath.

9. In cases where there is unacceptable background after hot low salt washes, the following standard formamide washes should be used:

(i) 3×5 min in 50% formamide, $2 \times$ SSC at 42°C.

(ii) 3×5 min in $2 \times$ SSC at 42°C.

(iii) 1×5 min in $4 \times$ SSCT at room temperature.

10. The following are commonly encountered problems with FISH and some possible solutions:

(i)   *No hybridization signal.* This may be due to inadequate denaturation of probe and/or chromosomes. Each batch of slides should be subjected to a time course to determine the optimum denaturation time. It is also possible that increasing the amount of probe in the hybridization mixture will improve the FISH signal, but bear in mind that when there is a large excess of probe over target, the probe may self-anneal.

(ii) *High background.* High background with strong specific signal may be due to low stringency of hybridization or post-hybridization washes. The stringency of hybridization can be increased by either increasing the hybridization temperature, increasing the formamide concentration of the hybridization mix, and/or post-hybridization washes to 60%, or decreasing the SSC concentration to 0.1% in the post-hybridization washes. In general, a greater effect is observed by increasing the stringency of the hybridization than of the washes.

(iii) *Brightly fluorescent signal all over the slide.* This may occur if the probe mixture is old or has been improperly stored and can be due to de-conjugation of the fluorochrome from the probe. A short spin in a microcentrifuge will precipitate the free fluorochrome (use the supernatant).

(iv) *Cells lost from slide.* Handle slides with care at all stages especially during removal of coverslips. Always tip the slides and allow the coverslip to slide off – never pull them off.

11. Alternative denaturation of probe and chromosomes:

(i)   Heat 70% formamide in $2 \times$ SSC to 72°C ($+/-1$ °C) in a coplin jar under a fume hood for at least 30 min before required. Place the slides in the heated formamide for 3 min.

(ii) Transfer the slides to ice-cold 70% ethanol. Leave for 4 min. Transfer to cold 90% ethanol and then 100% ethanol for 4-min each.

(iii) Air-dry the slides.

(iv) Denature the probe mixture (10 μL of SpectraVysion probe in an eppendorf tube) at 72°C in a waterbath for 3 min. Time this to coincide with denaturation of the slides.

(v) Centrifuge the probe mixture quickly to get the liquid to bottom of tube. Place this mixture on the previously treated slide containing denatured chromosomes and cover with a 22×22 mm^2 coverslip (do not let the drop dry). Seal the coverslip with rubber solution and place the slides in a humid chamber at 37°C for 1–2 days.

12. The following are potential problems encountered with M-FISH hybridizations and some possible solutions:

(i) The main problem leading to incorrect assignment of chromosomes is the poor hybridization of one or more fluorochromes. Poor signal to noise ratio will make it difficult to distinguish the specific signal from non-specific background. This may be due to a number of factors, some of which are common to all FISH experiments (*see* **Note 10**). However, cellular debris or bright background speckles are more of a problem for M-FISH than for ordinary FISH, as the software will not be able to assign the correct chromosome identification. Always apply pepsin pre-treatment to minimize background due to cellular debris.

(ii) *Poor chromosome morphology.* If the chromosomes look "blown", this may be due to overdenaturation. Carry out a denaturation time course for each batch of slides and use the shortest time that gives good hybridization. If chromosomes are overdenatured with 1 min denaturation, it may be necessary to age the slides for longer before hybridizing.

(iii) *Weak staining of all fluorochromes:* This may be due to a number of factors including old or improperly stored slides. Slides can be stored at –20°C in a sealed box with desiccant for many years. Avoid repeated thawing and re-freezing. Allow box to come up to room temperature before opening, and replace desiccant that has turned pink. Weak staining may also be due to overdenaturation, leading to loss of DNA. This may be due to overtreatment with pepsin and can be minimized by longer postfixation with formaldehyde. Weak staining may also be due to exposure to light, either to the probe, or the slides. Hybridized slides should be kept in the dark, and exposure to the fluorescence light on the microscope should be for no longer than is necessary in capturing the image.

(iv) *Weak staining of Spectrum Aqua, Spectrum FRed:* Weak staining of selected fluorochromes may be due to exposure to DAPI excitation. Always capture the fluorochromes in the order recommended.

(v) *Low signal/noise (weak specificity) of any (or all) of the fluorochromes:* This may be due to the incorrect filter sets. For example, we have found that the standard FITC filter set gives low specificity for Spectrum Green.

Acknowledgements

This work was supported by the Leukaemia Research Fund, Medical Research Council (UK), Kay Kendall Leukaemia Fund, and Children with Leukaemia Trust.

References

1. Mori H, Colman SM, Xiao Z, Ford AM, Healy LE, Donaldson C, et al. (2002) Chromosome translocations and covert leukemic clones are generated during normal fetal development. *Proc Natl Acad Sci USA.* **99**, 8242–8247.

2. Hong D, Gupta R, Ancliff P, Atzberger A, Brown J, Soneji S, et al. (2008) Initiating and cancer-propagating cells in TEL-AML1-associated childhood leukemia. *Science.* **319**, 336–339.

3. Speicher M, Ballard SG, Ward DC. (1996) Karyotyping human chromosomes by combinatorial multi-fluor FISH. *Nat Genet.* **12**, 368–375.

4. Schröck E, du Manoir S, Veldman T, Schoell B, Wienberg J, Ferguson-Smith MA, et al. (1996) Multicolor spectral karyotyping of human chromosomes. *Science.* **273**, 494–497.

5. Tanke HJ, Wiegant J, van Gijlswijk RP, Bezrookove V, Pattenier H, Heetebrij RJ, et al. (1999) New strategy for multi-colour fluorescence in situ hybridisation: COBRA: COmbined Binary RAtio labelling. *Eur J Hum Genet.* **7**, 2–11.

6. Karhu R, Ahlstedt-Soini M, Bittner M, Meltzer P, Trent JM, Isola JJ. (2001) Chromosome arm-specific multicolor FISH. *Genes Chromosomes Cancer.* **30**, 105–109.

7. Muller S, O'Brien PC, Ferguson-Smith MA, Wienberg J. (1998) Cross-species colour segmenting: a novel tool in human karyotype analysis. *Cytometry.* **33**, 445–452.

8. Chudoba I, Plesch A, Lorch T, Lemke J, Claussen U, Senger G. (1999) High resolution multicolor-banding: a new technique for refined FISH analysis of human chromosomes. *Cytogenet Cell Genet.* **84**, 156–160.

9. Nietzel A, Rocchi M, Starke H, Heller A, Fiedler W, Wlodarska I, et al. (2001) A new multicolor-FISH approach for the characterization of marker chromosomes: centromere-specific multicolor-FISH (cenM-FISH). *Hum Genet.* **108**, 199–204.

10. Brown J, Saracoglu K, Uhrig S, Speicher MR, Eils R, Kearney L. (2001) Subtelomeric chromosome rearrangements are detected using an innovative 12-color FISH assay (M-TEL). *Nat Med.* **7**, 497–501.

11. Fauth C, Zhang H, Harabacz S, Brown J, Saracoglu K, Lederer G, et al. (2001) A new strategy for the detection of subtelomeric rearrangements. *Hum Genet.* **109**, 576–583.

12. Bolzer A, Kreth G, Solovei I, Koehler D, Saracoglu K, Fauth C, et al. (2005) Three-dimensional maps of all chromosomes in human male fibroblast nuclei and prometaphase rosettes. *PLoS Biol.* **3**, e157.

13. Le Beau MM, Davis EM, Patel B, Phan VT, Sohal J, Kogan SC. (2003) Recurring chromosomal abnormalities in leukemia in PML-RARA transgenic mice identify cooperating events and genetic pathways to acute promyelocytic leukemia. *Blood.* **102**, 1072–1074.

14. Horsley SW, Mackay A, Iravani M, Fenwick K, Valgeirsson H, Dexter T, et al. (2006) Array CGH of fusion gene-positive leukemia-derived cell lines reveals cryptic regions of genomic gain and loss. *Genes Chromosomes Cancer.* **45**, 554–564.

15. Korac P, Jones M, Dominis M, Kusec R, Mason DY, Banham AH, et al. (2005) Application of the FICTION technique for the simultaneous detection of immunophenotype and chromosomal abnormalities in routinely fixed, paraffin wax embedded bone marrow trephines. *J Clin Pathol.* **58**, 1336–1338.

16. Fauth C, Speicher MR. (2001) Classifying by colors: FISH-based genome analysis. *Cytogenet Cell Genet.* **93**, 1–10.

17. Weber-Matthiesen K, Winkemann M, Muller-Hermelink A, Schlegelberger B, Grote W. (1992) Simultaneous fluorescence immunophenotyping and interphase cytogenetics: a contribution to the characterization of tumor cells. *J Histochem Cytochem.* **40**, 171–175.

18. Martin-Subero JI, Chudoba I, Harder L, Gesk S, Grote W, Novo FJ, et al. (2002) Multicolor-FICTION: expanding the possibilities of combined morphologic, immunophenotypic, and genetic single cell analyses. *Am J Pathol.* **161**, 413–420.

Chapter 5

LDI-PCR: Identification of Known and Unknown Gene Fusions of the Human *MLL* Gene

Claus Meyer and Rolf Marschalek

Summary

The human *MLL* gene is one of the most promiscuous recombination hot spots of our genome with regard to the onset of malignant diseases. With the exception of gene internal partial-tandem duplications involving several exons located in the 5′-end of *MLL*, all recombination events occur in a small genomic region flanked by *MLL* exons 8–14, designated as the *MLL* breakpoint cluster region. Efforts from different laboratories, including our own, have led to the identification of more than 50 *MLL* fusion partners that were characterized at the molecular level. The common theme of recombination events involving the human *MLL* gene is the creation of "functional" fusion genes that are translated into oncoproteins. Many different labs have already demonstrated that these MLL fusion proteins have the capability to instruct hematopoietic stem/precursor cells to convert into a preleukemic state, which finally leads to the onset of leukemia in experimental model systems.

Here we have focused on the identification of *MLL* fusion partners by using the genomic DNA of acute leukemia patients. After initial screening using for example split signal FISH experiments (as an example for technologies to identify *MLL* rearrangements), genomic DNA from leukemia patients is analyzed by long-distance-inverse (LDI)-PCR. LDI-PCR is based on the hydrolysis of patient DNA using distinct combinations of restriction enzymes, self-ligation of the resulting DNA fragments and a subsequent PCR reaction using a specific set of oligonucleotides. This strategy allows in principle any investigator to identify known and unknown *MLL* fusion partner genes. Furthermore, the genomic fusion site in *MLL* rearrangements represent a unique and reliable molecular marker that allows the tracing of minimal residual disease (MRD) in these patients before, during, and after therapy.

Key words: *MLL*, Chromosomal translocations, Genetic rearrangements, Fusion partner genes, Acute leukemia, LDI-PCR, Genomic DNA, Molecular marker, MRD

1. Introduction

Chromosomal translocations involving the human *MLL* gene were identified more than 15 years ago. The first chromosomal translocations of the human *MLL* gene (also designated as *ALL-1*

C.W.E. So (ed.), Leukemia, *Methods in Molecular Biology, vol. 538*
© Humana Press, a part of Springer Science + Business Media, LLC 2009
DOI: 10.1007/978-1-59745-418-6_5

or *HRX*) that were molecularly characterized were the reciprocal translocations t(4;11) and t(11;19) *(1, 2)*. Since then more than 50 additional fusion partners have been identified *(3, 4)*. So far, 55 translocation partner genes have been characterized at the molecular level *(5)*. It is interesting to note that only very few of these translocation partner genes were recurrently identified in leukemia patients. Of the latter, the six translocation partner genes *AF4* (*MLLT2*), *AF9* (*MLLT3*), *ENL* (*MLLT1*), *AF10* (*MLLT10*) *ELL, and AF6* (*MLLT4*) are the most frequent ones (~80%). With the exception of the *AF6* (*MLLT4*) gene, the gene products of the remaining five genes are part of a protein machinery that stimulates RNA polymerase II complex elongation and chromatin remodeling *(6–8)*. The remaining 20% comprise partner genes such as *EPS15*, *AF1Q (MLLT11)*, *SEPT9*, and *AF17* (*MLLT6*) or genes that have been identified so far only once *(5)*.

From cytogenetic studies, we can only estimate the final number of *MLL* translocation partner genes, designated as the "*MLL* recombinome." The final number will presumably be >100. Thus, many of these translocation partner genes are yet unidentified. Therefore, efforts in various laboratories are ongoing in order to unravel the remaining fusion partners in individual leukemia patients.

Genetic rearrangements of the human *MLL* gene are quite diverse. About 80% of the currently known *MLL* rearrangements are created by a balanced reciprocal chromosomal translocation involving *MLL* translocation partner genes. About 5% are inversions or deletions occurring on the long arm of chromosome 11, and thus, no other chromosome is involved. In case of 11q inversions, two genes with different transcriptional orientation are involved, leading to two fusion genes, while 11q deletions leads to *MLL* fusions with a telomer located gene with the same transcriptional orientation. The remaining 15% are complex recombination events mostly based on insertions of a small portion of chromosome 11 material (including *MLL* gene material) into another chromosome, or vice versa, by the insertion of chromatin material into the *MLL* gene. These "cut and paste" mechanisms lead to the generation of two chimerized genes on the recipient chromosome (one is the MLL fusion allele), and the reciprocal MLL fusion allele on the donor chromosome. In some patients, the reciprocal exchange of two larger chromosomal segments leads to the generation three or four independent fusion genes (summarized in *(4,5)*. *MLL* translocation partner genes known to be involved in these complex rearrangements are *LAF4, FKSG14, AF5Q31, FNBP1, CIP29, CREBBP, ACACA, SEPT6*, and the most prominent one, the *AF10* (*MLLT10*) gene. Complex rearrangements of the *MLL* gene can also be created by three-way translocations. In these cases, three different genes located on three different chromosomes are involved and three independent fusion genes are created of which only two are *MLL* fusions.

Therefore, investigators have to choose the right methodology in order to investigate known and unknown *MLL* rearrangements. An important question is whether the analysis should be done at the RNA or DNA level.

1.1. Analysis at the mRNA Level

Analyses at the mRNA level can be straight forward. Known *MLL* rearrangements can be analyzed by RT-PCR experiments using oligonucleotides specific to exons of the *MLL* gene and the translocation partner gene of interest. To investigate unknown *MLL* rearrangements different techniques are required to identify fused gene sequences.

- The rapid amplification of cDNA ends (RACE) technique allows the identification of cDNA sequences linked to known exonic sequences of the *MLL* gene. In principle, this method can be used not only to identify 3'-fusions encoded by the *der (11)* chromosome, but also 5'-fused sequences encoded on the reciprocal allele. RACE kits are commercially available, but the RACE technique is not that easy to handle, and thus, does not necessarily lead to a result. This is presumably due to mispriming and/or the presence of mRNA sequences derived from the wildtype allele. To our knowledge, 16 translocation partner genes were identified in the past 15 years by applying this particular technique.

- Another successful technique is panhandle-PCR, subject of Chapter "Panhandle-PCR Approaches to Cloning *MLL* Genomic Breakpoint Junctions and Fusion Transcript Sequences." This technique allows the identification of unknown and known fusion partners. To our knowledge, 14 translocation partner genes have been identified in the past years by applying this method (*see* **ref.** *9, 10)*. Moreover, panhandle-PCR can also be performed at the level of genomic DNA (see below).

- Additional six translocation partner genes have been cloned and characterized by using genomic and cDNA libraries that were established from individual leukemia patients. However, this is not a standard technique, and thus, this method has only been successfully performed in laboratories familiar with the technique.

1.2. Analysis at the Genomic DNA Level

The genomic DNA level is often seen as technically more complicated but offers several advantages over the RNA approach:

(1) DNA is more stable than RNA, and thus is more accessible for analysis.

(2) Genomic fusion sites are single-copy per cell (as the intact allele). This is important when both alleles (rearranged and germline) are being analyzed in the same PCR experiment. It is far easier to judge your results when you visually analyze

your PCR amplimers (no differences of gene expression level have to be taken into account).

(3) Genomic fusion sites are idiosyncratic for each patient (not the case on the RNA level, as many leukemia patients share the same exon–exon junctions of their fusion genes). Therefore, a given genomic fusion site is a perfect MRD marker, because it is single-copy per tumor cell and can be robustly quantified down to a dilution of 10^{-5} *(11)*. There is only one situation where the use of the patient-specific genomic fusion site can not be recommended for MRD experiments: repetitive sequences at the breakpoint junction. However, according to our own experience this happens very rarely (<1%). To ensure single copy sequences for MRD studies, the sequence of interest should be checked with the Repeat-Masker server available on the internet.

The genomic DNA level offers three different methods. Each of these methods has their advantages and disadvantages:

- *Direct long-range PCR*. If you expect to find one of the most frequent *MLL* fusion partners, design oligonucleotides according to the breakpoint cluster regions and go straight ahead with long-range PCR using the recommended conditions of your kit manufacturer *(12, 13)*. Nested long-range PCR can be used as well.

- *Genomic panhandle-PCR*. Panhandle-PCR is also applicable to genomic DNA experiments. Details of genomic panhandle-PCR experiments are discussed in the Chapter "Panhandle-PCR Approaches to Cloning *MLL* Genomic Breakpoint Junctions and Fusion Transcript Sequences" of this book *(9)*.

- *LDI-PCR (14)*. LDI-PCR method is the topic of this chapter and will be discussed in more detail. LDI-PCR allows "large-scale analyses" of known and unknown *MLL* fusion partner genes when universal *MLL*-specific oligonucleotides are used (see below). The other benefit is the short time required to obtain results. Using this method, 13 novel *MLL* fusion partner genes were identified within 36 months when 800 leukemia patients were analyzed. The details of the LDI-PCR method – as performed at the Diagnostic Center of Acute Leukemia (DCAL, **Note 1**) – are presented in the following sections.

2. Materials

2.1. Isolation of Genomic DNA

We recommend using standard DNA isolations kits from Qiagen (Qiagen blood kit) or equivalent kits to isolate genomic DNA of sufficient length and quality. The amount of DNA is quantified by UV spectroscopy and 1 μg genomic DNA will be used throughout the method (*see* **Note 2**).

2.2. Oligonucleotide Sequences (Fig.1a)

1. Use the following control primer specific for the *MLL* break-point cluster region:

   CF1 5′-CGAGGAAAAGAGTGAAGAAGGGAAGTCTC-GG-3′

   CF2 5′-GAAAAACCACCTCCGGTCAATAAGCAGGAGAATG-3′

   CR1 5′-CCTAGGCTAGAACATGTGG-3′

   CR2 5′-GTCCCAGGCACTCAGGGTGATAGCTGTTTCGG-3′

2. Use the following forward primers specific for the *MLL* break-point cluster region:

   F1 5′-GCAGCCTCCACCACCAGAATCAGGTGAGTG-3′

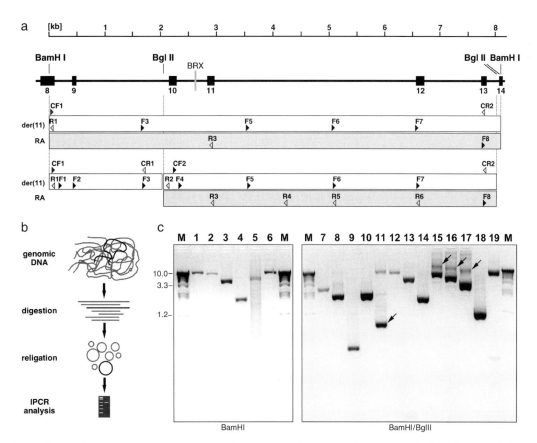

Fig. 1. Schematic outline, workflow, and results of the LDI-PCR technique. (**a**) Scheme of the *MLL* breakpoint cluster region and the position of all oligonucleotides used for the above mentioned LDI-PCR method using *Bam*HI or *Bam*HI/*Bgl*II digests. BRX marks the breakpoint of the t(9;11) translocation. *RA* reciprocal allele. Restriction fragments for BamHI and BamHI/BglII are indicated. (**b**) Workflow of the LDI-PCR analysis. (**c**) Analysis of a patient carrying a t(9;11) translocation. Lanes 1–19: see **Subheading 3.4.** *M* size marker. Beside the germline amplimers, several nongermline PCR amplimers (indicated by an *arrow*) were observed; their molecular identification was performed by DNA sequencing. No band was obtained for primer pair R1 × F3 with the *Bam*H I digest as the size of the nongermline PCR amplimer was too large in that patient.

F2 5′-GTGGCTCCCCGCCCAAGTATCCCTGTAAAAC-3′

F3 5′-CCCACATGTTCTAGCCTAGGAATCTGC-3′

F4 5′-GCTGGGAGAGCTTTGGTCAGTGTTGTTAGG-3′

F5 5′-ATCCTGAATAAATGGGACCTTTCTGTTGGTGG-3′

F6 5′-CTCTTTTCCGTCTTAATACAGTGCTTTGCACC-3′

F7 5′-TTGTGAGCCCTTCCACAAGTTTTGTTTAGAGG-3′

F8 5′-GTGTAATAAGTGCCGAAACAGCTATCACCCTG-3′

3. Use the following reverse primers specific for the *MLL* breakpoint cluster region:

R1 5′-GACATTCCCTTCTTCACTCTTTTCCTC-3′

R2 5′-GCCTTCACATTTGCAACAGATAATAATGC-3′

R3 5′-CATCTCCCACACATTTTCTGCTTCACAATCC-3′

R4 5′-CACTCAGTGATATGTCATGGACATCTTTCC-3′

R5 5′-GCAAAGCACTGTATTAAGACGGAAAAGAGG-3′

R 6 5′-CAAAACTTGTGGAAGGGCTCACAACAGACTTG G-3′

2.3. Reagents

1. Long-range PCR kit from Qiagen, according to the manufacturers recommendations.

2. Standard agarose gels in 1× TBE buffer with a concentration 1.0% agarose for the separation of PCR amplimers.

3. LowTE buffer (10 mM Tris–HCl pH 8.0, 0.1 mM EDTA pH 8.0).

4. 3 M sodium acetate pH 7.0.

5. 10× buffers for restrictions enzymes provided by manufacturer (New England Biolabs).

6. High concentrated BamHI (100 U/µl) and BglII (100 U/µl) from New England Biolabs.

7. T4 DNA ligase (400 U/µl) from New England Biolabs.

8. Thermal cycler 9700 from Applied Biosystems.

3. Methods

A flow chart of the methodology is shown in **Fig. 1b**.

3.1. Isolation and Quantification of Genomic DNA

1. Biopsy material (either peripheral blood or bone marrow aspirates) should be Ficoll-purifed and mononuclear cells (MNC) should be used for DNA isolation. Use $2–5 \times 10^6$ cells according to the purification protocol of the manufacturer.

2. Elute bound DNA from the column with LowTE buffer.

3. Quantify the amount of isolated DNA by UV spectroscopy (1×10^6 cells should result in about 6.6 µg DNA).

3.2. Restriction and Religation of Genomic DNA

1. One microgram of genomic DNA is digested for 4 h at 37°C with 50 U *Bam*HI in a 100 µl reaction.

2. One microgram genomic DNA is digested for 4 h at 37°C with 50 U *Bam*HI and 50 U *Bgl*II in a 100 µl reaction.

3. Both reactions are incubated for 10 min at 60°C to heat-inactivate the two restriction enzymes.

4. Perform a standard phenol extraction (phenol/chloroform/isoamyl alcohol = 25/24/1 w/w) followed by a standard chloroform extraction (chloroform/isoamyl alcohol = 24/1 w/w) (*see* **Note 3**).

5. Precipitate nucleic acids by using a standard ethanol precipitation with 1/10 volume 3 M sodium acetate pH 7.0; freeze for 1 h at –80°C and spin for 10 min at full speed in a centrifuge ($14,000 \times g$); decant the supernatant and briefly dry the nucleic acids.

6. Dissolve precipitated nucleic acids in 80 µl 1× ligation buffer and perform a DNA ligase reaction using 400 U T4 DNA ligase in a 80 µl reaction overnight at 2–8°C.

7. Incubate both reactions for 10 min at 60°C to heat-inactivate the T4 DNA ligase.

3.3. Quality Assessment of the Procedure

1. For first time users, we recommend establishing a small test system to control the reactions mentioned above. The test system can be designed for any genomic region with appropriate restriction recognition sites and should look as shown in **Fig. 2**.

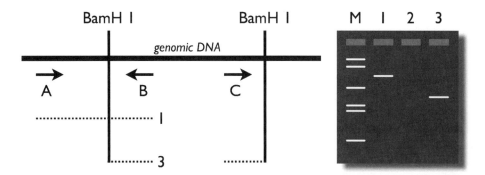

Fig. 2. Quality assessment. Any genomic DNA sequence with known restriction sites can be used for quality assessment. Two *Bam*HI restriction sites located adjacent to each other will be used to design a primer A located in a distance of about 300 bp upstream of *Bam*HI restriction site 1, a reverse primer B located about 200 bp downstream of *Bam*HI restriction site 1, and a primer C located about 200 bp upstream of *Bam*HI restriction site 2. PCR reactions will be performed always in the presence of all three primers A–C, respectively. Use undigested genomic DNA (1), digested genomic DNA (2), and digested and religated DNA (3) to quality control the workflow. *M* size marker.

2. Use an aliquot (20–50 pg) of undigested [1], digested [2] and religated DNA [3] in combination with a 3-primer PCR reaction (A–C). Fragment A–B should be in the range of 500 bp, while fragment B–C should be in the range of 400 bp. If the subsequent analysis on an agarose gel does not look like that schematically shown above, the restriction and ligation reactions must be improved (incubation times, test restriction enzymes from different companies, etc.). Go ahead only if all three test PCR reactions are working, i.e., that you have a product in lane 1 (A–B), no product in lane 2, and the inverse PCR product (B–C) in lane 3 (*M* size marker).

3.4 Long-Distance-Inverse PCR

1. For *Bam*HI-restricted and religated DNA, the following PCR reactions should be used:

   (a) R1 × F3 (der11)

   (b) R1 × F5 (der11)

   (c) R1 × F6 (der11)

   (d) R1 × F7 (der11)

   (e) R3 × F8 (derTP)

   (f) CF1 × CR2 (internal control)

2. For *Bam*HI/*Bgl*II-restricted and religated DNA, the following PCR reactions should be used:

   (g) R1 × F1 (der11)

   (h) R1 × F2 (der11)

   (i) R1 × F3 (der11)

   (j) CF1 × CR1 (internal control)

   (k) R2 × F4 (der11)

   (l) R2 × F5 (der11)

   (m) R2 × F6 (der11)

   (n) R2 × F7 (der11)

   (o) R6 × F8 (derTP)

   (p) R5 × F8 (derTP)

   (q) R4 × F8 (derTP)

   (r) R3 × F8 (derTP)

   (s) CF2 × CR2 (internal control)

3. The PCR program is set-up according to the recommendations of the manufacturer. Briefly, we recommend using the following conditions:
All PCR reactions should be carried out on an ABI 9700 PCR or equivalent cycler. All reactions should have a final volume of 50 µl. Run the PCR program overnight.

1 cycle	180 s	93°C
10 cycles	15 s	93°C
	30 s	62°C
	18 min	68°C
25 cycles	10 s	93°C
	30 s	62°C
	18 min	68°C (+20 s for each cycle)

3.5. Interpretation of Results

1. Load all 19 PCR reactions (50 μl) on 1.0% agarose gel and run it with 100 V (80 mA) for 2–3 h (*see* **Note 4**). Visualize the PCR amplimers under UV (365 nm) and photograph the gel. One should expect PCR amplimers of distinct sizes even if no *MLL* rearrangement is present, because the germline alleles produce a distinct PCR amplimer pattern which is your "internal control." Additional bands not corresponding to the expected germline PCR amplimers should be cut-out of the gel, extracted, and subjected to direct sequencing. An example of such an analysis is shown in **Fig. 1c**.

2. In a first attempt to identify putative *MLL* rearrangements by analyzing the nongermline PCR amplimers, use primer R1 as the sequencing primer for PCR reactions 1–4, primer F8 for PCR reaction 5, primer R1 for PCR reactions 7–9, primer R2 for PCR reactions 11–14 and primer F8 for PCR reactions 16–19. After all sequencing reactions have been carried out, blast your non-*MLL* sequences to identify the chromosome and the gene involved in the recombination event.

3. To identify the breakpoint (chromosomal fusion site) of the rearranged allele, you need to design several additional sequencing primers binding to *MLL* sequences in between your long-range primers to narrow down and finally to identify the fusion site between *MLL* and the translocation partner gene (*see* **Note 5**).

3.6. Troubleshooting Your Results

1. If you don't see any difference between your negative control (e.g., DNA extracted from a cell line without *MLL* rearrangement) and your sample under investigation, it does not necessarily tell you that there is no *MLL* rearrangement present in your patient sample. Although *Bam*HI and *Bgl*II should digest genomic DNA statistically every 4,096 bp, there are genomic areas with no such sites and lengths of more than 20 kb. In some cases, the rearranged allele is too long to obtain a positive PCR result. Depending on your type of prescreening (cytogenetics, split-signal FISH, or Southern blot), you should trust your prescreening data and try other enzyme

combinations to repeat the experiment. In that case, you have to design novel primers to quality control your initial reactions as outlined under **Subheading 3.3**

2. Run the agarose gel as long as possible to obtain a good separation. A good separation should help you also to see small differences between the germline and nongermline PCR amplimers.

3. If you see additional PCR amplimers beside the germline fragments, it does not necessarily mean that you have successfully identified a rearranged MLL allele. It might be that you have produced a PCR artifact. Only the subsequent sequencing of such a PCR amplimer will give you a result. Moreover, rearranged alleles – depending on where the breakpoint is actually located within the *MLL* breakpoint cluster region – will always give you a pattern similar to your germline PCR pattern – but at different sizes. If your breakpoint is, for example, located between the primer binding sites F6 and F7 you should see additional PCR amplimers of decreasing sizes in your PCR reactions 1–3, but no additional bands in PCR reaction 4.

4. If you have successfully identified a *der (11)* or *der(TP)* allele, it could be that you have not seen the reciprocal derivative allele in your PCR analyses. This does not necessarily tell you that there is no reciprocal derivative allele. To our experience, reciprocal alleles exist in most – if not all – leukemia patients, and can be found by direct long-range PCR experiments. It should be mentioned that nearly all *MLL* rearrangements are characterized by duplications (two to several hundred basepairs), inversions (<100 bp), and deletions (several basepair up to several kilobasepairs) at the chromosomal fusion site *(15, 16)*. Therefore, any reciprocal allele should be amplified by direct PCR using oligonucleotides that are several kilobasepairs away from your identified breakpoint on either derivative allele.

4. Notes

1. The "Diagnostic Center of Acute Leukemia" (DCAL) is a diagnostic unit situated at the Goethe-University in Frankfurt, Germany. It offers cost-free analysis for biopsy senders on a collaborative basis. The list of all partner institutions or clinical study centers is summarized in the Acknowledgement. Leukemia patients should be prescreened for *MLL* rearrangements by cytogenetic experiments, preferentially by split-signal FISH. Further

information can be obtained from our website (web.uni-frankfurt.de/fb14/dcal).

2. A human cell contains about 6.6 pg DNA; each cell of a leukemia patient carrying an *MLL* rearrangement contains only one copy of the rearranged allele; thus, 1 μg genomic DNA is equal to about 300,000 genomes of which only 150,000 genomes (or less depending on the blast count) carry your allele of interest. Assuming a 100% blast count, a PCR reaction using 50 ng genomic DNA contains not more than 7,500 copies of the rearranged allele. According to our experience, a 30% blast count (about 2,200 copies) is sufficient for a positive identification.

3. Alternatives for chlorofom/phenol extractions: use the QIAquick Nucleotide Removal Kit protocol to remove enzymes from your samples. Elute your DNA with elution buffer in a final volume of 30 μl.

4. We recommend adding 2 μl of a 10 mg/ml ethidiumbromide solution directly after the 1% agarose gel (100 ml) has been heated and dissolved in 1× TBE buffer. This enables visualization directly after the separation step and does not require additional steps such as staining and destaining of your gel for analysis.

5. We have a whole panel of oligonucleotides, separated by about 200 nucleotides for the coding and noncoding strand of the *MLL* breakpoint cluster region. After initial sequencing using the long-range primers mentioned earlier (*see* **Subheading 3.5**), we use these sequencing primers to identify the *MLL* fusion site in a straightforward procedure. Based on the length of the new amplimer and the approximate location of the breakpoint, about 2–3 sequencing reactions are normally necessary to finally identify the primary sequence of the genomic fusion site. You may need to adjust this, depending on the PCR reaction(s) that gave you a positive result.

Acknowledgements

We are grateful for the collaboration of many colleagues throughout Europe in the framework of the I-BFM, GMALL, and AMLCG study groups. Special thanks to M. den Boer and R. Pieters, Sophia Children's Hospital, Rotterdam; M.W.J.C. Jansen and J.J.M van Dongen, Erasmus MC, Rotterdam; H. Kempski and H. Brady, ICH, London; E. Delabesse, INSERM U563, Toulouse; E. Macintyre, INSERM EMIU210, Paris; C. Preud'Homme, Department of Paediatrics, Lille; F. Niggli and

B. Schäfer, Department of Oncology, Zürich; A. Attarbaschi, S. Strehl and O.A. Haas, CCRI, Vienna; T. Szczepanski, Silesian Academy of Medicine, Zabrze; J. Zuna and J. Trka, Charles University, Prague; L. Lo Nigro, University of Catania, Catania; A. Biondi, University of Milano-Bicocca, Monza; T. Te Kronnie, Department of Paediatrics, Padova; M.G. Ennas, University of Cagliari; E. Angelucci, Haematology and Oncology Hospital "A. Businco," Cagliari; M. Stanulla, Medical School of Hannover; Anja Möricke, André Schrauder, Gunnar Cario and M. Schrappe, Pediatric Hematology and Oncology, Kiel; J. Greil, Department of Pediatric Hematology and Oncology, Heidelberg; U. Köhl and T. Klingebiel, Pediatric Hematology and Oncology, Frankfurt; U. zur Stadt, Eppendorf, Hamburg; C. Eckert, Charité – Virchow Campus, Berlin; S. Schnittger and C. Schoch, Munich Leukemia Laboratory, Munich; F. Griesinger, Department of Pediatric Hematology, Göttingen; T. Burmeister, Charité – Benjamin Franklin Campus, Berlin.

This work was supported by grant 107819 from the Deutsche Krebshilfe.

References

1. Gu, Y., Nakamura, T., Alder, H., Prasad, R., Canaani, O., Cimino, G., et al. (1992) The t(4;11) chromosome translocation of human acute leukemias fuses the ALL-1 gene, related to Drosophila trithorax, to the AF-4 gene. Cell 71, 701–708.

2. Tkachuk, D. C., Kohler, S., Cleary, M. L. (1992) Involvement of a homolog of Drosophila trithorax by 11q23 chromosomal translocations in acute leukemias. Cell 71, 691–700.

3. Meyer, C., Schneider, B., Reichel, M., Angermüller, S., Strehl, S., Schnittger, S., et al. (2005) A new diagnostic tool for the identification of MLL rearrangements including unknown partner genes. Proc. Natl. Acad. Sci. USA 102, 449–454.

4. Meyer, C., Schneider, B., Jakob, S., Strehl, S., Schnittger, S., Schoch, C., et al. (2006) The MLL recombinome of acute leukemias. Leukemia 20, 777–784.

5. Meyer, C., Kowarz, E., Schneider, B., Oehm, C., Klingebiel, T., Dingermann, T., et al. (2006) Genomic DNA of leukemia patients: target for clinical diagnosis of MLL rearrangements. Biotechnol. J. 1, 656–663.

6. Estable, M. C., Naghavi, M. H., Kato, H., Xiao, H., Qin, J., Vahlne, A., et al. (2002) MCEF, the newest member of the AF4 family of transcription factors involved in leukemia, is a positive transcription elongation factor-b-associated protein. J. Biomed. Sci. 9, 234–245.

7. Zeisig, D. T., Bittner, C. B., Zeisig, B. B., Garcia-Cuellar, M. P., Hess, J. L., and Slany, R. K. (2005) The eleven-nineteen-leukemia protein ENL connects nuclear MLL fusion partners with chromatin. Oncogene 24, 5525–5532.

8. Bitoun, E., Oliver, P. L., and Davies, K. E. (2007) The mixed-lineage leukemia fusion partner AF4 stimulates RNA polymerase II transcriptional elongation and mediates coordinated chromatin remodeling. Hum. Mol. Genet. 16, 92–106.

9. Felix, C. A., Kim, C. S., Megonigal, M. D., Slater, D. J., Jones, D. H., Spinner, N. B., et al. (1997) Panhandle polymerase chain reaction amplifies MLL genomic translocation breakpoint involving unknown partner gene. Blood 90, 4679–4686.

10. Jones, D. H., Winistorfer, S. C. (1992) Sequence specific generation of a DNA panhandle permits PCR amplification of unknown flanking DNA. Nucleic Acids Res. 20, 595–600.

11. Burmeister, T., Marschalek, R., Schneider, B., Meyer, C., Gökbuget, N., Schwartz, S., et al. (2006) Monitoring minimal residual disease

by quantification of genomic chromosomal breakpoint sequences in acute leukemias with *MLL* aberrations. *Leukemia* **20**, 451–457.

12. Reichel, M., Gillert, E., Angermüller, S., Hensel, J. P., Heidel, F., Lode, M., et al. (2001) Biased distribution of chromosomal breakpoints involving the *MLL* gene in infants versus children and adults with t(4;11) ALL. *Oncogene* **20**, 2900–2907.

13. Langer, T., Metzler, M., Reinhardt, D., Viehmann, S., Borkhardt, A., Reichel, M., et al. (2003) Analysis of t(9;11) chromosomal breakpoint sequences in childhood acute leukemia: almost identical *MLL* breakpoints in therapy-related AML after treatment without etoposides. *Genes Chrom. Cancer* **36**, 393–401.

14. Ochman, H., Gerber, A. S., and Hartl, D. L. (1988) Genetic applications of an inverse polymerase chain reaction. *Genetics* **120**, 621–623.

15. Reichel, M., Gillert, E., Nilson, I., Siegler, G., Greil, J., Fey, G. H., et al. (1998) Fine structure of translocation breakpoints in leukemic blasts with chromosomal translocation t(4;11): the DNA damage-repair model of translocation. *Oncogene* **17**, 3035–3044.

16. Gillert, E., Leis, T., Repp, R., Reichel, M., Hösch, A., Breitenlohner, I., et al. (1999) A DNA damage repair mechanism is involved in the origin of chromosomal translocations t(4;11) in primary leukemic cells. *Oncogene* **18**, 4663–4671.

Chapter 6

Panhandle PCR Approaches to Cloning *MLL* Genomic Breakpoint Junctions and Fusion Transcript Sequences

Blaine W. Robinson and Carolyn A. Felix

Summary

Translocations and other rearrangements of the *MLL* gene at chromosome band 11q23 are biologically and clinically important molecular abnormalities in infant acute leukemias, leukemias associated with chemotherapeutic topoisomerase II poisons and, less often, acute leukemias in adults or myelodysplastic syndrome. Depending on the disease and the regimen, *MLL*-rearranged leukemias may be associated with inferior prognosis, and *MLL* rearrangements with some of the more than 60 known *MLL*–partner genes confer especially adverse effects as response to treatment (Blood 108:441–451, 2006). *MLL* rearrangements are usually evident as overt balanced chromosomal translocations by conventional cytogenetic analysis but up to one-third are cryptic rearrangements and occur in leukemias with del(11)(q23), a normal karyotype, or trisomy 11, the latter two of which sometimes are associated with partial tandem duplications of *MLL* itself (Proc Natl Acad Sci U S A 97:2814–2819, 2000; Proc Natl Acad Sci U S A 94:3899–3902, 1997). In addition, subsets of *MLL* rearrangements are complex at a cytogenetic level and/or molecular level, and fuse *MLL* with two different partner genes. Rapid and accurate methods to identify and characterize genomic breakpoint junctions and fusion transcripts resulting from the many types of *MLL* rearrangements are essential for risk group stratification, treatment protocol assignments, new partner gene discovery, understanding leukemia etiology and pathogenesis, and elucidating the impact of less common *MLL*–partner genes on biology and prognosis. Due to the vast heterogeneity in partner genes, typical gene-specific PCR based methods are not practical, especially when cytogenetics are normal or do not suggest involvement of a known partner gene of *MLL*. We have advanced seven different panhandle PCR based methods for cloning 5′-*MLL*–*partner gene*-3′ and 5′-*partner gene*–*MLL*-3′ genomic breakpoint junctions and identifying 5′-*MLL*–*partner gene*-3′ fusion transcripts, all of which employ a stem-loop template shaped schematically like a pan with a handle and amplify the template without knowledge of the unknown partner sequence using primers all derived from *MLL* alone.

Key words: *MLL*, Leukemia, Infant, Secondary, Partner gene, Panhandle PCR, 11q23

C.W.E. So (ed.), Leukemia, *Methods in Molecular Biology, vol. 538*
© Humana Press, a part of Springer Science + Business Media, LLC 2009
DOI: 10.1007/978-1-59745-418-6_6

1. Introduction

Although *MLL* is an extreme example of a gene involved in translocations with many different, often unknown partner genes, approaches for cloning both genomic breakpoint junctions are a prerequisite for determining the involvement and alterations of specific sequences in native *MLL* and its partner genes in the translocations. To circumvent the cloning difficulties from the many partner genes, we developed six different genomic and one cDNA panhandle PCR approaches *(1–8)*. Usually the 5′-*MLL–partner gene*-3′ genomic breakpoint junction is formed on the der(11) chromosome whereas the 5′-*partner gene–MLL*-3′ rearrangement forms on the other derivative chromosome. However, complex *MLL* rearrangements involving >2 genes or chromosomes may result in the formation of the 5′-*MLL–partner gene*-3′ junction on a different derivative chromosome. In instances where oppositely oriented partner genes (telomere to centromere) fuse with *MLL* via splitting of the MLL breakpoint cluster region (bcr) and inversion/insertion into band 11q23, both breakpoint junctions may form on the der(11) chromosome. Therefore, for the sake of clarity, the specific breakpoint junctions targeted by particular panhandle PCR approaches will be referred to as 5′-*MLL–partner gene*-3′ or 5′-*partner gene–MLL*-3′ even though the former usually forms on the der(11) and the latter on the other derivative chromosome. The salient differences between the various panhandle methods and their applications are summarized in **Table 1**.

MLL translocation breakpoints are distributed in an 8.3-kb bcr defined by the *Bam*HI fragment between exons 5 and 11. In each of the six genomic panhandle methods, Southern blot analysis of the *MLL* bcr in the leukemia DNA informs the rearrangement sizes, which approximate the sizes of potential target amplicons and guides the specific method used *(1, 3–8)*. Hence, the original panhandle PCR *(1, 4, 5)* and panhandle variant PCR *(3, 6)* methods for cloning 5′-*MLL–partner gene*-3′ breakpoint junctions, the earliest of these methods, and two different reverse panhandle PCR methods for cloning 5′-*partner gene–MLL*-3′ breakpoint junctions *(7, 9)* attach known *MLL* sequence to the partner sequence in *Bam*HI-digested DNA and thereby target rearranged *Bam*HI genomic fragments for the PCR. Genomic panhandle PCR approaches may be impeded when the targeted restriction fragment that contains the breakpoint junction is too large to amplify. Panhandle variant PCR and reverse panhandle PCR (single primer), which both employ single-primer PCR, have the theoretical advantage of inhibiting short products *(6)*. However, it has not been established whether one method is advantageous over the other method.

Table 1
Summary of panhandle PCR approaches

Target sequence	5'-*MLL–partner gene*-3' genomic breakpoint junction			5'-*Partner gene–MLL*-3' genomic breakpoint junction			5'-*MLL–partner gene*-3' fusion transcript
Method	Panhandle	Panhandle variant	*Bgl*II panhandle	Reverse panhandle (single primer)	Reverse panhandle (two primer)	*Bgl*II reverse panhandle	cDNA panhandle
Requires *Bam*HI cleavage	Yes	Yes	No	Yes	Yes	No	No
Requires *Bgl*II cleavage	No	No	Yes	No	No	Yes	No
Uses phosphorylated oligonucleotide to build template	Yes	No	Yes	Yes	Yes	Yes	No
Uses bridging oligonucleotide to build template	No	Yes	No	No	No	No	No
Uses exonuclease I digestion	No	Yes	No	No	No	No	No
Length of handle (short <70, long ≥70)	Long	Short	Short	Short	Long	Short	Short
DNA strand used for panhandle formation	Sense	DNA strand generated by primer 1 extension off of antisense strand	Sense	Antisense	Antisense	Antisense	Second-strand cDNA
Number of primers per PCR	2	1	2	1	2	2	2
PCR primer orientation	Sense	Sense	Sense	Antisense	Antisense	Antisense	Sense
# PCRs	2	3	2	3	2	2	2
Inhibits formation of short products	No	Yes	No	Yes	No	No	No
References	(1, 4, 5)	(3, 6)	(8)	(7)	(9)	(8)	(2, 3, 10)

Despite heterogeneity in *MLL* translocation breakpoint distribution, many *MLL* translocation breakpoints are 3′ in the bcr *(11, 12)*. Foreshortening the target amplicon for panhandle PCR by removal of more 5′-sequence could increase the feasibility of cloning genomic breakpoint junctions with more 3′-translocation breakpoints provided that there is a relevant restriction enzyme site proximal to the breakpoint in the partner gene. *Bgl*II panhandle PCR for 5′-*MLL–partner gene*-3′ breakpoint junctions takes advantage of the *Bgl*II restriction site at position 2,253 of the bcr in intron 6 to create the stem-loop template *(8)*. In addition, we devised a reverse panhandle PCR strategy to amplify the 5′-*partner gene–MLL*-3′ genomic breakpoint junction that makes use of the *Bgl*II restriction site at position 8,234 of the bcr in intron 10 *(8)*.

Stem-loop templates are created in all of these genomic methods by attaching known *MLL* bcr sequence to the unknown partner sequence at the site of restriction enzyme cleavage such that primers, all from *MLL*, can amplify the genomic breakpoint junction contained within the loop.

1.1. Original Panhandle PCR

This was the first panhandle PCR method adapted to clone 5′-*MLL–partner gene*-3′ genomic breakpoint junctions *(1, 4, 5)*. Ligation of a phosphorylated oligonucleotide complementary to known *MLL* exon 5 sequence 5′ in the bcr, to the unknown partner sequence at the 3′-end of *Bam*HI-digested DNA enables the formation of the stem-loop template. The loop contains the translocation breakpoint and unknown partner DNA; the "handle" contains known *MLL* bcr sequence and its complement. *MLL* exon 5 sense primers are used to amplify the breakpoint junction in two sequential two-primer two-sided PCRs (**Fig. 1**).

1.2. Panhandle Variant PCR

In panhandle variant PCR (**Fig. 2**), an *MLL* exon 5 sense oligonucleotide (Primer 3) is ligated to the 5′-ends of *Bam*HI-digested DNA through a bridging oligonucleotide comprised of a GATC sequence at the 5′-end and the complement of the 3′-end of Primer 3 at the 3′-end. The purpose of the bridging oligonucleotide is to position the 3′-end of Primer 3 for ligation to the 5′-ends of the *Bam*HI-digested DNA, after which excess unligated Primer 3 as well as the bridging oligonucleotide are eliminated by exonuclease I digestion *(3, 6)*. The stem-loop template is formed from the DNA strand resulting from primer extension of the antisense strand, and the 5′-*MLL–partner gene*-3′ breakpoint junction is amplified in three sequential two-sided PCRs using single *MLL* exon 5 sense primers, which anneal to both ends of the template, the last of which (Primer 3) is the same as the ligated oligonucleotide *(3, 6)*. Panhandle variant PCR is simpler and has fewer steps than the original panhandle PCR.

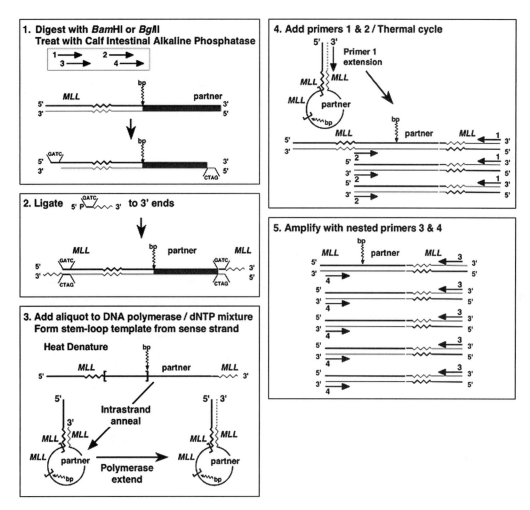

Fig. 1. General steps in original and *Bgl*I panhandle PCR for 5′-*MLL–partner gene*-3′ genomic breakpoint junctions. *Bold lines* indicate sense DNA strand containing *MLL* and partner gene sequence from which the template is created, and sense orientations of the primers. The 5′-phosphorylated oligonucleotide contains a GATC overhang at the 5′-end and the complement of sense sequence in *MLL* at the 3′-end. The GATC overhang at the 5′-end of the phosphorylated oligonucleotide promotes attachment of the complement of sequence in *MLL* at the restriction site in the sense strand of the partner gene (step 2) to create the template (step 3) for amplification with initial (step 4) and nested (step 5) *MLL* primers. Modified from *(8)* with permission from Wiley-Liss, Inc.

1.3. BgllI Panhandle PCR

This method to amplify 5′-*MLL–partner gene*-3′ genomic breakpoint junctions is accomplished by ligating a phosphorylated oligonucleotide containing a *Bgl*II overhang and *MLL* exon 7 complementary sequence to the 3′-ends of *Bgl*II-digested DNA and formation of the stem-loop template from the sense strand of the DNA followed by two sequential two-primer PCRs similar to the original panhandle PCR *(8)* (**Fig. 1**). The primers in *Bgl*II panhandle PCR are all 'sense' with respect to *MLL* exon 7 *(8)*.

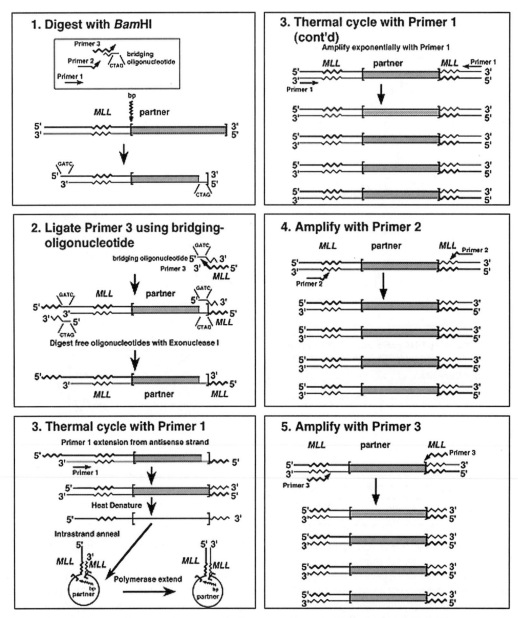

Fig. 2. Steps in panhandle variant PCR for 5′-*MLL–partner gene*-3′ genomic breakpoint junctions. All sequences in sense orientation are *bold* and all sequences in antisense orientation are shown as *thin lines* throughout all parts of the figure. The primers all are sense with respect to *MLL* exon 5. *Bam*HI digestion places the translocation breakpoint junction in a double stranded *Bam*HI fragment with *MLL* at the 5′-end and the unknown partner sequence at the 3′-end relative to the sense strand of the DNA (step 1). The bridging oligonucleotide contains a GATC at the 5′-end, which is complementary to the 4-base 5′ overhang of a *Bam*HI site, and the complement of the 3′-end of Primer 3 at the 3′-end, which can anneal to Primer 3. Thus, the GATC at the 5′-end of the bridging oligonucleotide promotes the ligation of Primer 3 to the *Bam*HI restriction site in the partner gene at the 5′-end of the antisense strand of the *Bam*HI-digested, double-stranded DNA (step 2). After the ligation, the bridging oligonucleotide and excess Primer 3 are removed by exonuclease I digestion. The new sense-strand template (*bold* in step 3) begins to be generated by Primer 1 extension off of the antisense strand containing Primer 3 attached at the 5′-end, resulting in a sense-strand template with the complement of Primer 3 at the 3′-end. After heat denaturation makes the DNA single stranded, an intrastrand loop is formed when the region in *MLL* exon 5 that corresponds to Primer 3 anneals to its complement at the 3′-end of the single strand. Polymerase extension of the recessed 3′-end completes the formation of the "handle" in the stem-loop template. This enables Primer 1 to anneal to its newly formed complement at the 3′-end to generate a new double-stranded template for the PCR. The ensuing steps all entail exponential amplification with the single primers, Primer 1 (step 3), Primer 2 (step 4) and Primer 3 (step 5), all of which anneal to both ends of the double-stranded template.

1.4. Reverse Panhandle PCR (Single Primer)

A full understanding of the translocation process requires sequencing of the genomic breakpoint junctions on both derivative chromosomes. Reverse panhandle PCR was devised for the 5′-*partner gene–MLL*-3′ genomic breakpoint junctions *(7)*, and has features of both panhandle PCR *(1, 4, 5)* and panhandle variant PCR *(3, 6)*. The steps include ligation of a sense phosphorylated oligonucleotide from *MLL* intron 10/exon 11, 3′ in the bcr, to the 3′-ends of *Bam*HI-digested DNA and formation of a stem-loop template from the antisense strand of DNA. Unknown partner sequence, the genomic breakpoint junction and *MLL* sequence are contained within the loop. *MLL* sequence and its complement at either end of the "handle" enable amplification of the breakpoint junction in three sequential single-primer, two-sided PCRs with primers that are all antisense with respect to exon 11 or intron 10/exon 11 sequences 3′ in the bcr.

1.5. Reverse Panhandle PCR (Two Primer)

A two-primer adaptation of reverse panhandle PCR for 5′-*partner gene–MLL*-3′ genomic breakpoint junctions *(9)* utilizes a template formed from *Bam*HI-digested DNA similar to single-primer reverse panhandle PCR, but two sequential two-primer PCRs are employed with primers that are all antisense with respect to exon 11, intron 10/exon 11 or exon 10 sequences 3′ in the bcr.

1.6. BglII Reverse Panhandle PCR

In *Bgl*II reverse panhandle PCR a phosphorylated oligonucleotide containing a *Bgl*II overhang and complementary sequence to the antisense strand of *MLL* exon 10 is ligated to the 3′-ends of *Bgl*II-digested DNA, and the stem-loop template, which is formed from the antisense strand of the DNA, is amplified in two sequential two-primer PCRs with primers that are antisense with respect to exon 10/intron 10 or exon 10 sequences in the 3′-bcr *(8)*.

1.7. cDNA Panhandle PCR

As the number of partner genes of *MLL* continued to increase, we developed cDNA panhandle PCR to identify 5′-*MLL–partner gene*-3′ fusion transcripts *(2, 3, 10)*. The occurrence of *MLL* genomic translocation breakpoints within an 8.3-kb bcr between exons 5 and 11 also enables targeting fusion transcripts from the corresponding 859-bp *MLL* bcr mRNA *(13)* regardless of the partner gene by cDNA panhandle PCR. The 5′-*MLL–partner gene*-3′ transcripts are of interest because the corresponding fusion proteins are leukemogenic *(14)*. By reverse transcribing first-strand cDNAs with an oligonucleotide mixture containing the coding sequence from *MLL* exon 5 at the 5′-end and random hexamers at the 3′-ends, known *MLL* sequence is attached to the unknown partner sequence during synthesis of first-strand cDNA. This enables the formation of stem-loop templates with the fusion point of the chimeric transcript in the loop, and the use of *MLL* primers for two-primer, two-sided PCR. cDNA panhandle PCR can lead readily to the discovery of the coding sequences of partner genes in smaller amplicons than genomic panhandle

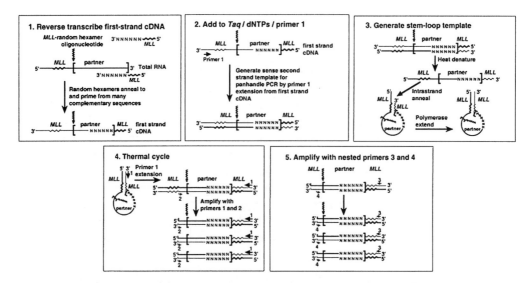

Fig. 3. Steps in cDNA panhandle PCR. *Corkscrew arrow* indicates fusion point in *MLL* chimeric transcript. A population of first-strand cDNAs of various sizes is expected because of *MLL*-random hexamer oligonucleotide design (step 1). Sense second-strand template is generated for panhandle PCR by primer 1 extension (step 2) to create the template (step 3) for amplification with initial (step 4) and nested (step 5) *MLL* primers. Transcripts from normal *MLL* allele also would be amplified. Reproduced from (2) with permission from National Academy of Sciences.

PCR approaches and is practical when genomic amplicons are particularly large or the DNA is of poor quality for PCR (**Fig. 3**). This method can identify an entire spectrum of normal and *MLL* fusion transcripts in the same reaction, which is germane to characterizing exon scrambling, alternative splicing and incompletely processed transcripts.

2. Materials

2.1. Original Panhandle PCR and BglII Panhandle PCR

2.1.1. DNA Digestion/ Ligation

1. *Bam*HI Enzyme (10 U/μl) (Invitrogen, Carlsbad, CA).
   (a) OR *Bgl*II Enzyme (10 U/μl) (Invitrogen).
2. REact 3 Buffer (Invitrogen).
3. DEPC Treated Water (Ambion, Austin, TX).
4. Calf Intestinal Alkaline Phosphatase (CIAP) (1 U/μl) (Roche, Indianapolis, IN) (*see* **Note 1**).
5. TE buffer (1×): 10 mM Tris–HCl, 1 mM EDTA, pH 8.0.
6. GeneClean III Kit (Qbiogene Inc., Carlsbad, CA).
7. Phosphorylated Oligonucleotide (P-oligo) with *Bam*HI overhang (250 ng/μl) (5′-*GAT CGA* AGC TGG AGT GGT GGC CTG TTT GGA TTC AGG-3′).

(a) Or Phosphorylated Oligo (P-oligo) with *Bgl*II overhang (250 ng/μl) (5′-*GAT* CGA ACT ATT GCC ATT GGA GAG AGT GCT GAG GAT-3′).

8. T4 DNA Ligase (1 U/μl) (Roche).

9. T4 Ligase Buffer (10×) (Roche).

2.1.2. PCR Amplification

1. GeneAmp Thin-Walled Reaction Tube with Flat Cap (Applied Biosystems, Foster City, CA).

2. DNA Polymerase Mix (Taq/Tgo) (5 U/μl) (Roche).

3. 25 mM dNTP Mix (1:1:1:1 mixture of 100 mM dATP, dCTP, dGTP, and dTTP).

4. Expand Long Template PCR System, Buffer I (10×) (Roche).

5. Primer #1 (5 pmol/μl) (5′-TCC TCC ACG AAA GCC CGT CGA G-3′).

6. Primer #2 (5 pmol/μl) (5′-TCA AGC AGG TCT CCC AGC CAG CAC-3′).

7. Primer #3 (5 pmol/μl) (5′-GGA AAA GAG TGA AGA AGG GAA TGT CTC GG-3′).

8. Primer #4 (5 pmol/μl) (5′-GTG GTC ATC CCG CCT CAG CCA C-3′).

9. *Bgl*II Primer #1 (5 pmol/μl) (5′-AAC CAC CTC CGG TCA ATA AGC AGG A-3′).

10. *Bgl*II Primer #2 (5 pmol/μl) (5′-AAT TCC AGC AGA TGG AGT CCA CAG GA-3′).

11. *Bgl*II Primer #3 (5 pmol/μl) (5′-CAG GAG AAT GCA GGC ACT TTG AAC-3′).

12. *Bgl*II Primer #4 (5 pmol/μl) (5′-CCA CAG GAT CAG AGT GGA CTT TAA G-3′).

2.1.3. Transformation

1. GeneClean III Kit (Qbiogene).

2. 14-ml Polypropylene Round-Bottom Tube (17 × 100 mm) (Becton Dickinson Labware, Franklin Lakes, NJ).

3. OneShot Max Efficiency DH5α-T1[R] Chemically Competent Cells (Invitrogen).

4. pCR® 2.1-TOPO® TA Cloning Vector (Invitrogen).

5. Salt Solution: 1.2 M NaCl, 0.06 M $MgCl_2$ (Invitrogen).

6. S.O.C. Medium (Invitrogen).

7. Carbenicillin (Sigma, St. Louis, MO). (Prepare 1-ml aliquots of carbenicillin stock solution of 100 mg/ml in water and store aliquots at −20°C.)

8. Miller's LB Broth (Mediatech Inc., Herndon, VA). (Prepare LB broth by adding 1 ml of carbenicillin (100 mg/ml) to each liter for a final concentration of 100 μg/ml.)

9. LB Agar Plates. (Prepare LB agar plates by adding 1 ml of carbenicillin (100 mg/ml) to each liter for a final concentration of 100 µg/ml.)

2.1.4. PCR Colony Screen

1. GeneAmp Thin-Walled Reaction Tube with Flat Cap (Applied Biosystems).

2. DNA Polymerase Mix (Taq/Tgo) (5 U/µl) (Roche).

3. 25 mM dNTP Mix (1:1:1:1 mixture of 100 mM dATP, dCTP, dGTP, and dTTP).

4. Expand Long Template PCR System, Buffer I (10×) (Roche).

5. Primer #3 (5 pmol/µl) (5′-GGA AAA GAG TGA AGA AGG GAA TGT CTC GG-3′).

6. Primer #4 (5 pmol/µl) (5′-GTG GTC ATC CCG CCT CAG CCA C-3′).

7. *Bgl*II Primer #3 (5 pmol/µl) (5′-CAG GAG AAT GCA GGC ACT TTG AAC-3′).

8. *Bgl*II Primer #4 (5 pmol/µl) (5′-CCA CAG GAT CAG AGT GGA CTT TAA G-3′).

2.2. Panhandle Variant PCR

1. *Bam*HI Enzyme (10 U/µl) (Invitrogen).

2. REact 3 Buffer (Invitrogen).

2.2.1. DNA Digestion/ Ligation

3. DEPC Treated Water (Ambion).

4. Bridging Oligo with *Bam*HI overhang (5 pmol/µl) (5′-*GAT CGA* GAC ATT CCC TTC T-3′).

5. Primer #3 (5 pmol/µl) (5′-TCG AGG AAA AGA GTG AAG AAG GGA ATG TCT C-3′).

6. T4 DNA Ligase (1 U/µl) (Roche).

7. T4 Ligase Buffer (10×) (Roche).

8. Exonuclease I (20 U/µl) (Epicentre Biotechnologies, Madison, WI).

2.2.2. PCR Amplification

1. GeneAmp Thin-Walled Reaction Tube with Flat Cap (Applied Biosystems).

2. DNA Polymerase Mix (Taq/Tgo) (5 U/µl) (Roche).

3. 25 mM dNTP Mix (1:1:1:1 mixture of 100 mM dATP, dCTP, dGTP, and dTTP).

4. Expand Long Template PCR System, Buffer I (10×) (Roche).

5. Primer #1 (5 pmol/µl) (5′-TCC TCC ACG AAA GCC CGT CGA G-3′).

6. Primer #2 (5 pmol/µl) (5′-CCA CGA AAG CCC GTC GAG GAA AAG-3′).

7. Primer #3 (5 pmol/µl) (5′-TCG AGG AAA AGA GTG AAG AAG GGA ATG TCT C-3′).

2.2.3. Transformation

1. GeneClean III Kit (Qbiogene).

2. 14-ml Polypropylene Round-Bottom Tube (17×100 mm) (Becton Dickinson Labware).

3. OneShot Max Efficiency DH5α-T1^R Chemically Competent Cells (Invitrogen).

4. pCR® 2.1-TOPO® TA Cloning Vector (Invitrogen).

5. Salt Solution: 1.2 M NaCl, 0.06 M MgCl$_2$ (Invitrogen).

6. S.O.C. Medium (Invitrogen).

7. Carbenicillin (Sigma). (Prepare 1-ml aliquots of carbenicillin stock solution of 100 mg/ml in water and store aliquots at –20°C.)

8. Miller's LB Broth (Mediatech). (Prepare LB broth by adding 1 ml of carbenicillin (100 mg/ml) to each liter for a final concentration of 100 µg/ml.)

9. LB Agar Plates. (Prepare LB agar plates by adding 1 ml of carbenicillin (100 mg/ml) to each liter for a final concentration of 100 µg/ml.)

2.2.4. PCR Colony Screen

1. GeneAmp Thin-Walled Reaction Tube with Flat Cap (Applied Biosystems).

2. DNA Polymerase Mix (Taq/Tgo) (5 U/µl) (Roche).

3. 25 mM dNTP Mix (1:1:1:1 mixture of 100 mM dATP, dCTP, dGTP, and dTTP).

4. Expand Long Template PCR System, Buffer I (10×) (Roche).

5. Primer #3 (5 pmol/µl) (5′-TCG AGG AAA AGA GTG AAG AAG GGA ATG TCT C-3′).

2.3. Reverse Panhandle PCR (Single Primer)

1. *Bam*HI Enzyme (10 U/µl) (Invitrogen).

2. REact 3 Buffer (Invitrogen).

2.3.1. DNA Digestion/ Ligation

3. DEPC Treated Water (Ambion).

4. Calf Intestinal Alkaline Phosphatase (CIAP) (1 U/µl) (Roche) (*see* **Note 1**).

5. TE buffer (1×): 10 mM Tris–HCl, 1 mM EDTA, pH 8.0.

6. GeneClean III Kit (Qbiogene).

7. Reverse (single primer) Phosphorylated Oligo (P-oligo) with *Bam*HI overhang (250 ng/µl) (5′-*GAT* CGA GAC ATT CCC TTC T-3′).

8. T4 DNA Ligase (1 U/µl) (Roche).

9. T4 Ligase Buffer (10×) (Roche).

2.3.2. PCR Amplification

1. GeneAmp Thin-Walled Reaction Tube with Flat Cap (Applied Biosystems).

2. DNA Polymerase Mix (Taq/Tgo) (5 U/µl) (Roche).

3. 25 mM dNTP Mix (1:1:1:1 mixture of 100 mM dATP, dCTP, dGTP, and dTTP).

4. Expand Long Template PCR System, Buffer I (10×) (Roche).

5. Primer #1 (5 pmol/μl) (5′-GGA TCC ACA GCT CTT ACA GCG AAC ACA C-3′).

6. Primer #2 (5 pmol/μl) (5′-ACA GCT CTT ACA GCG AAC ACA CTT GGT ACA GA-3′).

7. Primer #3 (5 pmol/μl) (5′-GCT CTT ACA GCG AAC ACA CTT GGT ACA GAT CTA GA-3′).

2.3.3. Transformation

1. GeneClean III Kit (Qbiogene).

2. 14-ml Polypropylene Round-Bottom Tube (17 × 100 mm) (Becton Dickinson Labware).

3. OneShot Max Efficiency DH5α-T1^R Chemically Competent Cells (Invitrogen).

4. pCR® 2.1-TOPO® TA Cloning Vector (Invitrogen).

5. Salt Solution: 1.2 M NaCl, 0.06 M MgCl$_2$ (Invitrogen).

6. S.O.C. Medium (Invitrogen).

7. Carbenicillin (Sigma). (Prepare 1-ml aliquots of carbenicillin stock solution of 100 mg/ml in water and store aliquots at –20°C.)

8. Miller's LB Broth (Mediatech). (Prepare LB broth by adding 1 ml of carbenicillin (100 mg/ml) to each liter for a final concentration of 100 μg/ml.)

9. LB Agar Plates. (Prepare LB agar plates by adding 1 ml of carbenicillin (100 mg/ml) to each liter for a final concentration of 100 μg/ml.)

2.3.4. PCR Colony Screen

1. GeneAmp Thin-Walled Reaction Tube with Flat Cap (Applied Biosystems).

2. DNA Polymerase Mix (Taq/Tgo) (5 U/μl) (Roche).

3. 25 mM dNTP Mix (1:1:1:1 mixture of 100 mM dATP, dCTP, dGTP, and dTTP).

4. Expand Long Template PCR System, Buffer I (10×) (Roche).

5. Primer #3 (5 pmol/μl) (5′-GCT CTT ACA GCG AAC ACA CTT GGT ACA GAT CTA GA-3′).

2.4. Reverse Panhandle PCR (Two Primer) and BglII Reverse Panhandle PCR

2.4.1. DNA Digestion/ Ligation

1. *Bam*HI Enzyme (10 U/μl) (Invitrogen).

   (a) OR *Bgl*II Enzyme (10 U/μl) (Invitrogen).

2. REact 3 Buffer (Invitrogen).

3. DEPC Treated Water (Ambion).

4. Calf Intestinal Alkaline Phosphatase (CIAP) (1 U/μl) (Roche) (*see* **Note 1**).

5. TE buffer (1×): 10 mM Tris–HCl, 1 mM EDTA, pH 8.0.

6. GeneClean III Kit (Qbiogene).

7. Reverse (two-primer) Phosphorylated Oligo (P-oligo) with *Bam*HI/*Bgl*II overhang (250 ng/μl) (5′-*GAT* CAC CCT GAG TGC CTG GGA CCA AAC TAC CCC ACC-3′).

8. T4 DNA Ligase (1 U/μl) (Roche).

9. T4 Ligase Buffer (10×) (Roche).

2.4.2. PCR Amplification

1. GeneAmp Thin-Walled Reaction Tube with Flat Cap (Applied Biosystems).

2. Elongase Enzyme Mix (1 U/μl) (Invitrogen).

3. 10 mM dNTP Mix (Invitrogen).

4. Buffer A (5×) (Invitrogen).

5. Buffer B (5×) (Invitrogen).

6. Primer #1 (5 pmol/μl) (5′-GGA TCC ACA GCT CTT ACA GCG AAC ACA C-3′).

7. *Bgl*II Primer #1 (5 pmol/μl) (5′-TAA AAG AGC ATC ATG TGT ATA ACT CAC-3′).

8. Primer #2 (5 pmol/μl) (5′-CAG GCA CTC AGG GTG ATA GCT GTT TCG-3′).

9. Primer #3 (5 pmol/μl) (5′-TAC AGC GAA CAC ACT TGG TAC AGA TCT AGA AAA GAA G-3′).

10. *Bgl*II Primer #3 (5 pmol/μl) (5′-CCA GAC TTT CTT CTT CTT TGT GGG TTT-3′).

11. Primer #4 (5 pmol/μl) (5′-AGC TGT TTC GGC ACT TAT TAC ACT CCA GCA-3′).

2.4.3. Transformation

1. GeneClean III Kit (Qbiogene).

2. 14-ml Polypropylene Round-Bottom Tube (17 × 100 mm) (Becton Dickinson Labware).

3. OneShot Max Efficiency DH5α-T1^R Chemically Competent Cells (Invitrogen).

4. pCR® 2.1-TOPO® TA Cloning Vector (Invitrogen).

5. Salt Solution: 1.2 M NaCl, 0.06 M $MgCl_2$ (Invitrogen).

6. S.O.C. Medium (Invitrogen).

7. Carbenicillin (Sigma). (Prepare 1-ml aliquots of carbenicillin stock solution of 100 mg/ml in water and store aliquots at –20°C.)

8. Miller's LB Broth (Mediatech). (Prepare LB broth by adding 1 ml of carbenicillin (100 mg/ml) to each liter for a final concentration of 100 μg/ml.)

9. LB Agar Plates. (Prepare LB agar plates by adding 1 ml of carbenicillin (100 mg/ml) to each liter for a final concentration of 100 μg/ml.)

2.4.4. PCR Colony Screen

1. GeneAmp Thin-Walled Reaction Tube with Flat Cap (Applied Biosystems).
2. Elongase Enzyme Mix (1 U/μl) (Invitrogen).
3. 10 mM dNTP Mix (Invitrogen).
4. Buffer A (5×) (Invitrogen).
5. Buffer B (5×) (Invitrogen).
6. Primer #3 (5 pmol/μl) (5′-TAC AGC GAA CAC ACT TGG TAC AGA TCT AGA AAA GAA G-3′).
7. *Bgl*II Primer #3 (5 pmol/μl) (5′-CCA GAC TTT CTT CTT CTT TGT GGG TTT-3′).
8. Primer #4 (5 pmol/μl) (5′-AGC TGT TTC GGC ACT TAT TAC ACT CCA GCA-3′).

2.5. cDNA Panhandle PCR

2.5.1. First-Strand cDNA Synthesis

1. GeneAmp Thin-Walled Reaction Tube with Flat Cap (Applied Biosystems).
2. DNase I, Amplification Grade (1 U/μl) (Invitrogen).
3. DNase I Reaction Buffer (10×) (Invitrogen).
4. DEPC Treated Water (Ambion).
5. 25 mM EDTA (Invitrogen).
6. *MLL* Random Hexamer Primer (50 ng/μl) (5′-CCT GAA TCC AAA CAG GCC ACC ACT CCA GCT TCN NNN NN-3′).
7. First Strand Buffer (5×) (Invitrogen).
8. 10 mM dNTP Mix, PCR Grade (Invitrogen).
9. 0.1 M DTT (Invitrogen).
10. SuperScript II Reverse Transcriptase (200 U/μl) (Invitrogen).
11. RNase H (2 U/μl) (Invitrogen).

2.5.2. PCR Amplification

1. GeneAmp Thin-Walled Reaction Tube with Flat Cap (Applied Biosystems).
2. DNA Polymerase Mix (Taq/Tgo) (5 U/μl) (Roche).
3. 25 mM dNTP Mix (1:1:1:1 mixture of 100 mM dATP, dCTP, dGTP, and dTTP).
4. Expand Long Template PCR System, Buffer I (10×) (Roche).
5. Primer #1 (5 pmol/μl) (5′-TCC TCC ACG AAA GCC CGT CGA G-3′).
6. Primer #2 (5 pmol/μl) (5′-TCA GCA GGT CTC CCA GCA GCA C-3′).
7. Primer #3 (5 pmol/μl) (5′-GGA AAA GAG TGA AGA AGG GAA TGT CTC GG-3′).
8. Primer #4 (5 pmol/μl) (5′-GTG GTC ATC CCG CCT CAG CCA C-3′).

2.5.3. Transformation

1. GeneClean III Kit (Qbiogene).

2. 14-ml Polypropylene Round-Bottom Tube (17×100 mm) (Becton Dickinson Labware).

3. OneShot Max Efficiency DH5α-T1[R] Chemically Competent Cells (Invitrogen).

4. pCR® 2.1-TOPO® TA Cloning Vector (Invitrogen).

5. Salt Solution: 1.2 M NaCl, 0.06 M $MgCl_2$ (Invitrogen).

6. S.O.C. Medium (Invitrogen).

7. Carbenicillin (Sigma). (Prepare 1-ml aliquots of carbenicillin stock solution of 100 mg/ml in water and store aliquots at –20°C.)

8. Miller's LB Broth (Mediatech). (Prepare LB broth by adding 1 ml of carbenicillin (100 mg/ml) to each liter for a final concentration of 100 μg/ml.)

9. LB Agar Plates. (Prepare LB agar plates by adding 1 ml of carbenicillin (100 mg/ml) to each liter for a final concentration of 100 μg/ml.)

2.5.4. PCR Colony Screen

1. GeneAmp Thin-Walled Reaction Tube with Flat Cap (Applied Biosystems).

2. DNA Polymerase Mix (Taq/Tgo) (5 U/μl) (Roche).

3. 25 mM dNTP Mix (1:1:1:1 mixture of 100 mM dATP, dCTP, dGTP, and dTTP).

4. Expand Long Template PCR System, Buffer I (10×) (Roche).

5. Primer #3 (5 pmol/μl) (5′-GGA AAA GAG TGA AGA AGG GAA TGT CTC GG-3′).

6. Primer #4 (5 pmol/μl) (5′-GTG GTC ATC CCG CCT CAG CCA C-3′).

3. Methods

The salient features of all of these methods include attachment of a known *MLL* sequence to the unknown partner sequence, which leads to the formation of the stem-loop structure, and PCR amplification of the genomic breakpoint junction or, in the case of cDNA panhandle PCR, the fusion point of the chimeric transcript, contained within the loop via sequential two-sided PCRs with either one or two primers all from the *MLL* bcr. Panhandle PCR methods offer the advantage of amplifying *MLL* translocation breakpoint junctions and fusion transcript sequences without any primers from the partner genes or knowledge of their sequences, thus enabling identification of involvement and alterations of specific sequences in native *MLL* and its partner genes with knowledge of the sequence of the *MLL* bcr alone.

The original panhandle PCR *(1, 4, 5)* and panhandle variant PCR *(3, 6)* approaches for amplification of 5′-*MLL–partner gene*-3′ genomic breakpoint junctions were adaptations of technologies originally advanced by Jones et al. to exploit PCR to amplify genomic regions containing unknown 3′-flanking sequences *(15, 16)*. We further developed panhandle PCR approaches not only to amplify genomic regions containing unknown 5′-flanking sequences comprising partner genes in 5′-*partner gene–MLL*-3′ rearrangements *(7, 8)* but also to identify the fusion point in 5′-*MLL–partner gene*-3′ fusion transcripts *(2, 3, 10)*. The positions and orientations of the primers and, where applicable, phosphorylated oligonucleotide, bridging oligonucleotide or 5′-*MLL*-NNNNNN-3′ utilized in each specific method are summarized in **Fig. 4**. The original iterations incorporated conventional subcloning and, later, recombination PCR was utilized for recovery of the products. However, in more recent iterations we have used TOPO TA cloning (Invitrogen) as an expeditious means for recovery of the products coupled with PCR screening with the same primers used in the last reaction for identification of the subclones of interest *(8)*. The methods have proved practical when applied by others to characterize the partner genes in various *MLL* rearrangements *(19–23)* and they have been

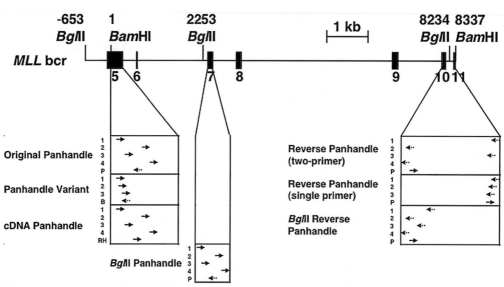

Fig. 4. Primer locations in panhandle PCR methods. *Line drawing* depicts the *MLL* bcr between *Bam*HI sites at positions 1 and 8,337. *Bgl*II restriction sites in the *MLL* bcr are also shown. Exons are shown as *black boxes*. *Black arrows* represent sense orientation, *dashed arrows* represent antisense orientation. *P* P-oligo; *B* bridging oligo; *RH* 5′-*MLL*-random hexamer-3′ primer. The exon numbering system is that originally proposed by Rasio et al. *(17)* In a later *MLL* exon numbering system, the same exons defined by the *Bam*HI genomic fragment are designated exons 8–14 *(18)*.

exploited further to characterize different leukemia-associated chromosomal translocations not involving *MLL (24)*.

It is recommended to perform genomic Southern blot analysis and select the most appropriate genomic panhandle PCR approach or approaches based on the number and size(s) of *MLL* bcr rearrangements. In some cases, the 3′-portion of the *MLL* bcr is deleted during the translocation and only the 5′-*MLL–partner gene*-3′ rearrangement is detectable on the Southern blot and by panhandle PCR. In addition, for every PCR performed during any step of a panhandle PCR method, a reagent control without any template should also be included.

3.1. Original Panhandle PCR and BglII Panhandle PCR

3.1.1. DNA Preparation (Digestion, Dephosphorylation, Extraction, and Ligation)

1. Approximately 5 µg of genomic DNA is digested to completion with 40 U of either *Bam*HI or *Bgl*II and 10 µl of REact 3 buffer (1× final concentration) for 2 h at 37°C. DEPC water is used to bring the total volume to 100 µl.

2. A portion of each digested sample (5 µl) is electrophoresed on a 0.8% agarose gel to check for complete digestion.

3. The digested DNA is dephosphorylated by adding 5 µl of CIAP (0.01 U/µl), gently mixed and collected by brief centrifugation. The dephosphorylation reactions are incubated at 37°C for 30 min.

4. The digested, dephosphorylated DNA is purified using a GeneClean III kit (*see* **Note 2**). The DNA is resuspended in 25 µl DEPC water. The DNA is stored at 4°C.

5. The P-oligo appropriate to the restriction enzyme used in **step 1** is ligated to the purified, digested, dephosphorylated DNA (25 µl) by adding 16.9 µl of DEPC water, 2.1 µl of P-oligo, 5 µl of (10×) T4 ligase buffer and 1 µl of T4 DNA ligase per reaction. The ligation reactions are gently mixed and collected by brief centrifugation and incubated overnight at 4°C.

6. The ligated DNA is purified using a GeneClean III kit (*see* **Note 2**). The DNA is resuspended in 25 µl DEPC water. The DNA is stored at 4°C.

3.1.2. Initial and Nested PCR Amplification

1. A PCR cocktail mixture is prepared for the initial PCR (0.5 µl of DNA polymerase mix, 0.7 µl of 25 mM dNTPs, 5 µl of (10×) Expand Long Buffer I and 36.8 µl of DEPC water per reaction). The PCR cocktail is mixed gently and 43.0 µl of PCR mix is aliquoted to each thin-walled PCR tube and briefly centrifuged. The tubes are preheated at 80°C for 5 min.

2. Two microliters of purified, ligated DNA is added to each tube and the panhandle is formed by incubating at 94°C for 1 min, followed by a 2 min ramp to 72°C and holding at 72°C for 30 s. The reaction is then maintained at 80°C while 2.5 µl of each of the appropriate primers 1 and 2 are added (*Bam*HI:

Primer #1 and Primer #2; OR for *Bgl*II panhandle PCR: *Bgl*II Primer #1 and *Bgl*II Primer #2).

3. Once the primers have been added to each initial PCR tube, an initial denaturation is performed at 94°C for 1 min, followed by 10 cycles at 94°C for 10 s and 68°C for 7 min, then an additional 20 cycles at 94°C for 10 s and 68°C for 7 min (increment, 20 s/cycle) and a final elongation at 68°C for 7 min. The reactions are maintained at 4°C before proceeding to the nested PCR.

4. A PCR cocktail mixture is prepared for the nested PCR (0.5 µl of DNA polymerase mix, 0.7 µl of 25 mM dNTPs, 5 µl of (10×) Expand Long Buffer I, 2.5 µl of Primer #3 (*Bam*HI or *Bgl*II), 2.5 µl of Primer #4 (*Bam*HI or *Bgl*II) and 37.8 µl of DEPC water per reaction). The PCR cocktail is mixed gently and 49.0 µl of PCR mix is aliquoted to each thin-walled PCR tube and briefly centrifuged. The tubes are preheated at 80°C for 5 min. One microliter of the initial PCR products is added to each respective tube to serve as a template DNA for the nested PCR.

5. Once the template DNA has been added, an initial denaturation is performed at 94°C for 1 min, followed by 10 cycles at 94°C for 10 s and 68°C for 7 min, then an additional 20 cycles at 94°C for 10 s and 68°C for 7 min (increment, 20 s/cycle) and a final elongation at 68°C for 7 min. The reactions are maintained at 4°C before proceeding to the analysis of the nested PCR products on an agarose gel.

6. Aliquots (5 µl) of each nested PCR are electrophoresed on a 0.8% agarose gel to determine the sizes of the products (*see* **Note 3**).

3.1.3. Transformation and PCR Screening of Colonies

1. The nested PCR products are purified using a GeneClean III kit (*see* **Note 2**). The DNA is resuspended in 10 µl of DEPC water. The purified DNA is stored at 4°C.

2. A 2.5-µl aliquot of the products of each nested PCR is combined with 1 µl of salt solution, 1.5 µl of DEPC water and 1 µl of TOPO TA cloning vector in a 1.5-ml centrifuge tube. The TOPO TA cloning reactions are incubated at room temperature for 15 min and then placed on ice to stop the reaction. The TOPO cloning reactions are stored at –20°C for future use (*see* **Note 4**).

3. The competent cells are thawed on ice and added (50 µl) to pre-chilled polypropylene tubes. A 2-µl aliquot of each TOPO TA cloning reaction is added to the competent cells and gently mixed. The cells are incubated on ice for 10–30 min before they are heat-shocked by incubating the chilled tubes in a 42°C water bath for 30 s. The tubes are placed on ice for 2 min before 300 µl of S.O.C. medium is added. The cells are shaken at 225 rpm at 37°C for 1 h to allow for recovery.

4. While the cells are recovering, LB agar plates are warmed at room temperature. The entire mixtures are plated onto LB agar plates and spread over the plates with sterilized glass rods. The plates are incubated upright at 37°C overnight. The plates are stored at 4°C once colonies have grown to a suitable size.

5. Colonies are picked using 10-μl pipet tips (*see* **Note 5**) and placed into 2 ml of LB broth (with carbenicillin). The cultures are shaken at 225 rpm and incubated at 37°C for 4–6 h. The cultures are stored at 4°C for future use.

6. A PCR cocktail mixture is prepared for PCR screening of the colonies (0.5 μl of DNA polymerase mix, 0.7 μl of 25 mM dNTPs, 5 μl of (10×) Expand Long Buffer I, 2.5 μl of Primer #3 (*Bam*HI or *Bgl*II), 2.5 μl of Primer #4 (*Bam*HI or *Bgl*II) and 36.8 μl of DEPC water per reaction). The PCR cocktail is mixed gently and 48.0 μl of PCR mix is aliquoted to each thin-walled PCR tube and briefly centrifuged. The tubes are preheated at 80°C for 5 min.

7. Two microliters of inoculated culture is added to each respective tube for individual colony screening using PCR.

8. Once each inoculated culture aliquot has been added to the tubes containing pre-heated PCR mixture, an initial denaturation is performed at 94°C for 1 min, with 10 cycles at 94°C for 10 s and 68°C for 7 min, then an additional 20 cycles at 94°C for 10 s and 68°C for 7 min (increment, 20 s/cycle) followed by a final elongation at 68°C for 7 min. The reactions are maintained at 4°C before proceeding to the analysis of the PCR screen reaction products on an agarose gel.

9. Aliquots (5 μl) of each PCR screen reaction are electrophoresed on a 0.8% agarose gel to determine the sizes of the products (*see* **Note 3**). Subclones of interest are selected and prepared for automated sequencing (*see* **Note 6**).

10. Sequences of the breakpoint junctions are validated experimentally (*see* **Note 7**).

3.2. Panhandle Variant PCR

3.2.1. DNA Preparation (Digestion and Ligation)

1. Approximately 2.4 μg of genomic DNA is digested to completion with 30 U of *Bam*HI and 4.8 μl of REact 3 buffer (1× final concentration) for 2 h at 37°C. DEPC water is used to bring the total volume to 48 μl.

2. A portion of each digested sample (5 μl) is electrophoresed on an 0.8% agarose gel to check for complete digestion.

3. With the aid of a bridging oligo, Primer #3 is ligated to an aliquot of the digested DNA (0.5 μg, 10 μl) by adding 7.3 μl of DEPC water, 1.6 μl of Primer #3, 1.7 μl of bridging oligo, 2.4 μl of (10×) T4 ligase buffer and 1 μl of T4 DNA ligase per reaction. The ligation reactions are gently mixed and collected by brief centrifugation. The ligation reactions are incubated overnight at 4°C.

4. The bridging oligo and excess Primer #3 are removed from the ligation reaction mixture by exonuclease digestion. One microliter of exonuclease I (20 U) is added to each reaction and incubated at 37°C for 30 min, followed by heat inactivation at 75°C for 15 min.

3.2.2. Initial and Nested PCR Amplification

1. A PCR cocktail mixture is prepared for the initial PCR (0.5 μl of DNA polymerase mix, 0.7 μl of 25 mM dNTPs, 5 μl of (10×) Expand Long Buffer I and 40.3 μl of DEPC water per reaction). The PCR cocktail is mixed gently and 46.5 μl of PCR mix is aliquoted to each thin-walled PCR tube and briefly centrifuged. The tubes are preheated at 80°C for 5 min.

2. While the reaction is maintained at 80°C, 1 μl of digested, ligated, exonuclease I-treated DNA and 2.5 μl of Primer #1 are added to each reaction tube.

3. Once the primer has been added, an initial denaturation is performed at 94°C for 1 min, followed by 10 cycles at 94°C for 10 s and 68°C for 7 min, then an additional 20 cycles at 94°C for 10 s and 68°C for 7 min (increment, 20 s/cycle) and is followed by a final elongation at 68°C for 7 min. The reactions are maintained at 4°C before proceeding to the first nested PCR.

4. A PCR cocktail mixture is prepared for the first nested PCR (0.5 μl of DNA polymerase mix, 0.7 μl of 25 mM dNTPs, 5 μl of (10×) Expand Long Buffer I, 2.5 μl of Primer #2 and 40.3 μl of DEPC water per reaction). The PCR cocktail is mixed gently and 49.0 μl of PCR mix is aliquoted to each thin-walled PCR tube and briefly centrifuged. The tubes are preheated at 80°C for 5 min. One microliter of the initial PCR products is added to each respective tube to serve as a template DNA for the first nested PCR.

5. Once the initial PCR template DNA has been added, an initial denaturation is performed at 94°C for 1 min, followed by 10 cycles at 94°C for 10 s and 68°C for 7 min, then an additional 20 cycles at 94°C for 10 s and 68°C for 7 min (increment, 20 s /cycle) and a final elongation at 68°C for 7 min. The reactions are maintained at 4°C before proceeding to the second nested PCR.

6. A PCR cocktail mixture is prepared for the second nested PCR (0.5 μl of DNA polymerase mix, 0.7 μl of 25 mM dNTPs, 5 μl of (10×) Expand Long Buffer I, 2.5 μl of Primer #3 and 40.3 μl of DEPC water per reaction). The PCR cocktail is mixed gently and 49.0 μl of PCR mix is aliquoted to each thin-walled PCR tube and briefly centrifuged. The tubes are preheated at 80°C for 5 min. One microliter of the first nested PCR products is added to each respective tube to serve as a template DNA for the second nested PCR.

7. Once the first nested PCR template DNA has been added, an initial denaturation is performed at 94°C for 1 min, followed by 10 cycles at 94°C for 10 s and 68°C for 7 min, then an additional 20 cycles at 94°C for 10 s and 68°C for 7 min (increment, 20 s/cycle) and a final elongation at 68°C for 7 min. The reactions are maintained at 4°C before proceeding to the analysis of the second nested PCR products on an agarose gel.

8. Aliquots (5 µl) of each second nested PCR are electrophoresed on a 0.8% agarose gel to determine the sizes of the products (*see* **Note 3**).

3.2.3. Transformation and PCR Screening of Colonies

1. To subclone the products of the second nested panhandle variant PCR, **Steps 1–5** should be performed exactly as per **Subheading 3.1.3**.

2. A PCR cocktail mixture is prepared for PCR screening of the colonies (0.5 µl of DNA polymerase mix, 0.7 µl of 25 mM dNTPs, 5 µl of (10×) Expand Long Buffer I, 2.5 µl of Primer #3, and 39.3 µl of DEPC water per reaction). The PCR cocktail is mixed gently and 48.0 µl of PCR mix is aliquoted to each thin-walled PCR tube and briefly centrifuged. The tubes are preheated at 80°C for 5 min.

3. The PCR screen of colonies for plasmids containing inserts of the desired size is performed exactly as per **Steps 7–10** in **Subheading 3.1.3**.

3.3. Reverse Panhandle PCR (Single Primer)

3.3.1. DNA Preparation (Digestion, Dephosphorylation, Extraction, and Ligation)

1. Approximately 2.5 µg of genomic DNA is digested to completion with 20 U of *Bam*HI and 10 µl of REact 3 buffer (1× final concentration) for 2 h at 37°C. DEPC water is used to bring the total volume to 100 µl.

2. A portion of each digested sample (5 µl) is electrophoresed on a 0.8% agarose gel to check for complete digestion.

3. The digested DNA is dephosphorylated by adding 5 µl of CIAP (0.01 U/µl), gently mixed and collected by brief centrifugation. The dephosphorylation reactions are incubated at 37°C for 30 min.

4. The digested, dephosphorylated DNA is purified using a GeneClean III kit (*see* **Note 2**). The DNA is resuspended in 25 µl DEPC water. The DNA is stored at 4°C.

5. The P-oligo is ligated to the purified, digested, dephosphorylated DNA (25 µl) by adding 16.9 µl of DEPC water, 2.1 µl of P-oligo, 5 µl of (10×) T4 ligase buffer and 1 µl of T4 DNA ligase per reaction. The ligation reactions are gently mixed and collected by brief centrifugation. The ligation reactions are incubated overnight at 4°C.

6. The ligated DNA is purified using a GeneClean III kit (*see* **Note 2**). The DNA is resuspended in 25 µl DEPC water and stored at 4°C.

1. A PCR cocktail mixture is prepared for the initial PCR (0.5 µl of DNA polymerase mix, 0.7 µl of 25 mM dNTPs, 5 µl of (10×) Expand Long Buffer I and 39.3 µl of DEPC water per reaction). The PCR cocktail is mixed gently and 45.5 µl of PCR mix is aliquoted to each thin-walled PCR tube and briefly centrifuged. The tubes are preheated at 80°C for 5 min.

2. Two microliters of purified, ligated DNA is added to each tube and the panhandle is formed by incubating at 94°C for 1 min, followed by a 2 min ramp to 72°C and holding at 72°C for 30 s. The reaction is then maintained at 80°C while 2.5 µl of Primer #1 is added.

3. Once the primer has been added to each tube, an initial denaturation is performed at 94°C for 1 min, followed by 10 cycles at 94°C for 10 s and 68°C for 7 min, then an additional 20 cycles at 94°C for 10 s and 68°C for 7 min (increment, 20 s/cycle) and a final elongation at 68°C for 7 min. The reactions are maintained at 4°C before proceeding to the first nested PCR.

4. A PCR cocktail mixture is prepared for the first nested PCR (0.5 µl of DNA polymerase mix, 0.7 µl of 25 mM dNTPs, 5 µl of (10×) Expand Long Buffer I, 2.5 µl of Primer #2 and 40.3 µl of DEPC water per reaction). The PCR cocktail is mixed gently and 49.0 µl of PCR mix is aliquoted to each thin-walled PCR tube and briefly centrifuged. The tubes are preheated at 80°C for 5 min. One microloiter of the initial PCR products is added to each respective tube to serve as template DNA for the first nested PCR.

5. Once the template DNA has been added to each respective tube, an initial denaturation is performed at 94°C for 1 min, followed by 10 cycles at 94°C for 10 s and 68°C for 7 min, then an additional 20 cycles at 94°C for 10 s and 68°C for 7 min (increment, 20 s/cycle) and a final elongation at 68°C for 7 min. The reactions are maintained at 4°C before proceeding to the second nested PCR.

6. A PCR cocktail mixture is prepared for the second nested PCR (0.5 µl of DNA polymerase mix, 0.7 µl of 25 mM dNTPs, 5 µl of (10×) Expand Long Buffer I, 2.5 µl of Primer #3 and 40.3 µl of DEPC water per reaction). The PCR cocktail is mixed gently and 49.0 µl of PCR mix is aliquoted to each thin-walled PCR tube and briefly centrifuged. The tubes are preheated at 80°C for 5 min. One microliter of the first nested PCR products is added to each respective tube to serve as template DNA for the second nested PCR.

7. Once the template DNA has been added to each respective tube, an initial denaturation is performed at 94°C for 1 min, followed by 10 cycles at 94°C for 10 s and 68°C for 7 min,

then an additional 20 cycles at 94°C for 10 s and 68°C for 7 min (increment, 20 s/cycle) and a final elongation at 68°C for 7 min. The reactions are maintained at 4°C before proceeding to analysis of the second nested PCR products on an agarose gel.

8. Aliquots (5 μl) of each second nested PCR are electrophoresed on a 0.8% agarose gel to determine the sizes of the products (*see* **Note 3**).

3.3.3. Transformation and PCR Screening of Colonies

1. To subclone the products of the second nested reverse panhandle PCR **Steps 1–5** should be performed exactly as per **Subheading 3.1.3**.

2. A PCR cocktail mixture is prepared for PCR screening of the colonies (0.5 μl of DNA polymerase mix, 0.7 μl of 25 mM dNTPs, 5 μl of (10×) Expand Long Buffer I, 2.5 μl of Primer #3, and 39.3 μl of DEPC water per reaction). The PCR cocktail is mixed gently and 48.0 μl of PCR mix is aliquoted to each thin-walled PCR tube and briefly centrifuged. The tubes are preheated at 80°C for 5 min.

3. The PCR screen of colonies for plasmids containing inserts of the desired size is performed exactly as per **Steps 7–10** in **Subheading 3.1.3**.

3.4. Reverse Panhandle PCR (Two Primer) and BglII Reverse Panhandle PCR

3.4.1. DNA Preparation (Digestion, Dephosphorylation, Extraction, and Ligation)

1. Approximately 5 μg of genomic DNA is digested to completion with 40 U of either *Bam*HI or *Bgl*II and 10 μl of REact 3 buffer (1× final concentration) for 2 h at 37°C. DEPC water is used to bring the total volume to 100 μl.

2. A portion of each digested sample (5 μl) is electrophoresed on an 0.8% agarose gel to check for complete digestion.

3. The digested DNA is dephosphorylated by adding 5 μl of CIAP (0.01 U/μl), gently mixed and collected by brief centrifugation. The dephosphorylation reactions are incubated at 37°C for 30 min.

4. The digested, dephosphorylated DNA is purified using a GeneClean III kit (*see* **Note 2**). The DNA is resuspended in 25 μl DEPC water and stored at 4°C.

5. The P-oligo is ligated to the purified, digested, dephosphorylated DNA (25 μl) by adding 16.9 μl of DEPC water, 2.1 μl of P-oligo, 5 μl of (10×) T4 ligase buffer and 1 μl of T4 DNA ligase per reaction. The ligation reactions are gently mixed and collected by brief centrifugation. The ligation reactions are incubated overnight at 4°C.

6. The ligated DNA is purified using a GeneClean III kit (*see* **Note 2**). The DNA is resuspended in 25 μl DEPC water and stored at 4°C.

<table>
<tr><td>

3.4.2. Initial and Nested PCR Amplification

</td><td>

1. A PCR cocktail mixture is prepared for the initial PCR (1.0 μl of Elongase enzyme mix, 1.0 μl of 10 mM dNTPs, 4 μl of (5×) Buffer A, 6 μl of (5×) Buffer B and 31.0 μl of DEPC water per reaction). The PCR cocktail is mixed gently and 43.0 μl of PCR mix is aliquoted to each thin-walled PCR tube and briefly centrifuged. The tubes are preheated at 80°C for 5 min.

</td></tr>
</table>

2. Two microliters of purified, ligated DNA is added to each respective tube and the panhandle is formed by incubating at 94°C for 1 min, followed by a 2 min ramp to 72°C and holding at 72°C for 30 s. The reaction is then maintained at 80°C while 2.5 μl of each primer is added to the appropriate reaction tube (*Bam*HI: Primer #1 and Primer #2; OR for *Bgl*II reverse panhandle PCR: *Bgl*II Primer #1 and Primer #2).

3. Once the primers have been added to each tube, an initial denaturation is performed at 94°C for 1 min, followed by 10 cycles at 94°C for 10 s and 68°C for 7 min, then an additional 20 cycles at 94°C for 10 s and 68°C for 7 min (increment, 20 s/cycle) and is followed by a final elongation at 68°C for 7 min. The reactions are maintained at 4°C before proceeding to the nested PCR.

4. A PCR mixture is prepared for the nested PCR (1.0 μl of Elongase enzyme mix, 1.0 μl of 10 mM dNTPs, 4 μl of Buffer A, 6 μl of Buffer B, 2.5 μl of Primer #3 (or *Bgl*II Primer #3), 2.5 μl of Primer #4 and 32.0 μl of DEPC water per reaction). The PCR cocktail is mixed gently and 49.0 μl of PCR mix is aliquoted to each thin-walled PCR tube and briefly centrifuged. The tubes are preheated at 80°C for 5 min. One microliter of the initial PCR products is added to each respective tube to serve as template DNA for the nested PCR.

5. Once the initial PCR template DNA has been added to each nested PCR tube, an initial denaturation is performed at 94°C for 1 min, followed by 10 cycles at 94°C for 10 s and 68°C for 7 min, then an additional 20 cycles at 94°C for 10 s and 68°C for 7 min (increment, 20 s/cycle) and a final elongation at 68°C for 7 min (*see* **Note 8**). The reactions are maintained at 4°C before proceeding to analysis of the nested PCR products on an agarose gel.

6. Aliquots (5 μl) of each nested PCR are electrophoresed on a 0.8% agarose gel to determine the sizes of PCR products (*see* **Note 3**).

<table>
<tr><td>

3.4.3. Transformation and PCR Screening of Colonies

</td><td>

1. To subclone the products of the nested reverse panhandle PCR **steps 1–5** should be performed exactly as per **Subheading 3.1.3**.

2. A PCR cocktail mixture is prepared for PCR screening of the colonies (1.0 μl of Elongase enzyme mix, 1.0 μl of 10 mM

</td></tr>
</table>

dNTPs, 4 μl of Buffer A, 6 μl of Buffer B, 2.5 μl of Primer #3 (or *Bgl*II Primer #3), 2.5 μl of Primer #4 and 31.0 μl of DEPC water per reaction). The PCR cocktail is mixed gently and 48.0 μl of PCR mix is aliquoted to each thin-walled PCR tube and briefly centrifuged. The tubes are preheated at 80°C for 5 min.

3. Two microliters of inoculated culture is added to each respective tube for individual colony screening using PCR.

4. Once each inoculated culture aliquot has been added to the tubes containing pre-heated PCR mixture, an initial denaturation is performed at 94°C for 1 min, with 10 cycles at 94°C for 10 s and 68°C for 7 min, then an additional 20 cycles at 94°C for 10 s and 68°C for 7 min (increment, 20 s/cycle) followed by a final elongation at 68°C for 7 min (*see* **Note 8**). The reactions are maintained at 4°C before proceeding to analysis of the PCR screen reaction products on an agarose gel.

5. Aliquots (5 μl) of each PCR screen reaction are electrophoresed on a 0.8% agarose gel to determine the sizes of the products (*see* **Note 3**). Subclones of interest are selected and prepared for automated sequencing (*see* **Note 6**).

6. Sequences of the breakpoint junctions are validated experimentally (*see* **Note 7**).

3.5. cDNA Panhandle PCR

3.5.1. Synthesis of First-Strand cDNA

1. Between 1 and 5 μg of total RNA (*see* **Note 9**) is placed in a thin-walled reaction tube and incubated with 1 μl of DNase I and (10×) DNase I reaction buffer for 15 min at room temperature. DEPC water is used to bring the total volume to 10 μl.

2. Following DNase I digestion of any possible contaminating DNA, 1 μl of 25 mM EDTA is added and the tubes are incubated at 70°C for 10 min to stop the reactions and then placed on ice.

3. Two microliters of 5'-*MLL*-random hexamer-3' primer is added to each tube containing the total RNA and the tubes are incubated at 70°C for 10 min and then placed on ice.

4. A reaction cocktail is prepared (4 μl of (5×) first strand buffer, 1 μl of 10 mM dNTPs and 2 μl of 0.1 M DTT per reaction) and then 7 μl of the cocktail is added to each tube containing the total RNA and 5'-*MLL*-random hexamer-3' primer. The reactions are mixed gently, collected by brief centrifugation and incubated at 25°C for 5 min.

5. One microliter of SuperScript II reverse transcriptase is added to each tube and mixed gently followed by brief centrifugation. The reaction is incubated at 25°C for 10 min, and then at 42°C for 50 min and 70°C for 15 min to generate the first-strand cDNA. The reaction is then placed on ice.

6. One microliter of RNase H is added to each tube, and the tubes are mixed gently followed by brief centrifugation to digest the RNA. The reaction is incubated at 37°C for 20 min. The first-strand cDNA is then stored at –20°C for future use.

3.5.2. Initial and Nested PCR Amplification

1. A PCR cocktail mixture is prepared for the initial PCR (0.5 μl of DNA polymerase mix, 0.7 μl of 25 mM dNTPs, 5 μl of (10×) Expand Long Buffer I, 2.5 μl of Primer #1 and 36.8 μl of DEPC water per reaction). The PCR cocktail is mixed gently and 45.5 μl of PCR mix is aliquoted to each thin-walled PCR tube and briefly centrifuged. The tubes are preheated at 80°C for 5 min.

2. Two microliters of cDNA is added to each respective tube, and primer 1 extension generates the second-strand cDNA after denaturation at 94°C for 1 min, followed by 94°C at 10 s and annealing/elongation at 68°C for 7 min. The reaction is then maintained at 80°C while 2.5 μl of Primer #2 is added.

3. Once Primer 2 has been added, an initial denaturation is performed at 94°C for 1 min, followed by 10 cycles at 94°C for 10 s and 68°C for 7 min, then an additional 20 cycles at 94°C for 10 s and 68°C for 7 min (increment, 20 s/cycle) and a final elongation at 68°C for 7 min. The reactions are maintained at 4°C before proceeding to the nested PCR.

4. A PCR cocktail mixture is prepared for the nested PCR (0.5 μl of DNA polymerase mix, 0.7 μl of 25 mM dNTPs, 5 μl of (10×) Expand Long Buffer I, 2.5 μl of Primer #3, 2.5 μl of Primer #4 and 37.8 μl of DEPC water per reaction). The PCR cocktail is mixed gently and 49.0 μl of PCR mix is aliquoted to each thin-walled PCR tube and briefly centrifuged. The tubes are preheated at 80°C for 5 min. One microliter of the initial PCR products is added to each respective tube to serve as a template DNA for the nested PCR.

5. Once the initial PCR template DNA has been added to each nested PCR tube, an initial denaturation is performed at 94°C for 1 min, followed by 10 cycles at 94°C for 10 s and 68°C for 7 min, then an additional 20 cycles at 94°C for 10 s and 68°C for 7 min (increment, 20 s/cycle) and a final elongation at 68°C for 7 min. The reactions are maintained at 4°C before proceeding to the analysis of the nested PCR products on an agarose gel.

6. Aliquots (5 μl) of each nested PCR are electrophoresed on a 2.0% agarose gel to determine the sizes of the products (*see* **Note 10**).

3.5.3. Transformation and PCR Screening of Colonies

1. The nested PCR products are purified using a GeneClean III kit (*see* **Note 2**). The DNA is resuspended in 10 µl of DEPC water. The purified DNA is stored at 4°C.

2. A 2.5-µl aliquot of the products of each nested PCR is combined with 1 µl of salt solution, 1.5 µl of DEPC water and 1 µl of TOPO TA cloning vector in a 1.5-ml centrifuge tube. The TOPO TA cloning reactions are incubated at room temperature for 5 min (*see* **Note 11**) and then placed on ice to stop reactions. The TOPO cloning reactions are stored at –20°C for future use (*see* **Note 4**).

3. The competent cells are thawed on ice and added (50 µl) to pre-chilled polypropylene tubes. A 2-µl aliquot of each TOPO TA cloning reaction is added to the competent cells and mixed gently. The cells are incubated on ice for 10–30 min before the cells are heat-shocked by incubating the chilled tubes in a 42°C water bath for 30 s. The tubes are placed on ice for 2 min before 300 µl of S.O.C. medium is added to the cells. The cells are shaken at 225 rpm and incubated at 37°C for 1 h to allow for recovery.

4. While the cells are recovering, LB agar plates are warmed at room temperature. The entire mixtures are plated onto LB agar plates and spread over the plates with sterilized glass rods. The plates are incubated upright at 37°C overnight. The plates are stored at 4°C once colonies have grown to a suitable size.

5. Colonies are picked using 10-µl pipet tips (*see* **Note 5**) and placed into 2 ml of LB broth (with carbenicillin). The cultures are shaken at 225 rpm and incubated at 37°C for 4–6 h. The cultures are stored at 4°C for future use.

6. A PCR cocktail mixture is prepared for PCR screening of the colonies (0.5 µl of DNA polymerase mix, 0.7 µl of 25 mM dNTPs, 5 µl of (10×) Expand Long Buffer I, 2.5 µl of Primer #3, 2.5 µl of Primer #4 and 36.8 µl of DEPC water per reaction). The PCR cocktail is mixed gently and 48.0 µl of PCR mix is aliquoted to each thin-walled PCR tube and briefly centrifuged. The tubes are preheated at 80°C for 5 min.

7. Two microliters of inoculated culture is added to each respective tube for individual colony screening using PCR.

8. Once each inoculated culture aliquot has been added to the tubes containing pre-heated PCR mixture, an initial denaturation is performed at 94°C for 1 min, with 10 cycles at 94°C for 10 s and 68°C for 7 min, then an additional 20 cycles at 94°C for 10 s and 68°C for 7 min (increment, 20 s/cycle) followed by a final elongation at 68°C for 7 min. The reactions are maintained at 4°C before proceeding to the analysis of the PCR screen reaction products on an agarose gel.

9. Aliquots (5 µl) of each PCR screen reaction are electrophoresed on a 2.0% agarose gel to determine the sizes of PCR products (*see* **Note 12**). Subclones of interest are selected and prepared for automated sequencing (*see* **Note 6**).

10. Sequences of the fusion transcripts are validated experimentally (*see* **Note 7**).

4. Notes

1. Dilute CIAP 1:100 with (1×) TE buffer to achieve a final concentration of 0.01 U/µl.

2. Follow GeneClean III kit protocol.

3. The PCR products are used for further steps if the sizes are consistent with the size of a rearrangement in the same DNA on Southern blot analysis with the same restriction enzyme.

4. Recombination PCR can be used as an alternative to TOPO TA cloning *(3, 6)*.

5. A quicker PCR screening alternative is to use a robotic colony picker and perform all subsequent steps in a 96-well plate format (colony picking, culture growth, PCR screen, miniprep, and sequencing) which may decrease time and cost.

6. Subclones can be sequenced in one of two ways: Purify PCR screen reaction products and directly sequence them with the same nested primer(s) used in the last PCR; or inoculate 4 ml of LB broth (with carbenicillin) with 50 µl of culture of interest, shake at 225 rpm overnight at 37°C, isolate plasmid DNA via miniprep of the culture, and sequence with common primers found in the TOPO TA cloning vector [M13 forward (–20) and M13 reverse (–48)].

7. Sequences are validated by either an independent panhandle PCR or PCR with gene-specific primers informed by the panhandle PCR.

8. For better nested *Bgl*II reverse panhandle PCR results, add an additional 55°C annealing step (30 s) between each denaturation and extension step for every cycle.

9. Use of more RNA to generate the cDNA will ensure a better contingency of products, thus making it easier to isolate the *MLL* fusion transcript sequences, but cDNA panhandle using nanogram quantities of starting RNA can still yield the fusion transcript sequence depending on the frequency of the transcript in question.

10. Nested cDNA panhandle PCR products appear as a smear of bands on the agarose gel ranging from ~200 to >1,000 bp in size due to the multiplicity of sites in the total RNA where the 5′-*MLL*-random hexamer-3′ primer anneals. In some cases several more discrete bands may appear on the gel in cases where the RNA is less abundant or the quality is poor, but *MLL* fusion transcript sequences can still be recovered.

11. cDNA panhandle PCR products tend to be <1,000 bp in size, such that less time is need for the TOPO TA cloning reaction to generate a sufficient number of colonies for PCR screening.

12. Typically, cDNA panhandle PCR products containing 5′-*MLL–partner gene*-3′ fusion transcript sequences are greater than 200 bp due to the position of the primers used in the PCR, but they may be ~400 to 600 bp in size depending on the point of fusion; however the reaction also generates larger products.

Acknowledgments

We wish to thank Maureen Megonigal, Diana Slater, Caroline Kim, Leslie Raffini, Luca Lo Nigro, Anna SechserPerl, Giuseppe Germano, the many other Felix lab members, and Douglas Jones and Eric Rappaport for their contributions to the methodologies of panhandle PCR. This work was supported by grants CA80175, CA77683 and CA85469 from the National Institutes of Health.

References

1. Megonigal MD, Rappaport EF, Jones DH, et al. (1997). Panhandle PCR strategy to amplify MLL genomic breakpoints in treatment-related leukemias. *Proc Natl Acad Sci U S A*;**94**:11583–8.

2. Megonigal MD, Rappaport EF, Wilson RB, et al. (2000). Panhandle PCR for cDNA: a rapid method for isolation of MLL fusion transcripts invol-ving unknown partner genes. *Proc Natl Acad Sci U S A*; **97**:9597–602.

3. Megonigal MD, Cheung NK, Rappaport EF, et al.(2000). Detection of leukemia-associated MLL-GAS7 translocation early during chemotherapy with DNA topoisomerase II inhibitors. *Proc Natl Acad Sci U S A*; **97**:2814–9.

4. Felix CA, Kim CS, Megonigal MD, et al. (1997). Panhandle polymerase chain reaction amplifies MLL genomic translocation breakpoint involving unknown partner gene. *Blood*; **90**:4679–86.

5. Felix CA, Jones DH. 1998 Panhandle PCR: a technical advance to amplify MLL genomic translocation breakpoints. *Leukemia*;**12**:976–81.

6. Megonigal MD, Rappaport EF, Jones DH, et al. (1998). t(11;22)(q23;q11.2) in acute myeloid leukemia of infant twins fuses MLL with hCDCrel, a cell division cycle gene in the genomic region of deletion in DiGeorge and velocardiofacial syndromes. *Proc Natl Acad Sci U S A*;**95**:6413–8.

7. Raffini LJ, Slater DJ, Rappaport EF, et al. (2002). Panhandle and reverse-panhandle PCR enable cloning of der(11) and der(other) genomic breakpoint junctions of MLL translocations and identify complex translocation of MLL, AF-4, and CDK6. *Proc Natl Acad Sci U S A*;**99**:4568–73.

8. Robinson BW, Slater DJ, Felix CA. (2006). *Bgl*II-based panhandle and reverse panhandle PCR approaches increase capability for cloning

der(II) and der(other) genomic breakpoint junctions of MLL translocations. *Genes Chromosomes Cancer*, **45**:740–53.

9. LoNigro L, Slater DJ, Mirabile E, Rappaport EF, Schiliro G, Felix CA. (2003). Reverse panhandle PCR identifies *RIBOSOMAL PROTEIN S3 (RPS3)* as a new partner gene of *MLL* in a three-way *MLL* rearrangement in infant acute monoblastic leukemia *Blood*; **102**:184–5b.

10. Pegram LD, Megonigal MD, Lange BJ, et al. (2000). t(3;11) translocation in treatment-related acute myeloid leukemia fuses MLL with the GMPS (GUANOSINE 5'-MONO-PHOSPHATE SYNTHETASE) gene. *Blood*; **96**:4360–2.

11. Reichel M, Gillert E, Angermuller S, et al. (2001). Biased distribution of chromosomal breakpoints involving the MLL gene in infants versus children and adults with t(4;11) ALL. *Oncogene*; **20**:2900–7.

12. Whitmarsh RJ, Saginario C, Zhuo Y, et al. (2003). Reciprocal DNA topoisomerase II cleavage events at 5'-TATTA-3' sequences in MLL and AF-9 create homologous single-stranded overhangs that anneal to form der(11) and der(9) genomic breakpoint junctions in treatment-related AML without further processing. *Oncogene*; **22**:8448–59.

13. Gu Y, Nakamura T, Alder H, et al. (1992). The t(4;11) chromosome translocation of human acute leukemias fuses the *ALL-1* gene, related to Drosophila *Trithorax*, to the *AF-4* gene. *Cell*; **71**:701–8.

14. Ayton PM, Cleary ML. MLL in normal and malignant hematopoiesis. In: Ravid K, Licht JD, eds. (2001). Transcription Factors: Normal and Malignant Development of Blood Cells. New York: Wiley-Liss.

15. Jones DH, Winistorfer SC. (1992). Sequence specific generation of a DNA panhandle permits PCR amplification of unknown flanking DNA. *Nucleic Acids Res*; **20**:595–600.

16. Jones DH, Winistorfer SC. (1997). Amplification of 4-9-kb human genomic DNA flanking a known site using a panhandle PCR variant. *Biotechniques*; **23**:132–8.

17. Rasio D, Schichman SA, Negrini M, Canaani E, Croce CM. (1996). Complete exon structure of the *ALL1* gene. *Cancer Res*; **56**:1766–9.

18. Nilson I, Lochner K, Siegler G, et al. (1996). Exon/intron structure of the human ALL-1 (MLL) gene involved in translocations to chromosomal region 11q23 and acute leukaemias. *Br J Haematol*; **93**:966–72.

19. Wechsler DS, Engstrom LD, Alexander BM, Motto DG, Roulston D. (2003). A novel chromosomal inversion at 11q23 in infant acute myeloid leukemia fuses MLL to CALM, a gene that encodes a clathrin assembly protein. *Genes Chromosomes Cancer*; **36**:26–36.

20. Fu JF, Hsu JJ, Tang TC, Shih LY. (2003). Identification of CBL, a proto-oncogene at 11q23.3, as a novel MLL fusion partner in a patient with de novo acute myeloid leukemia. *Genes Chromosomes Cancer*; **37**:214–9.

21. Imamura T, Morimoto A, Ikushima S, et al. (2002). A novel infant acute lymphoblastic leukemia cell line with MLL-AF5q31 fusion transcript. *Leukemia*; **16**:2302–8.

22. Suzukawa K, Shimizu S, Nemoto N, Takei N, Taki T, Nagasawa T. (2005). Identification of a chromosomal breakpoint and detection of a novel form of an MLL-AF17 fusion transcript in acute monocytic leukemia with t(11;17) (q23;q21). *Int J Hematol*; **82**:38–41.

23. Fu JF, Hsu HC, Shih LY. (2005). MLL is fused to EB1 (MAPRE1), which encodes a microtubule-associated protein, in a patient with acute lymphoblastic leukemia. *Genes Chromosomes Cancer*; **43**:206–10.

24. Taketani T, Taki T, Shibuya N, et al. (2002). The HOXD11 gene is fused to the NUP98 gene in acute myeloid leukemia with t(2;11) (q31;p15). *Cancer Res*; **62**:33–7.

Chapter 7

MRD Detection in Acute Lymphoblastic Leukemia Patients Using Ig/TCR Gene Rearrangements as Targets for Real-Time Quantitative PCR

Vincent H.J. van der Velden and Jacques J.M. van Dongen

Summary

Minimal residual disease (MRD) diagnostics has proven to be clinically relevant for evaluation of treatment effectiveness in patients with acute lymphoblastic leukemia (ALL). In most ALL treatment protocols, MRD diagnostics is performed by real-time quantitative PCR (RQ-PCR) analysis of the junctional regions of rearranged immunoglobulin (Ig) and T-cell receptor (TCR) genes.

MRD diagnostics via Ig/TCR genes is broadly applicable (>95% of ALL patients) and can reach a good sensitivity ($\leq 10^{-4}$). However, the technique is complex and requires extensive knowledge and experience, because the junctional regions of each leukemia have to be identified before the patient-specific RQ-PCR assays can be designed for MRD monitoring. This chapter provides all relevant background information and technical aspects for the complete laboratory process from detection of the clonal Ig/TCR gene rearrangements in ALL cells at diagnosis to the actual MRD measurements in clinical follow-up samples. This information aims at facilitating the PCR-based MRD diagnostics in ALL patients. However, it should be noted that MRD diagnostics for clinical treatment protocols has to be accompanied by regular international quality control rounds to ensure the reproducibility and reliability of the MRD results.

Key words: Minimal residual disease (MRD), Acute lymphoblastic leukemia (ALL), Immunoglobulin (Ig), T-cell receptor (TCR), Real-time quantitative PCR (RQ-PCR), Junctional region, IGH IGK, IGL, TCRB, TCRG, TCRD, Quantitative range, sensitivity

1. Introduction

Several studies have shown that detection of minimal residual disease (MRD) in childhood acute lymphoblastic leukemia (ALL) is clinically relevant, both in de novo ALL and relapsed ALL as well as in ALL patients undergoing stem cell transplan-

C.W.E. So (ed.), Leukemia, *Methods in Molecular Biology, vol. 538*
© Humana Press, a part of Springer Science + Business Media, LLC 2009
DOI: 10.1007/978-1-59745-418-6_7

tation *(1–5)*. Based on these results, MRD diagnostics is now implemented in many front-line ALL treatment protocols, in which patients are stratified according to MRD levels in bone marrow (BM) samples obtained during and after induc-

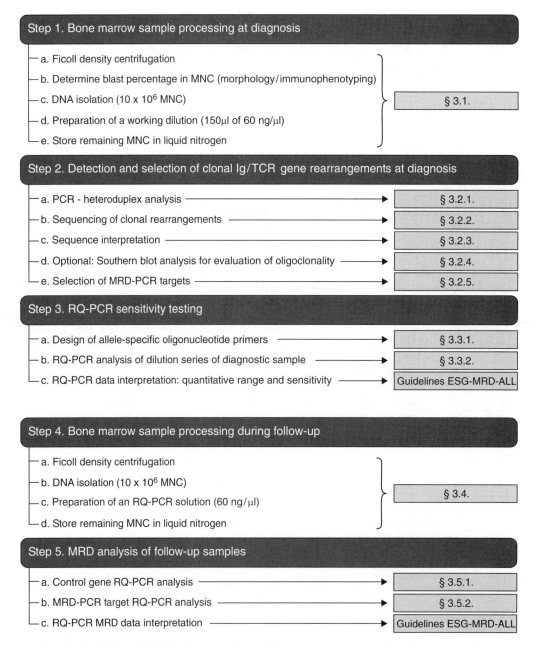

Fig. 1. Steps in RQ-PCR based MRD detection employing Ig/TCR gene rearrangements. Steps 1–3 represent the processing of the diagnostic cell sample, the MRD-PCR target identification and selection, and the RQ-PCR design. Steps 4 and 5 represent the processing of the follow-up samples and the actual MRD measurements.

tion therapy *(6)*. In most of these MRD-based stratification studies, MRD diagnostics is performed by RQ-PCR analysis of immunoglobulin (Ig) and T-cell receptor (TCR) gene rearrangements *(7–9)*.

During early B- and T-cell differentiation the germline V, (D,) and J gene segments of the Ig and TCR gene complexes rearrange, and each lymphocyte thereby obtains a specific combination of V-(D-)J segments that codes for the variable domains of Ig or TCR molecules. The random insertion and deletion of nucleotides at the junction sites of V, (D,) and J gene segments make the junctional regions of Ig and TCR genes into "fingerprint-like" sequences, which are most probably different in each lymphocyte and thus also in each lymphoid malignancy. Therefore, junctional regions can be used as tumor-specific targets for MRD-PCR analysis. Such targets can be identified (e.g., by PCR heteroduplex analysis or GeneScan analysis) at initial diagnosis in >98% of lymphoid malignancies *(8)*. Subsequently, the precise nucleotide sequence of the junctional regions can be determined. This sequence information allows the design of junctional region-specific oligonucleotides (either probes or primers), which can be used for sensitive detection of low frequencies of malignant cells, down to one malignant cell in 10^4–10^5 normal cells (10^{-4}–10^{-5}).

In this chapter, we have described all the relevant background information and technical aspects needed for RQ-PCR-based MRD detection using Ig/TCR gene rearrangements as MRD-PCR targets in ALL patients (**Fig. 1**). The approach described here detects virtually all "classical" Ig/TCR gene rearrangements and identifies MRD-PCR targets in >95% of ALL patients. Consequently, the vast majority of ALL patients can be monitored for treatment effectiveness.

2. Materials

2.1. Bone Marrow Sample Processing at Diagnosis

1. Ficoll Hypaque™ Plus (GE Healthcare BioSciences AB, Uppsala, Sweden). Store in the dark at room temperature.
2. Cell storage medium: 10% Dimethyl sulfoxide (DMSO), 40% fetal calf serum (FCS), 50% RPMI-1640 medium.

2.2. PCR Detection of Clonal Ig/TCR Targets at Diagnosis

2.2.1. PCR-Heteroduplex Analysis

1. 1× TBE buffer: 90 mM Tris–HCl 90 mM H_3BO_3, 2.5 mM EDTA, in Milli-Q water.
2. Bromophenol Blue (BPB) loading buffer: 30% (v/v) glycerol, 0.25% (w/v) bromophenol blue (electrophoresis purity rea-

gent), 0.25% (w/v) xylene cyanole FF (electrophoresis purity reagent), in Milli-Q water.

3. Ethidium bromide 1%.

4. MgCl$_2$ (25 mM).

5. Deoxynucleotide (dNTP) mix (20 mM each).

6. Bovine serum albumin (BSA, 20 mg/ml): 20% (w/v) BSA (Fraction V) in Milli-Q water.

7. Orange G: 20% Ficoll, 10 mM Tris–HCl, pH 7.6, 1 mg/ml Orange G, in Milli-Q water.

8. DNA ladders.

9. TaqGOLD (5 U/µl) (Applied Biosystems, Foster City, CA).

10. PE buffer II (10×) (Applied Biosystems).

11. Agarose gel (1%).

12. Criterion Precast gels, 5% (BioRad, Veenendaal, The Netherlands).

13. Forward and reverse primers for the various Ig/TCR gene rearrangements.

14. Electrophoresis cells.

15. DNA isolated from peripheral blood (PB) mononuclear cells (MNCs) obtained from five to ten healthy individuals (10 ng/µl).

16. DNA from cell lines or patients known to be positive for certain Ig/TCR gene rearrangements (10 ng/µl).

2.2.2. Sequencing of Clonal Rearrangements

1. 96% Ethanol.

2. 2 M NaAc (pH 5.6).

3. 70% Ethanol.

4. Sephadex G-50, 6% (w/v) fine DNA grade in Milli-Q water.

5. 10× Buffer with EDTA (Applied Biosystems).

6. Elution buffer: 0.5 M Ammoniumacetate, 10 mM magnesiumacetate, 1 mM EDTA, 0.1% SDS, in Milli-Q water.

7. Big Dye® Terminator cycle sequencing ready reaction kit version 3.1 (Applied Biosystems). Store stock at −15 to −25°C; store working dilution at 4°C and protect it from light.

8. Forward and reverse primers for the various Ig/TCR gene rearrangements.

9. ABI Prism® 3100 Genetic Analyzer with POP-4™ or POP-6™ polymer (Applied Biosystems).

**2.3. RQ-PCR
Sensitivity Testing**

1. 1× TE buffer: 10 mM Tris–HCl pH 7.6, 1 mM EDTA, in Milli-Q water.
2. Spectrophotometer (Nanodrop, Wilmington).

*2.3.1. Design of
Allele-Specific
Oligonucleotide Primers*

1. BSA (0.2%, w/v) (RIA grade).

*2.3.2. RQ-PCR Analysis
of Dilutions of Diagnostic
Sample*

2. Universal Master mix (2×) (Applied Biosystems).
3. Forward primer (30 pmole/µl).
4. Reverse primer (30 pmole/µl).
5. TaqMan probe (5 pmole/µl).
6. DNA isolated from PB MNCs obtained from five to ten healthy individuals (60 ng/µl).

**2.4. Bone Marrow
Sample Processing
During Follow-Up**

See **Subheading 2.1** for materials needed.

**2.5. MRD Analysis of
Follow-Up Samples**

See **subheading 2.3.2** for materials needed.

3. Methods

**3.1. Bone Marrow
Sample Processing
at Diagnosis**

1. Perform Ficoll density centrifugation of the bone marrow (BM) sample obtained at diagnosis to isolate MNCs.
2. Assess the percentage of ALL blast cells in the MNCs fraction by cytomorphology or, preferably, by flow cytometric immunophenotyping *(10, 11)*, because this information is needed for correction of the tumor load in the standard curve (*see* **Subheading 3.3**) (*see* **Note 1**).
3. For reasons of standardization and prediction of DNA recovery, use a fixed number of 10×10^6 MNCs for DNA extraction using column-based DNA extraction procedures (*see* **Notes 2** and **3**).
4. Determine the concentration of the DNA stock solution by analyzing the optical density at 260 and 280 nm in duplicate on the Nanodrop (*see* **Note 4**).
5. Prepare 150 µl of a DNA working solution of 60 ng/µl in sterile Milli-Q water; this working dilution will be used for the PCR analyses and RQ-PCR analyses (*see* below).

6. Check the DNA concentration by analyzing the optical density at 260 and 280 nm in duplicate on the Nanodrop. The acceptable range is 55–65 ng/μl.

7. Store the stock solution and working dilution at 4°C (or –20°C) for short periods of time (<3 months), or at –80°C for long-term storage.

8. Store remaining MNCs at diagnosis in cell-storage medium for later studies; store in liquid nitrogen.

3.2. Detection and Selection of Clonal Ig/TCR Gene Rearrangements at Diagnosis

3.2.1. PCR-Heteroduplex Analysis

By applying PCR-heteroduplex analysis (see **Fig. 2a**) *(12)* with appropriate primer-sets, Ig/TCR gene rearrangements can be detected in virtually all precursor-B-ALL and T-ALL patients. In **Table 1**, the frequency of the various types of Ig/TCR gene rearrangements in childhood ALL are indicated *(13–29)*. The number and type of Ig/TCR rearrangements is however dependent on the age of the patient and the presence of fusion gene transcripts, such as *TEL-AML1* and *MLL-AF4 (21–25, 27)*. Based on the frequencies of the various gene rearrangements, we developed an approach in which the most common Ig/TCR gene rearrangements are being identified first. This will result in the identification of at least two Ig/TCR gene rearrangements in >95% of ALL patients. For those few patients in whom less than two Ig/TCR gene rearrangements have been identified, a second set of primers can be applied, focusing on additional rearrangements.

1. Prepare a 10 ng/μl dilution of the diagnostic DNA sample by mixing 50 μl of the working dilution (60 ng/μl) with 250 μl of Milli-Q water.

2. For precursor-B-ALL patients, perform 30 PCR reactions (see **Table 2**). For T-ALL, perform 22 PCR reactions (see **Table 3**). The reaction mixes for these tubes are shown in **Table 4**. Use Milli-Q water as a negative control, normal MNCs DNA as a polyclonal control, and an appropriate positive control (see **Table 2** (precursor-B-ALL) and **Table 3** (T-ALL)).

3. PCR conditions are: 95°C, 7 min; 35 cycles of 94°C, 30 s; 60°C, 45 s; 72°C, 90 s; 72°C, 10 min; hold 15°C.

4. Prepare a 1% agarose gel.

5. For each of the positive and negative controls, mix 10 μl of the control with 10 μl of Orange G and load these samples on the agarose gel; run for 1 h at 150 V. The positive controls should give a clear band of the expected size, whereas the negative controls should be negative. If this is not the case, repeat the PCR assays with insufficient results.

6. Heat the PCR products of the patient samples and controls tested for 5 min at 94°C in a PCR machine.

7. Cool the PCR products for 60 min at 4°C in a PCR machine.

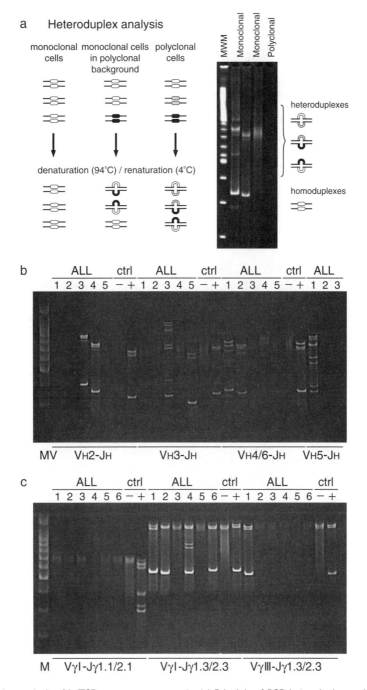

Fig. 2. Heteroduplex analysis of Ig/TCR gene rearrangements. (**a**) Principle of PCR-heteroduplex analysis. Examples of PCR-heteroduplex analysis are presented for several *IGH* (VH-JH) rearrangements and (**b**) *TCRG* gene rearrangements (**c**) ALL patients were evaluated for the presence of *IGH* or *TCRG* rearrangements by PCR analysis followed by heteroduplex analysis. Mononuclear cells from healthy donors were used as negative control (ctrl–), whereas cell lines were used as positive controls (ctrl +). Clonal *IGH* rearrangements can be seen in ALL patient 3, 4 (VH2-JH), 5 (VH3-JH), 1 and 2 (VH4/6-JH) (only homoduplexes visible). In ALL patient 3 (VH3-JH), bi-allelic rearrangements can be seen (both homoduplexes and heteroduplexes present). In ALL patient 1 (VH5-JH) an oligoclonal pattern can be seen, with several heteroduplexes (some with weaker intensity) present. Clonal *TCRG* gene rearrangements can be seen for Vγl-Jγ1.3/2.3 in ALL patient 1, 2, and 6 and for VγlII-Jγ1.3/2.3 in ALL patient 1. A bi-allelic Vγl-Jγ1.3/2.3 rearrangement can be detected in ALL patient 4. Note that in the latter patient the two homoduplexes appear as a single band on the gel.

Table 1
Frequency of Ig/TCR gene rearrangements in childhood ALL

Gene	Type of rearrangement	Precursor-B-ALL (%)	T-ALL (%)
IGH	V_H-J_H	80–85	~5
	D_H-J_H	~20	~20
	Total *IGH*	>95	20–25
IGK	Vκ-Kde	45	0
	Intron-Kde	15–25	0
	Vκ-Jκ	30	NT
	Total *IGK*-Kde	60–75	0
IGL	Vλ-Jλ	15–20	NT
TCRB	Vβ-Jβ	25–30	80
	Dβ-Jβ	15	55
	Total *TCRB*	35	90
TCRG	Vγ-Jγ	50–60	95
TCRD	Vδ2-Dδ3 or Dδ2-Dδ3	40	5–10
	Vδ-Jδ1 or Dδ2-Jδ1	<1	50
	Total *TCRD*	40	55
TCRD/A	Vδ2-Jα	40–45	NT

8. Use Criterion Precast gels (*see* **Note 5**); remove the white strip at the bottom of the cassette and place the Criterion Precast gel in the electrophoresis cell.

9. Fill the buffer chamber of the gel cassette with 60 ml TBE buffer (1×) and fill both sides of the electrophoresis cell with 1× TBE buffer till the indicated bar (~800 ml).

10. Remove the comb.

11. Mix 10 µl denaturated and renatured PCR product with 2 µl BFB loading buffer in a 96-well plate.

12. Pipet the mixture immediately in one of the gel slots.

13. Load the DNA ladder on the gel.

14. Cover the electrophoresis cell, place the electrodes, and run the gel for 60 min at 150 V (the exact time depends on the size of the PCR products that are loaded on the gel).

15. After turning of the power, remove the cover and carefully take out the gel cassette.

Table 2
Primer combinations for detection of Ig and TCR gene rearrangements in precursor-B-ALL

Tube	Forward primer	Reverse primer	Positive control	Product size (bp)	Protocol[a]	Reference
1	VγI	Jγ1.1/2.1	Molt-3/ Molt-4	329	A	(30)
2	VγI	Jγ1.3/2.3	ALL-1	533	A	(30)
3	VγII	Jγ1.1/2.1	Patient	318	A	(30)
4	VγII	Jγ1.3/2.3	HSB2	522	A	(30)
5	VγIV	Jγ1.1/2.1	Patient	353	A	(30)
6	VγIV	Jγ1.3/2.3	Jurkat	557	A	(30)
7	Vδ2	Dδ3	REH	501	A	(30)
8	Dδ2	Dδ3	Nalm16	608	A	(30)
9	VκI	Kde	ROS15	433	A	(30)
10	VκII	Kde	380	443	A	(30)
11	VκIII	Kde	REH	429	A	(30)
12	VκIV	Kde	ROS5	445	A	(30)
13	Intron-F1-B1	Kde	Nalm1	511	A	(30)
14	VH1/7	JH	Nalm6	300–400	A	(31)
15	VH2	JH	Patient	300–400	A	(31)
16	VH3	JH	REH	300–400	A	(31)
17	VH4/6	JH	ROS16	300–400	A	(31)
18	VH5	JH	VH5-TL	300–400	A	(31)
19	23xVβ: 2, 4, 5, 6a, 6b, 6c, 7a, 8a, 9, 10, 11, 13a, 13b, 14, 16, 17, 18, 19, 20, 21, 22, 23, 24	Jβ: 1.1, 1.2, 1.3, 1.4, 1.5, 1.6, 2.2, 2.6, 2.7	Jurkat/ ALL-1	240–280	B	(32)
20	23xVβ: 2, 4, 5, 6a, 6b, 6c, 7a, 8a, 9, 10, 11, 13a, 13b, 14, 16, 17, 18, 19, 20, 21, 22, 23, 24	Jβ: 2.1, 2.3, 2.4, 2.5	Peer/ CMLT1	240–280	C	(32)
21	Dβ1 + Dβ2	Jβ: 1.1, 1.2, 1.3, 1.4, 1.5, 1.6, 2.1, 2.2, 2.3, 2.4, 2.5, 2.6, 2.7	Jurkat	170–200 (Dβ2) 290–310 (Dβ1)	D	(32)

(continued)

Table 2
(continued)

Tube	Forward primer	Reverse primer	Positive control	Product size (bp)	Protocol[a]	Reference
22	Vδ2	Jα29	Patient	200–350	E	*(13)*
23	Vδ2	Jα9, 30, 48, 49, 52, 54, 55, 56, 57, 58, 59, 61	Patient	200–350	F	*(13)*
24	DH1	JH	Patient	130	A	*(16)*
25	DH2	JH	Patient	240	A	*(16)*
26	DH3	JH	Patient	160	A	*(16)*
27	DH4	JH	Patient	180	A	*(16)*
28	DH5	JH	Patient	300	A	*(16)*
29	DH6	JH	Patient	200	A	*(16)*
30	DH7	JH	Patient	230	A	*(16)*

[a]*See* **Table 4** for detailed information about PCR mixture per protocol

Table 3
PCR primer combinations for detection of TCR and D_H-J_H rearrangements in T-ALL

Tube	Forward primer	Reverse primer	Positive control	Product size (bp)	Protocol[a]	Reference
1	VγI	Jγ1.1/2.1	Molt-3/Molt-4	329	A	*(30)*
2	VγI	Jγ1.3/2.3	ALL-1	533	A	*(30)*
3	VγII	Jγ1.3/2.3	HSB2	522	A	*(30)*
4	VγIII	Jγ1.3/2.3	ALL-1	522	A	*(30)*
5	VγIV	Jγ1.3/2.3	Jurkat	557	A	*(30)*
6	Vδ1	Jδ1	Peer	452	A	*(30)*
7	Vδ2	Dδ3	REH	501	A	*(30)*
8	Vδ2	Jδ1	Patient	443	A	*(30)*
9	Vδ3	Jδ1	Patient	440	A	*(30)*
10	Dδ2	Dδ3	Nalm 16	608	A	*(30)*

(continued)

Table 3
(continued)

Tube	Forward primer	Reverse primer	Positive control	Product size (bp)	Protocol[a]	Reference
11	Dδ2	Jδ1	Loucy	550	A	*(30)*
12	Sil	Tal1db1	ALL-1	300	A	*(30)*
13	23xVβ: 2, 4, 5, 6a, 6b, 6c, 7a, 8a, 9, 10, 11, 13a, 13b, 14, 16, 17, 18, 19, 20, 21, 22, 23, 24	Jβ: 1.1, 1.2, 1.3, 1.4, 1.5, 1.6, 2.2, 2.6, 2.7	Jurkat/ ALL1	240–280	B	*(32)*
14	23xVβ2: 2, 4, 5, 6a, 6b, 6c, 7a, 8a, 9, 10, 11, 13a, 13b, 14, 16, 17, 18, 19, 20, 21, 22, 23, 24	Jβ: 2.1, 2.3, 2.4, 2.5	Peer/ CMLT1	240–280	C	*(32)*
15	Dβ1 + Dβ2	Jβ: 1.1, 1.2, 1.3, 1.4, 1.5, 1.6, 2.1, 2.2, 2.3, 2.4, 2.5, 2.6, 2.7	Jurkat	170–200 (Dβ2) 290–310 (Dβ1)	D	*(32)*
16	DH1	JH	Patient	130	A	*(16)*
17	DH2	JH	Patient	240	A	*(16)*
18	DH3	JH	Patient	160	A	*(16)*
19	DH4	JH	Patient	180	A	*(16)*
20	DH5	JH	Patient	300	A	*(16)*
21	DH6	JH	Patient	200	A	*(16)*
22	DH7	JH	Patient	230	A	*(16)*

[a] *See* **Table 4** for detailed information about PCR mixture per protocol

16. Open the gel cassette and rinse the gel of the cassette using 100 ml Milli-Q water.
17. Incubate the gel for 2–5 min in 100 ml Milli-Q water with 10 µl EtBr on a rocker platform.
18. Wash the gel for 2–5 min in 100 ml Milli-Q water on a rocker platform.
19. Analyse the gel using UV light, make a photograph of the gel.

Table 4
Composition of PCR mixture per protocol

Reaction mix per 50 µl reaction	Protocol							
	A	B	C	D	E	F	G	H
PE buffer II (10×)	5	5	5	5	5	5	5	5
MgCl2 (25 mM)	3	6	6	3	4	4	4	3
Milli-Q water	34	16.1	18.6	27.8	33.4	27.7	28.7/29.2/29.7	31.1/33.8
dNTP (20 mM)	0.5	0.5	0.5	0.5	0.5	0.5	0.5	0.5
BSA (20 mg/ml)	1	1	1	1	1	1	1	1
Forward primer (10 pmole/µl)	0.7							
Reverse primer (10 pmole/µl)	0.7							
Primer mix $TCRB$ tube 1 (23 × Vβ + 9× Jβ) (20 pmole/µl, 0.5 µl each)		16						
Primer mix $TCRB$ tube 2 (23× Vβ + 4x Jβ) (20 pmole/µl, 0.5 µl each)			13.5					
Primer mix $TCRB$ tube 3 (2× Dβ + 13× Jβ) (20 pmole/µl, 0.5 µl each)				7.5				
Forward primer (20 pmole/µl)					0.5			
Reverse primer (20 pmole/µl)					0.5			
Forward primer (20 pmole/µl)						0.5		
Reverse primers (20 pmole/µl, 0.5 µl each)						6		
Forward primer (20 pmole/µl)							0.5	
Reverse primer (20 pmole/µl; 0.5 µl each)							4/4.5/5	
Primer mix (20 pmole/µl; 0.5 µl each)								4 (Vκ-Jκ) 1.5 (Vλ-Jλ)
TaqGOLD (5 U/µl)	0.1	0.4	0.4	0.2	0.1	0.3	0.3	0.2
DNA (10 ng/µl)	5	5	5	5	5	5	5	5

Table 5
Additional (second phase) PCR reactions for precursor-B-ALL

Forward primer	Reverse primer	Positive control	Product size (bp)	Protocol[a]	References
Vδ2	Jα1,6,7,22,26,40,54,57	Patient	200–400	G	(13)
Vδ2	Jα2,3,5,8,11,12,13,19	Patient	200–400	G	(13)
Vδ2	Jα4,10,14,20,23, 29,42,48	Patient	200–400	G	(13)
Vδ2	Jα9,16,35,37,38,41,49,51,56,60	Patient	250–400	G	(13)
Vδ2	Jα15,18,28,34,36,43,44,45,46	Patient	200–400	G	(13)
Vδ2	Jα17,21,24,25,27,31,32,33,39	Patient	200–400	G	(13)
Vδ2	Jα30,47,50,52,53,55,58,59,61	Patient	200–400	G	(13)
Vκ1/6,2,3,4,5,7	Jκ1-4,5	ROS 15	200–650	H	(32)
Vλ1/2,3	Jλ1,2,3	ROS 5	140–165	H	(32)

[a]*See* **Table 4** for detailed information about PCR mixture per protocol

20. Interpret the gel (*see* **Fig. 2**). One band of expected size indicates one clonal rearrangement; two homoduplex bands plus two heteroduplex bands indicate two clonal rearrangements (bi-allelic or bi-clonal); >4 bands ("ladder pattern") indicate oligoclonal rearrangements; a smear indicates polyclonal rearrangements. Weak or very weak bands may indicate subclonal rearrangements.

21. If no (sufficient) MRD-PCR targets can be identified, perform the PCR reactions as indicated in **Table 5** according to the conditions indicated in **Table 4**. Continue from **step 4** onwards.**Table 4** Composition of PCR mixture per protocol

3.2.2. Sequencing of Clonal Rearrangements

After having identified clonal Ig/TCR gene rearrangements in the DNA sample of the patient at diagnosis, the precise sequences of these rearrangements have to be determined. By comparing the obtained sequences with the sequences of the germline gene segments, the exact composition of the patient-specific junctional regions can be obtained.

1. Select the source of material that should be used for the sequencing reaction; this depends on the PCR-heteroduplex analysis data:

    (a) Monoallelic rearrangements detected in single PCR reactions (thus not multiplex) can generally directly be sequenced from the PCR product. Use 1 µl of PCR product for the sequencing reaction.

    (b) In case of bi-allelic rearrangements, the relevant homoduplex bands need to be isolated. If the two homoduplexes are not well-separated, the relevant heteroduplex bands should be isolated. For isolation of the relevant bands, the heteroduplex analysis (*see* **Subheading 3.2.1**) is repeated with three lanes of 10 µl each. The bands of interest are cut from the gel (on an UV lamp), and each put in a microcentrifuge tube. 100 µl elution buffer is added to each tube and the tubes are incubated overnight at 37°C. The eluate is subsequently transferred to a new tube and 10 µl NaAc and 200 µl ice-cold 96% EtOH are added. After overnight incubation at –20°C (or 2× 45 min on dry ice), the tube is centrifuged for 20 min at 10,000 rpm. The pellet is washed with 200 µl of 70% EtOH, followed by centrifugation for 20 min at 10,000 rpm. After removal of the supernatant, the pellet is air-dried and dissolved in 10 µl Milli-Q water. Generally, 2 µl of PCR product can be used for the sequencing reaction. If the recovery of the excised DNA is low, a higher volume may however be necessary.

    (c) For multiplex reactions, isolation of the relevant PCR band is generally required. This can be done as described for bi-allelic rearrangements (*see* **step b**)

    (d) Exceptionally, if the above approaches are not successful, one might decide to clone the obtained PCR products, followed by sequencing of 10–15 clones.

2. Perform sequencing using the BigDye® Terminator (BDT) v3.1 Cycle Sequencing Kit (Applied Biosystems) in a total reaction volume of 20 µl. The reaction contains template DNA (PCR product; *see* **step 4**), 1 µl of BDT, 3.5 µl of sequencing buffer, 1.3 µl of primer (2.5 pmole/µl), and Milli-Q water (*see* **Note 6**). In case of multiplex sequencing reactions, use 0.5 µl of each primer (2 pmole/µl).

3. Use the same primers as used for the PCR reactions (**Tables 2** and **3**). In case of multiple primers in the first PCR reaction, use all forward or reverse primers for sequencing.

4. The amount of template DNA should be: singleplex PCR, strong band: 1 µl; weak band: 2 µl; very weak band: 3 µl; eluted homo- or heteroduplex band, strong: 2 µl; weak: 3 µl; very weak: 4 µl.

5. The PCR conditions are: 96°C, 1 min; 25 cycles of 96°C 10 s, 50°C 5 s, 60°C 3 min.

6. After the sequencing reaction, purify the samples, e.g., using Sephadex G-50 Superfine (*see* instructions of manufacturer).

7. Load and run the purified samples on the sequencing instrument, e.g., an ABI3100 (Applied Biosystems).

8. To obtain a reliable junctional region sequence, sequence the clonal PCR product always from both directions (i.e., using both a forward as well as a reverse primer). In case of doubt, a second (independent) clonal PCR product should be sequenced (*see* **Note 7**).

9. Analyze the sequence data using Sequence Navigator or comparable software programs.

3.2.3. Sequence Interpretation

The junctional regions of rearranged Ig/TCR genes can be considered as "DNA fingerprints" of the leukemic cells, which are used as MRD-PCR targets for sensitive detection of low frequencies of leukemic cells. Therefore, it is crucial to correctly assess the precise composition of the junctional region. To this end, the obtained sequence should be aligned with the germline V, D, and/or J gene segments, so that the exact number of deleted and inserted nucleotides can be determined. Alignment can be done using several databases freely available on the internet or using hard copies. Since some variations can be seen between different databases, it is advised to check the alignment of the sequence in at least two ways.

1. Identify sequences using DNAPLOT software by searching for homology with all known human germline sequences obtained from the VBASE directory of human Ig genes (http://www.mrc-cpe.cam.ac.uk/DNAPLOT.php?menu=901) and IMGT (http://imgt.cines.fr/imgt-vquest/share/textes/) for human Ig and TCR genes. Sequences can be confirmed by using BLAST sequence similarity searching tool (National Center for Biotechnology Information: http://www.ncbi.nlm.nih.gov/BLAST/ orhttp://www.ncbi.nlm.nih.gov/igblast/) (*see* **Note 8**).

2. First, try to assign the appropriate V, D, and/or J gene segment to the sequence. For recognition of D segments, a minimum length of 1/3 of the complete germline segment is required, with a minimum length of 5 bp (except for Dδ2: four nucleotides).

3. For *TCRB* gene rearrangements:

   (a) Use IMGT for recognition of Vβ gene segment usage and Jβ gene segment usage; use the IMGT nomenclature (corresponding to the Rowen nomenclature, although BIOMED primers are termed according to the Arden nomenclature).

   (b) Analysis of deletions/insertions is performed using the complete germline *TCRB* sequence published by Rowen (U66059, U66060, U66061).

4. After having identified the appropriate V, D, and/or J gene segments, determine the number of deletions at both sides of all joining sites, i.e., the number of nucleotides present in the germline V, D, and/or J gene segments that are lost in the patient's sequence. The remaining parts of the germline V, D, and/or J gene segments should give a 100% alignment with the patient's sequence. Lack of complete alignment may be due to somatic hypermutations (generally not present in ALL, potentially except for *BCR-ABL* positive patients *(33)*) or due to polymorphisms. Since such variations may impact RQ-PCR primer and/or probe binding, these variations should clearly be marked in the patient's sequence.

5. Subsequently, determine the number of insertions in the joining site(s).

6. Recognition of (second) D segments is often not done by software. Therefore, if the N region consists of >10 bp, check for D segment by hand (using hard copies) or use only the sequence around the N region for analysis in databases.

7. If sequencing of *TCRG* gene rearrangements (identified by using the VγI family primer) is not successful, one can decide to repeat the PCR-heteroduplex reaction using Vγ member-specific primers (*see* **Table 6**) using the conditions shown in **Table 4**.

Table 6
V-specific PCR reactions for detection of TCRG gene rearrangements

Forward primer	Reverse primer	Positive control	Product size (bp)	Protocol[a]	References
Vγ2	Jγ1.1/2.1	Karpas299	295	A	*(30)*
Vγ3	Jγ1.1/2.1	patient	221	A	*(30)*
Vγ4	Jγ1.1/2.1	Patient	216	A	*(30)*
Vγ5	Jγ1.1/2.1	Patient	214	A	*(30)*
Vγ7	Jγ1.1/2.1	Patient	223	A	*(30)*
Vγ8	Jγ1.1/2.1	Molt16, Molt17, H9	286	A	*(30)*
Vγ2	Jγ1.3/2.3	CEM, CMLT1	499	A	*(30)*
Vγ3	Jγ1.3/2.3	CEM, SUPT1	425	A	*(30)*
Vγ4	Jγ1.3/2.3	SUPT1	420	A	*(30)*
Vγ5	Jγ1.3/2.3	DND41, HUT78	418	A	*(30)*
Vγ7	Jγ1.3/2.3	Patient	427	A	*(30)*
Vγ8	Jγ1.3/2.3	Molt16, Peer, Jurkat	490	A	*(30)*

[a] *See* **Table 4** for detailed information about PCR mixture per protocol

3.2.4. Optional: Southern Blot Analysis for Evaluation of Oligoclonality

In a proportion of ALL patients, the leukemic cell population consists of two or more subpopulations in which the Ig/TCR gene rearrangements may differ, i.e., are oligoclonal. Since it is not know at diagnosis which subclone may eventually cause a relapse, *(34, 35)* oligoclonal rearrangements should preferably not be used as MRD-PCR target. Based on PCR-heteroduplex information, only limited information on the oligoclonal nature of the Ig/TCR gene rearrangements can be obtained, since the applied primer sets do not cover the full spectrum of possible Ig/TCR gene rearrangements. Furthermore, the identification of two *IGH* gene rearrangements by PCR-heteroduplex analysis does not prove a bi-allelic rearrangement, but may also be due to the presence of two subclones, each with one identified rearranged *IGH* allele. To more accurately determine the clonality status of the Ig/TCR gene rearrangements, Southern blot analysis can be performed (*see* **Note 9**) *(36)*. Although the information obtained by Southern blot analysis is very informative, most MRD-PCR laboratories do not (routinely) perform such analysis because of the relatively large amount of DNA needed and because the Southern blotting is technically demanding and time-consuming.

3.2.5. Selection of MRD-PCR Targets

To limit the risk of false-negative MRD results due to clonal evolution phenomena (e.g., ongoing rearrangements, loss of subclones) *(37, 38)*, preferably two MRD-PCR targets should be used for each ALL patient. These MRD-PCR targets should be selected based on: (1) expected stability and (2) expected sensitivity. In most current MRD-based ALL protocols, a sensitivity of at least 10^{-4} should be obtained.

Stability: There are two main causes for instability of Ig/TCR gene rearrangements during the disease course. First, the Ig/TCR rearrangement may only be present in a subclone of the leukemic population, whereas it is absent in another (therapy-resistant) subclone. Several studies indeed have shown that in precursor-B-ALL, monoclonal Ig/TCR gene rearrangements have a much higher stability (80–90%) than oligoclonal rearrangements (40–50%) (**Table 7**) *(25, 29, 39)*. Consequently, especially monoclonal rearrangements should be selected in such patients. In T-ALL, oligoclonality at diagnosis is rare and the stability of TCR gene rearrangements is high; particularly *TCRD* gene rearrangements are highly stable *(38)*. Second, Ig/TCR rearrangements may be prone to secondary or ongoing rearrangements. To limit the risk of loosing MRD-PCR targets by such processes, one should preferably select "end-stage" Ig/TCR rearrangements (e.g., *IGK*-Kde or Vγ-Jγ2.3 rearrangements).

Sensitivity: The sensitivity of MRD-PCR analysis of junctional regions is dependent on several factors, including the type of

Table 7
Stability of Ig/TCR gene rearrangements between diagnosis and relapse in childhood ALL patients

| PCR target | Monoclonality (%) | Stability at relapse (%) | | |
		Monoclonal	Oligoclonal	All
Precursor-B-ALL				
IGH	60–70	86	45	61
IGK-Kde	90	95	<50	90
Vκ-Jκ	60–70	>95	70	89
Vλ-Jλ	Nt	77	Nt	77
TCRB	90	Nt	Nt	73
TCRG	60–65	Nt	Nt	75
TCRD	60	86	26	63
Vδ2-Jα	65	83	44	66
T-ALL				
TCRB	>95	Nt	Nt	80
TCRG	>95	Nt	Nt	86
TCRD	>95	Nt	Nt	100

Nt not tested

rearrangement, the size of the junctional region, and the "background" of normal lymphoid cells with comparable Ig/TCR gene rearrangements *(7, 13, 20, 28, 29, 40, 41)*. If a relatively high proportion of leukemic cells is present, the MRD level can generally reliably be quantified, but in case of very low MRD levels the assay becomes less accurate. Thus, the variation in C_T values between replicates is generally less than 1.5 if the mean C_T value of the replicates is below 36, with greater variation between replicates if the mean C_T value of the replicates is higher *(7)*. Within the European Study Group on MRD detection in ALL (ESG-MRD-ALL; *see* **Note 10**) it therefore was decided to define the "quantitative range" and the "sensitivity". The "quantitative range" reflects the part of the standard curve in which the MRD levels can be quantified reproducibly and accurately, whereas the "sensitivity" reflects the lowest MRD level that still can be detected, although not reproducibly and accurately.

Generally, Ig/TCR gene rearrangements involving V, D, and J gene segments result in higher sensitivities than those rearrangements involving only two types of gene segments, e.g., V and J, V and D. In **Table 8** the expected quantitative range and sensitivity of randomly chosen Ig/TCR gene rearrangements are given.

Based on the expected stability and sensitivity, a general priority order can be made:

– In precursor-B-ALL, if no Southern blot data are available on clonality status: *IGK*-Kde → *IGH/TCRB*/Vδ2-Jα → *TCRD* → Vκ-Jκ/Vλ-Jλ → *TCRG*. In case of clear oligoclonality of a certain locus (e.g., by the identification of three or more unrelated rearrangements within one locus), one can decide to monitor all the identified rearrangements in this particular locus, thereby increasing the chance that the slowest-responding leukemic subclone will be followed.

– In precursor-B-ALL, if Southern blotting is performed: Choose monoclonal targets with best chance of obtaining a good sensitivity in the RQ-PCR analysis (**Table 8**).

Table 8
Overall sensitivities of Ig/TCR gene rearrangements in RQ-PCR assays

Rearrangement		Quantitative range of at least 10^{-4} (%)[a]	Sensitivity of at least 10^{-4} (%)[a]
IGH	DJ	50	75
	VDJ	80	95
IGK-Kde		80	90
IGK Vκ-Jκ		45	80
Vλ-Jλ		50	80
TCRD	Incomplete	45	90
	Complete	80	95
Vδ2-Jα		75	90
TCRB	VDJ	70	90
	DJ	55	90
TCRG	precursor-B-ALL	25	45
	T-ALL	70	80

[a]Percentage of rearrangements with quantitative range/sensitivity of at least 10^{-4}

– General priority order in T-ALL: *TCRB/TCRD → TCRG*. It should be noted that in about 15–20% of childhood T-ALL patients, *SIL-TAL1* fusion genes can easily be detected; these fusion genes can be used as stable and sensitive MRD-PCR targets a well *(42, 43)*.

3.3. RQ-PCR Sensitivity Testing

3.3.1. Design of Allele-Specific Oligonucleotide Primers

For RQ-PCR analysis of Ig/TCR gene rearrangements, generally the TaqMan (hydrolysis) probe approach is being used (*see* **Note 11**). Several primer-probe sets for RQ-PCR-based detection of tumor-specific *IGH (40)*, *IGK (25, 29)*, *IGL (25)*, *TCRG (28)*, *TCRD (13, 44)*, and *TCRB (20)* have been designed. Although both an ASO probe approach and ASO primer approach can be used, the ASO primer approach has the advantage that it is much cheaper as no patient-specific probes need to be ordered.

The germline primer and probe sets should be used in combination with a patient-specific allele-specific oligonucleotide (ASO) primer. This ASO primer should be positioned within and around the junctional region in such a way that it provides maximal specificity.

1. Enter the sequence of the Ig/TCR rearrangement in Primer Express software (Applied Biosystems).

2. Select an appropriate germline primer and probe, based on the sequence of the Ig/TCR gene rearrangement. In **Figs. 3–8** the primer-probe sets most commonly used in our laboratory are shown.

3. Mark the position of the germline primer and probe in the sequence

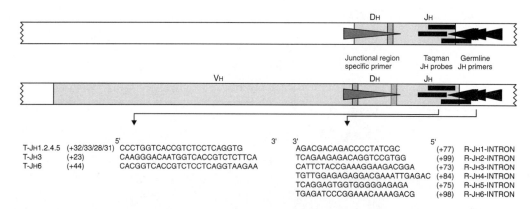

Fig. 3. RQ-PCR analysis of incomplete and complete *IGH* gene rearrangements. The diagrams summarize the positions of the germline J$_H$ TaqMan probes (*n* = 3) and germline J$_H$ primers (*n* = 6) which can be combined with junctional region specific primers for RQ-PCR analysis of D$_H$-J$_H$ and V$_H$-J$_H$ rearrangements. The probe and primer sequences are derived from Verhagen et al. *(40)* *R* reverse primer; *T* probe.

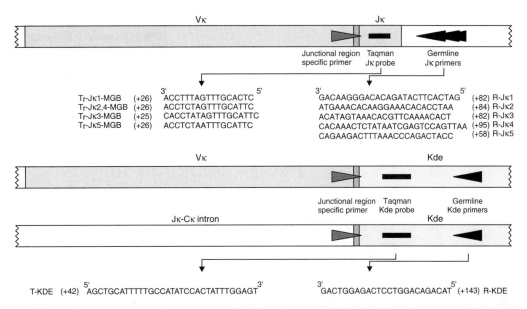

Fig. 4. RQ-PCR analysis of *IGK* gene rearrangements. The diagrams summarize the positions of the germline Kde TaqMan probe and germline Kde primer, which can be combined with junctional-specific primers for RQ-PCR analysis of Vκ-Kde and Intron-Kde rearrangements, and the positions of the germline Jκ TaqMan probes and germline Jκ primers, which can be combined with junctional-specific primers for RQ-PCR analysis of Vκ-Jκ rearrangements. The probe and primer sequences are derived from Van der Velden et al. *(25, 29) R* reverse primer; *T* probe; *Tr* reverse probe; *T–MGB* minor groove binding probe.

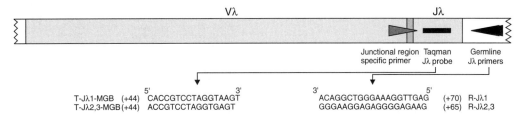

Fig. 5. RQ-PCR analysis of *IGL* gene rearrangements. The diagram summarizes the positions of the germline Jλ Taq-Man probes and germline Jλ primers, which can be combined with junctional-specific primers for RQ-PCR analysis of Vλ-Jλ rearrangements. The probe and primer sequences are derived from Van der Velden et al. *(25) R* reverse primer; *T-MGB* minor groove binding probe.

4. Design an allele-specific oligonlucleotide (ASO) primer using Primer Express and OLIGO6.0 software (Molecular Biology Insights, Inc., Cascade) according to the following guidelines (*see* **Note 12**):
   - Place the 3′ end of the primer in or just over the junctional region; maximum overlap with germline sequence: 2–6 nucleotides. In case of *IGH* gene rearrangements, the design of an ASO primer within the D_H-J_H junctional region

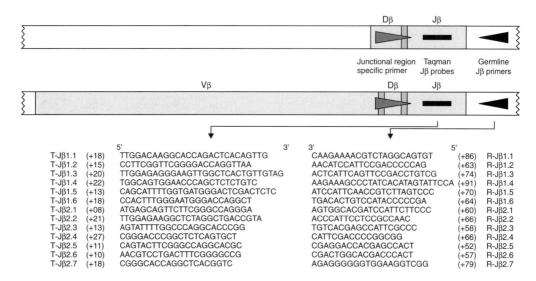

		5′	3′	3′		5′	
T-Jβ1.1	(+18)	TTGGACAAGGCACCAGACTCACAGTTG		CAAGAAAACGTCTAGGCAGTGT		(+86)	R-Jβ1.1
T-Jβ1.2	(+15)	CCTTCGGTTCGGGGACCAGGTTAA		AACATCCATTCCGACCCCCAG		(+63)	R-Jβ1.2
T-Jβ1.3	(+20)	TTGGAGAGGGAAGTTGGCTCACTGTTGTAG		ACTCATTCAGTTCCGACCTGTCG		(+74)	R-Jβ1.3
T-Jβ1.4	(+22)	TGGCAGTGGAACCCAGCTCTCTGTC		AAGAAAGCCCTATCACATAGTATTCCA		(+91)	R-Jβ1.4
T-Jβ1.5	(+13)	CAGCATTTTGGTGATGGGACTCGACTCTC		ATCCATTCAACCGTCTTAGTCCC		(+70)	R-Jβ1.5
T-Jβ1.6	(+18)	CCACTTTGGGAATGGGACCAGGCT		TGACACTGTCCATACCCCCGA		(+64)	R-Jβ1.6
T-Jβ2.1	(+08)	ATGAGCAGTCTTCGGGCCAGGGA		AGTGGCACGATCCATTCTTCCC		(+60)	R-Jβ2.1
T-Jβ2.2	(+21)	TTGGAGAAGGCTCTAGGCTGACCGTA		ACCCATTCCTCCGCCAAC		(+66)	R-Jβ2.2
T-Jβ2.3	(+13)	AGTATTTTGGCCCAGGCACCCGG		TGTCACGAGCCATTCGCCC		(+58)	R-Jβ2.3
T-Jβ2.4	(+27)	CGGGACCCGGCTCTCAGTGCT		CATTCGACCCCGGCGG		(+66)	R-Jβ2.4
T-Jβ2.5	(+11)	CAGTACTTCGGGCCAGGCACGC		CGAGGACCACGAGCCACT		(+52)	R-Jβ2.5
T-Jβ2.6	(+10)	AACGTCCTGACTTTCGGGGCCG		CGACTGGCACGACCCACT		(+57)	R-Jβ2.6
T-Jβ2.7	(+18)	CGGGCACCAGGCTCACGGTC		AGAGGGGGGTGGAAGGTCGG		(+79)	R-Jβ2.7

Fig. 6. RQ-PCR analysis of *TCRB* gene rearrangements. The diagrams summarize the position of the germline Dβ and Jβ TaqMan probes and germline Dβ and Jβ primers, which can be combined with junctional-specific primers for RQ-PCR analysis of Dβ-Jβ and Vβ-Jβ rearrangements. The probe and primer sequences are derived from Brüggemann et al. *(20)* *R* reverse primer; *T* probe.

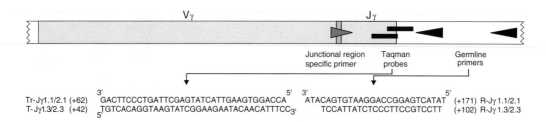

		3′		5′	3′		5′	
Tr-Jγ1.1/2.1	(+62)	GACTTCCCTGATTCGAGTATCATTGAAGTGGACCA			ATACAGTGTAAGGACCGGAGTCATAT		(+171)	R-Jγ1.1/2.1
T-Jγ1.3/2.3	(+42)	TGTCACAGGTAAGTATCGGAAGAATACAACATTTCC_{3′} 5′			TCCATTATCTCCCTTCCGTCCTT		(+102)	R-Jγ1.3/2.3

Fig. 7. RQ-PCR analysis of *TCRG* gene rearrangements. The diagram summarizes the positions of germline Jγ TaqMan probes and germline Jγ primers, which can be used in combination with junctional region specific primers for RQ-PCR analysis of Vγ-Jγ rearrangements. The probe and primer sequences are derived from Van der Velden et al. *(28)* *R* reverse primer, *T* probe, *Tr* reverse probe.

has the advantages that it enables the simultaneous monitoring of potential subclones containing this common stem, and that it may avoid a false-negative MRD result that can occur due to ongoing clonal evolution.

- T_m = 57–60°C, according to the Primer Express nearest neighbor algorithm.
- Percentage of GC in the range of 20–80%.
- Check in OLIGO 6.0:
  - (a) Internal stability graph (if possible no more than two G/C's in the last five bases on 3′ end according to Primer Express): strong binding in middle part of primer; lower binding at 3′ end $(-\Delta G > -10)$.

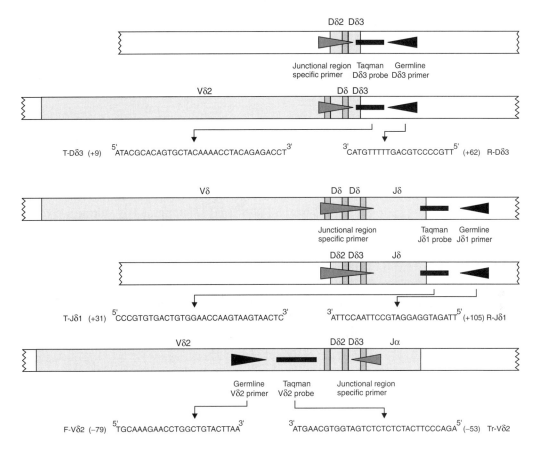

Fig. 8. RQ-PCR analysis of *TCRD* and Vδ2-Jα rearrangements. The diagrams summarize the positions of germline Jδ1 and Dδ3 TaqMan probes and primers, which can be combined with junctional region specific primers for RQ-PCR analysis of the various types of *TCRD* gene rearrangements (Vδ-Jδ1, Dδ-Jδ1, Dδ2-Dδ3, and Vδ-Dδ3), and position of the germline Vδ2 TaqMan probe and primer, which can be combined with junctional region specific primers for RQ-PCR analysis of the various types of Vδ2-Jα rearrangements. The probe and primer sequences are derived from Szczepanski et al. *(13, 44)* and Langerak et al. *(45)* *F* forward primer; *R* reverse primer; *T* probe; *Tr* reverse probe.

(b) 3′-dimers forward–forward and forward–reverse primer (<5 kcal/mole)

(c) Dimers forward–forward and forward–reverse primer (preferably <10 kcal/mole)

(d) Hairpin stems 3′ ends (no hairpin with T_m within 10°C from T_m primer)

5. Order the primers (several companies available).

6. Upon receipt, dissolve the primer in 1× TE-buffer; prepare a concentration of ~100 pmole/μl. Check the concentration of the primer with the Nanodrop® (ND-1000 spectrophotometer) by measuring 1.0 μl primer (in duplicate).

7. Prepare 300 μl of a primer working dilution in milli-Q water with a concentration of 30 pmole/μl. Store the stock and working solution at –20°C.

To determine the specificity of the designed ASO primer and the
sensitivity of the RQ-PCR assay, serial dilutions of the diagnostic
sample should be used.

1. Based on the morphological or (preferably) immunophenotypically determined blast percentage in the diagnostic MNCs
   preparation, the diagnostic DNA sample (60 ng/µl) should
   be diluted in normal control MNCs DNA (60 ng/µl) to a
   blast percentage of 10% (*see* **Note 13**). Prepare 150 µl of this
   10^{-1} dilution (*see* **Note 14**).

2. Prepare a 10^{-2} dilution by mixing 15 µl of the 10^{-1} dilution
   with 135 µl normal control MNCs DNA (60 ng/µl). Compa-
   rably, prepare 150 µl of a 10^{-3}, 10^{-4}, and 10^{-5} dilution. Prepare
   a 5×10^{-4} dilution by mixing 7 µl of the 10^{-2} dilution with 133 µl
   of normal control MNCs DNA (60 ng/µl).

3. Perform an RQ-PCR reaction using the 10^{-1}–10^{-5} dilutions
   in duplicate as well as the normal control MNCs DNA in six-
   fold (*see* **Note 15**) and Milli-Q water in duplicate. 600 ng
   DNA should be used per well (equivalent to ~200,000 cells,
   required to obtain a theoretical sensitivity of 10^{-5}). Reaction
   mixes are shown in **Table 9**.

4. Thermal cycler conditions are: 50°C, 2 min; 95°C, 10 min; 50
   cycles of 95°C, 15 s, and 60°C, 1 min.

5. Analyze the RQ-PCR data using appropriate software.

6. The threshold of the RQ-PCR assay should always be set in
   the region of exponential amplification across all amplification plots. This region is depicted in the log view of
   amplification plots as the portion of the curve that is linear.

Table 9
RQ-PCR reaction mixtures

Reaction mix per 25 µl reaction	final concentration	µl/well
Universal Master mix (2×)	1×	12.5
Forward primer (30 pmole/µl)	300 nM	0.25
Reverse primer (30 pmole/µl)	300 nM	0.25
TaqMan probe (5 pmole/µl)	100 nM	0.5
BSA (0.2%, w/v)	0.04%	0.5
Milli-Q water		1
DNA (60 ng/µl)		10

Often the threshold automatically determined by the instrument software can be used. However, if the threshold appears to be positioned outside the linear part of (some of) the amplification curves, adjustments may be made *(7, 46)*.

7. By plotting the logarithmic value of the dilution series against the obtained cycle threshold (C_T), a standard curve can be obtained.

3.3.3. RQ-PCR Data Interpretation: Quantitative Range and Sensitivity

For defining the sensitivity, several criteria (including reproducibility of the measurement, the difference between specific and nonspecific amplification, slope and correlation coefficient of the standard curve) should be taken into account *(7)*. Furthermore, in order to compare data between different studies and/or different laboratories, it is essential to have uniform guidelines for RQ-PCR data interpretation *(9)*. For Ig/TCR-based MRD data in ALL, such guidelines have been developed within the ESG-MRD-ALL *(46)*; (*see* **Notes 16–18**).

3.4. Bone Marrow Sample Processing During Follow-Up

1. Obtain a total of 2.5–3 ml BM in one first aspirate (*see* **Note 19**).

2. Perform Ficoll density centrifugation for obtaining MNCs.

3. Extract DNA from 10×10^6 MNCs using a DNA-extraction column, generally resulting in 30–40 µg of DNA *(47)*. This is sufficient for standard RQ-PCR analysis (applying two MRD-PCR targets and one control gene) (*see* **Note 20**).

4. Make an RQ-PCR solution of 60 ng/µl and store at 4°C (or –20°C) (<3 months); long-term storage should be done at –80°C.

5. Store remaining MNCs of the BM follow-up samples in cell-storage medium for later studies; store in liquid nitrogen.

3.5. MRD Analysis of Follow-Up Samples

The actual MRD analysis includes three main steps: RQ-PCR analysis of a control gene for checking the quality and quantity of the DNA, RQ-PCR analysis of the Ig/TCR targets, and finally interpretation of the obtained data.

3.5.1. Control Gene RQ-PCR Analysis

To check for the quantity and quality of the DNA, RQ-PCR analysis of a control gene is required. For this purpose the albumin (*ALB*) gene on chromosome 4 can be used *(48)*.

1. Make dilutions of normal control MNCs DNA (100 ng/µl) in Milli-Q water, so that solutions of 50, 10, and 1 ng/µl are obtained.

2. Analyse the four normal control DNA samples (i.e., 100, 50, 10, and 1 ng/µl), the (undiluted) diagnostic DNA (60 ng/µl)

and the follow-up samples (60 ng/µl) in duplicate. Use Milli-Q water as a negative control (in duplicate). Use the reaction mix as indicated in **Table 9**.

3. Thermal cycler conditions (for ABI 7000; other platforms may require different optimal temperatures and times): 50°C, 2 min; 95°C, 10 min; 95°C, 15 s; 60°C, 1 min (50×).

4. Analyze the RQ-PCR data using appropriate software. It is advised to use a common threshold setting for all control gene RQ-PCR reactions, since this allows an easier comparison of data obtained in different RQ-PCR runs. The C_T values obtained for the standard curve wells can be used to monitor the performance of the RQ-PCR reaction over time.

5. Construct a standard curve by plotting the C_T values of the four normal control MNCs DNA against their C_T values.

6. Determine the DNA content of the diagnostic and follow-up DNA samples using their C_T value and the obtained standard curve (*see* **Note 21**).

3.5.2. MRD-PCR Target RQ-PCR Analysis

For the actual analysis of MRD in the follow-up samples, RQ-PCR analysis is performed for the selected Ig/TCR targets (generally two targets per patient).

1. For each MRD-PCR target, analyse the dilutions series (10^{-1}–10^{-5}; *see* **Subheading 3.3.2**) of the diagnostic DNA (60 ng/µl) in duplicate, the follow-up samples (60 ng/µl) in triplicate, and normal control MNCs DNA in sixfold. Use Milli-Q water as a negative control (in triplicate). Use the reaction mix as indicated in **Table 9**.

2. Of importance, the control gene PCR and MRD-PCR target PCRs should be performed using exactly the same DNA sample in identical reaction volumes and using identical amounts of DNA.

3. Thermal cycler conditions (for ABI 7000; other platforms may require different optimal temperatures and times): 50°C, 2 min; 95°C, 10 min; 95°C, 15 s; 60°C, 1 min (50×) (*see* **Note 22**).

4. Analyze the RQ-PCR data using appropriate software.

5. The threshold of the RQ-PCR assay should always be set in the region of exponential amplification across all amplification plots. This region is depicted in the log view of amplification plots as the portion of the curve that is linear. Often the threshold automatically determined by the instrument software can be used. However, if the threshold appears to be positioned outside the linear part of (some of) the amplification curves, adjustments may be made *(7, 46)*.

3.5.3. RQ-PCR MRD Data Interpretation

For interpretation of the MRD data, the guidelines of the ESG-MRD-ALL *(46)* should be used (*see* **Notes 23** and **24**).

The requirements for the MRD-PCR target(s) is dependent on the clinical protocol that is being used. Most current protocols require the availability of two targets, of which one should have a quantitative range of $\leq 10^{-4}$ and the second should have a quantitative range of $\leq 10^{-3}$ and a sensitivity of $\leq 10^{-4}$.

The MRD-PCR target with the highest MRD level should be regarded as the most reliable target because of the potential subclonal origin of the lower MRD value. So, always the highest MRD level per time point should be reported.

3.6. Conclusion

Whereas it is obvious that MRD diagnostics provides critical information for further improvement of treatment in ALL patients, it is also clear that the PCR-based MRD diagnostics via Ig/TCR genes is complex, requires extensive knowledge about Ig/TCR gene rearrangement processes, and needs regular internal and external quality control. Standardization, internationally accepted guidelines for interpretation of RQ-PCR results, and regular quality control rounds are essential for providing MRD results that are comparable between different MRD laboratories and between different treatment protocols. Since Autumn 2001, the ESG-MRD-ALL has served the European MRD laboratories in these aims. We hope that this chapter and the presented protocols further contribute to the quality and reliability of MRD diagnostics for ALL patients.

4. Notes

1. If no BM sample is available at diagnosis, one might decide to use a peripheral blood (PB) sample in patients with a sufficiently high percentage of ALL blasts in PB (preferably >25% of MNCs). The use of samples with lower percentages of blast cells may hamper the detection of Ig/TCR rearrangements and is therefore not recommended.

2. For DNA extraction, phenol–chloroform-based extraction methods should be avoided as this will generally result in high molecular weight DNA which is very hard to pipet in a reproducible way.

3. Extraction of DNA from 10×10^6 MNCs will generally result in 30–40 µg of DNA *(47)*, which is sufficient for all relevant PCR analyses at diagnosis, Southern Blot analysis, and preparation of a standard curve. Based on a theoretical recovery of 1 µg DNA per 160,000 cells, the efficiency of the DNA isolation is 50–65% when frozen MNCs are used *(47)*. If fresh samples are used, efficiencies up to 80% can be reached *(47)*.

4. For assessment of DNA concentration, the Nanodrop method is preferred over analysis using another type of spectrophotometer, since the results are more robust and accurate.

5. Instead of commercially available gels, also home-made 6% PAGE gels can be used.

6. Alternatively, comparable commercially available sequencing kits can be used.

7. If heteroduplexes are used as template, the sequence obtained with the forward and reverse primer should differ, but alignment with the sequences obtained for the second heteroduplex (forward 1 with reverse 2 and forward 2 with reverse 1) should give similar results.

8. Some sequences can also easily be analyzed using hard copies: these are available upon request (v.h.j.vandervelden@erasmusmc.nl).

9. Given the frequency of oligoclonality in the *IGH* (45%) *(27, 49)*, *IGK* (10%) *(27, 29, 50)* and *TCRD* (25%) loci *(14, 27, 51)*, and the frequent coincidence of oligoclonality in these three loci *(27)*, the priority order for Southern blotting is *IGH>TCRD>IGK*. Oligoclonality in the *TCRG* and *TCRB* loci occurs less frequently *(15)*. A *Bgl*II digest of 10–15 µg diagnostic material can be used for Southern blotting and subsequent hybridization with IGHJ6, IGKDE, and/or TCRDJ1 (and/or TCRDV2) probes *(36, 49–51)*. For analysis of oligoclonality in the *TCRB* or *TCRG* loci, *Eco*RI and *Hind*III digests or *Eco*RI digests can be used, respectively *(15, 36)*. Southern blot analysis is not needed for T-ALL, because the frequency of oligoclonality in this disease category is low *(51)*.

10. The European Study Group on MRD detection in ALL (ESG-MRD-ALL) is a consortium of 30 international MRD-PCR laboratories, coordinated by J.J.M. van Dongen and V.H.J. van der Velden. The main aims of the ESG-MRD-ALL are the organization of a quality control program twice per year, the collaborative development and clinical evaluation of new MRD strategies and techniques, and the development of guidelines for the interpretation of RQ-PCR-based MRD data.

11. For RQ-PCR analysis, other probe formats (e.g., hybridization probes) can also be used *(7)*. The use of nonspecific dyes, such as SYBR Green I, should be avoided, since this limits the sensitivity.

12. If no appropriate primer can be designed (e.g., because dimerformation with the standard germline primer-probe sets, too large number of deletions) or if the composition of the junctional region necessitates the design of a reverse ASO instead of a forward primer (or vice versa), alternative primer-probes sets can be used. In **Table 10** the most commonly used alternative sets are shown.

Table 10
Alternative primer-probe sets for RQ-PCR analysis of Ig/TCR gene rearrangements

Locus	Gene segment	Primer (5′ → 3′)[a]	Probe (5′ → 3′)[a]
IGK	Vκ2.30	F-Vκ2.30-cons2 (−89) GGT-CAGGCACTGATTTCACACT	T-Vκ2.30-cons1 (−61) CAGCAGGGT-GGAGGCTGAGGATGT
	Vκ3.20	F-Vκ3.20-cons2 (−79) AGACT-TCACTCTCACCATCAGCAG	Tr-Vκ3.20-cons1 (−52) GGAGCCTGAA-GATTTTGCAGTGTATACTGTCA
	Vκ4.1	F-Vκ4-cons1 (−116) GGGTC-CCTGACCGATTCAGT	T-Vκ4-cons1 (−93) AGCGGGTCT-GGGACAGATTTCACTCTC
	Intron	F-intron-cons3 (−74) GCCGCCTTGCCGCTA	T-intron-cons1 (−48) CCACCCTGT-GTCTGCCCGATTG
TCRB	Jβ2.5	R-Jβ2.5-cons2 (+102) CGCAAAAACCAGAC-CCAAG	Tr-Jβ2.5 −cons2 (+53) CTCACCGAG-CACCAGGAGCCG
	Jβ2.7	R-Jβ2.7-cons2 (+64) AGACGCCCGAATCT-CACCT	Tr-Jβ2.7-cons2 (+44) TGACCGT-GAGCCTGGTGCCC
	Dβ1	F-Dβ1 (−79) CACTCCCCT-CAAAGGAGCAG	T-Dβ1 (−51) CTCTGGTGGTCTCTC-CCAGGCTCTG
	Dβ2	F-Dβ2 (−56) CCGCGCCCAGT-GGTT	T-Dβ2 (−13) ACTAGCAGGGAGGAAA-CATTTTTGTATCATGG
TCRD	Dδ3	R-Dδ3-cons1 (+135) GGGAAGCTGCTTGCTGT-GTT	T-Dδ3-cons3 (+81) ATATCCTCAC-CCTGGGTCCCATGCC
	Vδ2	Vδ2-cons5 (−110) TCAAA-GACAATTTCCAAGGTGACA	Tr-Vδ2-cons1 (−85) ACTATAACGTT-TCTTGGACCGACATGAATTCTAT-GAAC
TCRG	Vγ2	F-Vγ2-cons1 (−92) CTTACG-CAAGCACAAGGAACAA	T-Vγ2-cons1 (−69) TTGAGATTGA-TACTGCGAAATCTAATTGAAAAT-GACTC
	Vγ3	F-Vγ3- cons2 (−145) CTCCAC-CGCAAGGGATGT	T-Vγ23-cons1 (−95) ACTCATACAC-CCAGGAGGTGGAGCTGGATATT
	Vγ4	F-Vγ4-cons2 (−96) GATACT-TACGGAAGCACAAG-GAAGA	T-Vγ4-cons2 (−70) CTTGAGAAT-GATACTGCGAAATCTTATT-GAAAATGA
	Vγ5	F-Vγ5-cons2 (−117) GGACT-CAGTCCAGGAAAGTAT-TATACTCAT	Tr-Vγ5-cons1 (−85) ATCAATATC-CAGCTCCACCTCCTGGGT
	Vγ9	F-Vγ9-cons2 (−120) GGCATTC-CGTCAGGCAAA	T-Vγ9-cons1 (−91) TAGGATACCT-GAAACGTCTACATCCACTCT-CACC

(continued)

Table 10
(continued)

Locus	Gene segment	Primer (5′ → 3′)[a]	Probe (5′ → 3′)[a]
	Vγ10	F-Vγ10-cons1 (−106) CAAAGT-GGAGGCAAGAAAGAATTC	T-Vγ10-cons1 (−68) CAATCCTTAC-CATCAAGTCCGTAGAGAAAGAA-GACAT
	Vγ11	F-Vγ11-cons0 (−159) CAT-GTCTTCTTGACAATCTCT-GCTC	Tr-Vγ11-cons0 (−133) TCAAGTTTCT-TAGTCTTCCCACCTGAGCAATCT
	Jγ2.1	R-Jγ2.1-new (+170) ACT-GGAATAAAAACA-GAAAAAAAATTACTT	Tr-Jγ2.1-cons2 (+62) ACCAGGCAAGT-TACTATGAGCCTAGTCCCT

[a]Position of the primer and probe upstream (−) or downstream (+) relative to the RSS of the gene segment with the primer included. *F* forward primer; *R* reverse primer; *T* probe; *Tr* reverse probe

13. Ideally MNCs obtained from normal BM samples should be used, but most MRD laboratories use PB MNCs due to the much easier collection of such material. To limit a potential skewed Ig/TCR repertoire in the MNCs DNA used, a pool of at least five healthy individuals should be used.

14. If only a limited amount of diagnostic DNA is available, one might decide to skip the 10^{-1} dilution and to use the 10^{-2} dilution as the lowest dilution of the standard curve.

15. Since nonspecific amplification is generally only detected at low levels and outside the reproducible range of the RQ-PCR, nonspecific amplification controls should be run at least in six-fold in each RQ-PCR analysis for each Ig or TCR marker.

16. The background of the RQ-PCR assay, i.e., the nonspecific amplification of comparable Ig/TCR gene rearrangements present in normal cells, is defined by the lowest C_T value obtained in the nonspecific amplification controls (normal MNCs DNA). One should, however, be aware that the "background" of normal lymphoid cells is not constant, but can differ per treatment phase. For example, high frequencies of normal T-cells can be detected in postinduction follow-up samples *(52)* and substantial expansions of normal precursor-B-cells can be detected in regenerating BM after cessation of therapy *(53, 54)*. Indeed, higher levels of nonspecific amplification can be observed for Ig targets in BM samples taken just after induction therapy and taken after end of therapy *(55)*. Of importance, these higher levels of nonspecific amplification virtually never reach the quantitative range of the assay.

17. If the quantitative range and/or sensitivity of the RQ-PCR test is not sufficient, the annealing temperature can be increased (up to 70°C) in order to improve specificity (26, 28, 29, 40). If this is not successful, one can decide to design an alternative ASO primer.

18. One should be aware that all MRD data below the quantitative range are nonreproducible. Indeed, comparative RQ-PCR analysis of follow-up samples in threefold and in tenfold clearly showed that MRD levels below 10^{-4} are not reproducible if triplicate analyses are performed, whereas data become more concordant if the analyses is performed in tenfold (56).

19. Usage of a second BM aspirate should be avoided, because of the high chance of dilution with PB. Monitoring of BM samples is strongly preferred over monitoring of PB samples, because MRD studies in paired BM-PB samples showed a poor correlation in precursor-B-ALL (twofold to more than 1,000-fold difference) (57). In contrast, MRD levels in BM and PB samples of T-ALL patients showed a better correlation (57). Nevertheless, from a logistical point of view it may be most convenient to use BM samples for both groups of patients, i.e., to make no exception for the small subset of T-ALL (about 15–20% of all ALL patients). Since MRD levels appear to be distributed homogeneously over the BM (at least during the initial phases of therapy) (56), obtaining a single BM aspirate is sufficient.

20. At least 2×10^6 MNCs should be used for DNA extraction since at least 5–8 μg of DNA should be available for RQ-PCR analysis.

21. If the RQ-PCR of the control gene shows a lower amount of template than expected, based on physical measurements (e.g., Nanodrop measurement), special caution is needed since this lower value can be the result of inhibition, which can be found in a substantial number of BM or PB samples (5–10%). Addition of bovine serum albumin (BSA) prevents inhibition (58) and the ESG-MRD-ALL therefore recommends the inclusion of 0.04% BSA in all RQ-PCR reactions (46). Since the addition of less amount of template will result in loss of sensitivity, the control gene values of all samples need to be within predefined ranges, that is between 250 and 1,000 ng/reaction. If the DNA amount appears to be higher, the follow-up sample should be diluted and retested because too high DNA concentrations may also result in PCR inhibition (58). If the DNA amount is lower, correct interpretation may not be possible. Consequently, reanalysis is recommended after adaptation of the amount of DNA (46).

22. The annealing temperature can be different, dependent on the results of the sensitivity testing.

23. The interpretation of RQ-PCR results obtained in follow-up samples is most difficult when MRD levels are outside the "quantitative range" of the assay. In these cases, it may not always be clear whether the signal observed is due to specific amplification from leukemic cell DNA or from nonspecific amplification of normal DNA. However, the decision to classify a follow-up sample to be "MRD positive" or "MRD negative" may have major clinical implications. Therefore, it was decided within the ESG-MRD-ALL to develop separate guidelines for (i) protocols that aim at therapy reduction and therefore wish to prevent false-negative results and (ii) for protocols directed towards therapy intensification, where false-positive results should be avoided *(46)*.

24. Logically, very low MRD levels (below the "quantitative range") should always be judged with caution; especially if only one well of the three replicates is positive. In such case, reanalysis of the doubtful sample(s) may be performed, but one should be aware that by definition the results will often not be reproducible.

Acknowledgement

We gratefully acknowledge Patricia Hoogeveen and Maaike de Bie for critically reviewing this manuscript and for their excellent technical support. We thank Marieke Comans-Bitter for preparing the figures.

References

1. van Dongen, J. J. M., Seriu, T., Panzer-Grumayer, E. R., Biondi, A., Pongers-Willemse, M. J., Corral, L., Stolz, F., Schrappe, M., Masera, G., Kamps, W. A., Gadner, H., van Wering, E. R., Ludwig, W. D., Basso, G., de Bruijn, M. A., Cazzaniga, G., Hettinger, K., van der Does-van den Berg, A., Hop, W. C., Riehm, H., and Bartram, C. R. (1998) Prognostic value of minimal residual disease in acute lymphoblastic leukaemia in childhood. *Lancet* **352**, 1731–1738.

2. Cave, H., van der Werff ten Bosch, J., Suciu, S., Guidal, C., Waterkeyn, C., Otten, J., Bakkus, M., Thielemans, K., Grandchamp, B., and Vilmer, E. (1998) Clinical significance of minimal residual disease in childhood acute lymphoblastic leukemia. European Organization for Research and Treatment of Cancer–Childhood Leukemia Cooperative Group. *New England Journal of Medicine* **339**, 591–598.

3. Coustan-Smith, E., Sancho, J., Hancock, M. L., Boyett, J. M., Behm, F. G., Raimondi, S. C., Sandlund, J. T., Rivera, G. K., Rubnitz, J. E., Ribeiro, R. C., Pui, C. H., and Campana, D. (2000) Clinical importance of minimal residual disease in childhood acute lymphoblastic leukemia. *Blood* **96**, 2691–2696.

4. Panzer-Grumayer, E. R., Schneider, M., Panzer, S., Fasching, K., and Gadner, H. (2000) Rapid molecular response during early induction chemotherapy predicts a good outcome in childhood acute lymphoblastic leukemia. *Blood* **95**, 790–794.

5. Goulden, N., Bader, P., Van Der Velden, V., Moppett, J., Schilham, M., Masden, H. O., Krejci, O., Kreyenberg, H., Lankester, A., Revesz, T., Klingebiel, T., and Van Dongen, J. (2003) Minimal residual disease prior to stem cell transplant for childhood acute lymphoblastic leukaemia. *British Journal of Haematology* **122**, 24–29.

6. Schrappe, M. (2002) Risk-adapted therapy: lessons from childhood acute lymphoblastic leukemia. *Hematological Journal* **3**, 127–132.

7. van der Velden, V. H. J., Hochhaus, A., Cazzaniga, G., Szczepanski, T., Gabert, J., and van Dongen, J. J. M. (2003) Detection of minimal residual disease in hematologic malignancies by real-time quantitative PCR: principles, approaches, and laboratory aspects. *Leukemia* **17**, 1013–1034.

8. Szczepanski, T., Flohr, T., van der Velden, V. H. J., Bartram, C. R., and van Dongen, J. J. M. (2002) Molecular monitoring of residual disease using antigen receptor genes in childhood acute lymphoblastic leukaemia. *Best Practice & Research. Clinical Haematology* **15**, 37–57.

9. van der Velden, V. H., Panzer-Grumayer, E. R., Cazzaniga, G., Flohr, T., Sutton, R., Schrauder, A., Basso, G., Schrappe, M., Wijkhuijs, J. M., Konrad, M., Bartram, C. R., Masera, G., Biondi, A., and van Dongen, J. J. (2007) Optimization of PCR-based minimal residual disease diagnostics for childhood acute lymphoblastic leukemia in a multicenter setting. *Leukemia* **21**, 706–713.

10. Szczepanski, T., van der Velden, V. H., and van Dongen, J. J. (2006) Flow-cytometric immunophenotyping of normal and malignant lymphocytes. *Clinical Chemistry and Laboratory Method* **44**, 775–796.

11. Szczepanski, T., van der Velden, V. H., and van Dongen, J. J. (2003) Classification systems for acute and chronic leukaemias. *Best Practice & Research. Clinical Haematology* **16**, 561–582.

12. Langerak, A. W., Szczepanski, T., van der Burg, M., Wolvers-Tettero, I. L., and van Dongen, J. J. (1997) Heteroduplex PCR analysis of rearranged T cell receptor genes for clonality assessment in suspect T cell proliferations. *Leukemia* **11**, 2192–2199.

13. Szczepanski, T., van der Velden, V. H. J., Hoogeveen, P. G., De Bie, M., Jacobs, D. C. H., Van Wering, E. R., and van Dongen, J. J. M. (2004) V{delta}2-J{alpha} gene rearrangements are frequent in precursor-B-acute lymphoblastic leukemia but rare in normal lymphoid cells. *Blood* **103**, 3798–3804.

14. Szczepanski, T., Langerak, A. W., Wolvers-Tettero, I. L., Ossenkoppele, G. J., Verhoef, G., Stul, M., Petersen, E. J., de Bruijn, M. A.,

van't Veer, M. B., and van Dongen, J. J. M. (1998) Immunoglobulin and T cell receptor gene rearrangement patterns in acute lymphoblastic leukemia are less mature in adults than in children: implications for selection of PCR targets for detection of minimal residual disease. *Leukemia* **12**, 1081–1088.

15. Szczepanski, T., Beishuizen, A., Pongers-Willemse, M. J., Hahlen, K., Van Wering, E. R., Wijkhuijs, A. J., Tibbe, G. J., De Bruijn, M. A., and Van Dongen, J. J. M. (1999) Cross-lineage T cell receptor gene rearrangements occur in more than ninety percent of childhood precursor-B acute lymphoblastic leukemias: alternative PCR targets for detection of minimal residual disease. *Leukemia* **13**, 196–205.

16. Szczepanski, T., Pongers-Willemse, M. J., Langerak, A. W., Harts, W. A., Wijkhuijs, A. J., van Wering, E. R., and van Dongen, J. J. M. (1999) Ig heavy chain gene rearrangements in T-cell acute lymphoblastic leukemia exhibit predominant DH6-19 and DH7-27 gene usage, can result in complete V-D-J rearrangements, and are rare in T-cell receptor alpha beta lineage. *Blood* **93**, 4079–4085.

17. Szczepanski, T., Willemse, M. J., van Wering, E. R., van Weerden, J. F., Kamps, W. A., and van Dongen, J. J. M. (2001) Precursor-B-ALL with D(H)-J(H) gene rearrangements have an immature immunogenotype with a high frequency of oligoclonality and hyperdiploidy of chromosome 14. *Leukemia* **15**, 1415–1423.

18. Beishuizen, A., Hahlen, K., Hagemeijer, A., Verhoeven, M. A., Hooijkaas, H., Adriaansen, H. J., Wolvers-Tettero, I. L., van Wering, E. R., and van Dongen, J. J. (1991) Multiple rearranged immunoglobulin genes in childhood acute lymphoblastic leukemia of precursor B-cell origin. *Leukemia* **5**, 657–667.

19. Beishuizen, A., de Bruijn, M. A., Pongers-Willemse, M. J., Verhoeven, M. A., van Wering, E. R., Hahlen, K., Breit, T. M., de Bruin-Versteeg, S., Hooijkaas, H., and van Dongen, J. J. (1997) Heterogeneity in junctional regions of immunoglobulin kappa deleting element rearrangements in B cell leukemias: a new molecular target for detection of minimal residual disease. *Leukemia* **11**, 2200–2207.

20. Bruggemann, M., van der Velden, V. H. J., Raff, T., Droese, J., Ritgen, M., Pott, C., Wijkhuijs, A., Goekbuget, N., Hoelzer, D., van Wering, E. R., van Dongen, J. J. M., and Kneba, M. (2004) Rearranged T-cell receptor beta genes represent powerful targets for quantification of minimal residual disease (MRD) in childhood and adult T-cell acute lymphoblastic leukemia (T-ALL). *Leukemia* **18**, 709–719.

21. Brumpt, C., Delabesse, E., Beldjord, K., Davi, F., Cayuela, J. M., Millien, C., Villarese, P.,

Quartier, P., Buzyn, A., Valensi, F., and Mac-intyre, E. (2000) The incidence of clonal T-cell receptor rearrangements in B-cell precursor acute lymphoblastic leukemia varies with age and genotype. *Blood* **96**, 2254–2261.

22. Huebner, S., Cazzaniga, G., Flohr, T., van der Velden, V. H. J., Konrad, M., Basso, G., Schrappe, M., van Dongen, J. J. M., Bartram, C., Biondi, A., and Panzer-Gruemayer, E. (2004) High incidence and unique features of antigen receptor gene rearrangements in TEL-AML1 positive leukemias. *Leukemia* **18**, 84–91.

23. Jansen, M. W., Corral, L., van der Velden, V. H., Panzer-Grumayer, R., Schrappe, M., Schrauder, A., Marschalek, R., Meyer, C., den Boer, M. L., Hop, W. J., Valsecchi, M. G., Basso, G., Biondi, A., Pieters, R., and van Dongen, J. J. (2007) Immunobiological diversity in infant acute lymphoblastic leukemia is related to the occurrence and type of MLL gene rearrangement. *Leukemia* **21**, 633–641.

24. Mann, G., Cazzaniga, G., van der Velden, V. H., Flohr, T., Csinady, E., Paganin, M., Schrauder, A., Dohnal, A. M., Schrappe, M., Biondi, A., Gadner, H., van Dongen, J. J., and Panzer-Grumayer, E. R. (2007) Acute lymphoblastic leukemia with t(4;11) in children 1 year and older: The 'big sister' of the infant disease? *Leukemia* **21**, 642–646.

25. van der Velden, V. H., de Bie, M., van Wering, E. R., and van Dongen, J. J. (2006) Immunoglobulin light chain gene rearrangements in precursor-B-acute lymphoblastic leukemia: characteristics and applicability for the detection of minimal residual disease. *Haematologica* **91**, 679–682.

26. van der Velden, V. H. J., Bruggemann, M., Hoogeveen, P. G., de Bie, M., Hart, P. G., Raff, T., Pfeifer, H., Luschen, S., Szczepanski, T., van Wering, E. R., Kneba, M., and van Dongen, J. J. M. (2004) TCRB gene rearrangements in childhood and adult precursor-B-ALL: frequency, applicability as MRD-PCR target, and stability between diagnosis and relapse. *Leukemia* **18**, 1971–1980.

27. Van Der Velden, V. H. J., Szczepanski, T., Wijkhuijs, J. M., Hart, P. G., Hoogeveen, P. G., Hop, W. C., Van Wering, E. R., and Van Dongen, J. J. M. (2003) Age-related patterns of immunoglobulin and T-cell receptor gene rearrangements in precursor-B-ALL: implications for detection of minimal residual disease. *Leukemia* **17**, 1834–1844.

28. van der Velden, V. H. J., Wijkhuijs, J. M., Jacobs, D. C., van Wering, E. R., and van Dongen, J. J. M. (2002) T cell receptor gamma gene rearrangements as targets for detection of minimal residual disease in acute lymphoblastic leukemia by real-time quantitative PCR analysis. *Leukemia* **16**, 1372–1380.

29. van der Velden, V. H. J., Willemse, M. J., van der Schoot, C. E., Hahlen, K., van Wering, E. R., and van Dongen, J. J. M. (2002) Immunoglobulin kappa deleting element rearrangements in precursor-B acute lymphoblastic leukemia are stable targets for detection of minimal residual disease by real-time quantitative PCR. *Leukemia* **16**, 928–936.

30. Pongers-Willemse, M. J., Seriu, T., Stolz, F., d'Aniello, E., Gameiro, P., Pisa, P., Gonzalez, M., Bartram, C. R., Panzer-Grumayer, E. R., Biondi, A., San Miguel, J. F., and van Dongen, J. J. M. (1999) Primers and protocols for standardized detection of minimal residual disease in acute lymphoblastic leukemia using immunoglobulin and T cell receptor gene rearrangements and TAL1 deletions as PCR targets: report of the BIOMED-1 CONCERTED ACTION: investigation of minimal residual disease in acute leukemia. *Leukemia* **13**, 110–118.

31. Kuppers, R., Zhao, M., Rajewsky, K., and Hansmann, M. L. (1993) Detection of clonal B cell populations in paraffin-embedded tissues by polymerase chain reaction. *American Journal of Pathology* **143**, 230–239.

32. van Dongen, J. J. M., Langerak, A. W., Bruggemann, M., Evans, P. A. S., Hummel, M., Lavender, F. L., Delabesse, E., Davi, F., Schuuring, E., Garcia Sanz, R., van Krieken, J. H. J. M., Droese, J., Gonzalez, D., Bastard, C., White, H. E., Spaargaren, M., Gonzalez Diaz, M., Parreira, A., Smith, J. L., Morgan, G. J., Kneba, M., and Macintyre, E. A. (2003) Design and standardization of PCR primers and protocols for detection of clonal immunogloulin and T-cell receptor gene recombinations in suspect lymphoproliferations. *Leukemia* **17**, 2257–2317.

33. Feldhahn, N., Henke, N., Melchior, K., Duy, C., Soh, B. N., Klein, F., von Levetzow, G., Giebel, B., Li, A., Hofmann, W. K., Jumaa, H., and Muschen, M. (2007) Activation-induced cytidine deaminase acts as a mutator in BCR-ABL1-transformed acute lymphoblastic leukemia cells. *The Journal of Experimental Medicine* **204**, 1157–1166.

34. de Haas, V., Verhagen, O. J., von dem Borne, A. E., Kroes, W., van den Berg, H., and van der Schoot, C. E. (2001) Quantification of minimal residual disease in children with oligoclonal B-precursor acute lymphoblastic leukemia indicates that the clones that grow out during relapse already have the slowest

rate of reduction during induction therapy. *Leukemia* **15**, 134–140.

35. Konrad, M., Metzler, M., Panzer, S., Ostreicher, I., Peham, M., Repp, R., Haas, O. A., Gadner, H., and Panzer-Grumayer, E. R. (2003) Late relapses evolve from slow-responding subclones in t(12;21)-positive acute lymphoblastic leukemia: evidence for the persistence of a preleukemic clone. *Blood* **101**, 3635–3640.

36. van Dongen, J. J. and Wolvers-Tettero, I. L. (1991) Analysis of immunoglobulin and T cell receptor genes. Part I: Basic and technical aspects. *Clinical Chimica Acta* **198**, 1–91.

37. Li, A., Zhou, J., Zuckerman, D., Rue, M., Dalton, V., Lyons, C., Silverman, L. B., Sallan, S. E., and Gribben, J. G. (2003) Sequence analysis of clonal immunoglobulin and T-cell receptor gene rearrangements in children with acute lymphoblastic leukemia at diagnosis and at relapse: implications for pathogenesis and for the clinical utility of PCR-based methods of minimal residual disease detection. *Blood* **102**, 4520–4526.

38. Szczepanski, T., van der Velden, V. H. J., Raff, T., Jacobs, D. C. H., van Wering, E. R., Brüggemann, M., Kneba, M., and van Dongen, J. J. M. (2003) Comparative analysis of T-cell receptor gene rearrangements at diagnosis and relapse of T-cell acute lymphoblastic leukemia (T-ALL) shows high stability of clonal markers for monitoring of minimal residual disease and reveals the occurrence of secondary T-ALL. *Leukemia* **17**, 2149–2156.

39. Szczepanski, T., Willemse, M. J., Brinkhof, B., van Wering, E. R., van der Burg, M., and van Dongen, J. J. M. (2002) Comparative analysis of Ig and TCR gene rearrangements at diagnosis and at relapse of childhood precursor-B-ALL provides improved strategies for selection of stable PCR targets for monitoring of minimal residual disease. *Blood* **99**, 2315–2323.

40. Verhagen, O. J., Willemse, M. J., Breunis, W. B., Wijkhuijs, A. J., Jacobs, D. C., Joosten, S. A., van Wering, E. R., van Dongen, J. J. M., and van der Schoot, C. E. (2000) Application of germline IGH probes in real-time quantitative PCR for the detection of minimal residual disease in acute lymphoblastic leukemia. *Leukemia* **14**, 1426–1435.

41. Bruggemann, M., Droese, J., Bolz, I., Luth, P., Pott, C., von Neuhoff, N., Scheuering, U., and Kneba, M. (2000) Improved assessment of minimal residual disease in B cell malignancies using fluorogenic consensus probes for real-time quantitative PCR. *Leukemia* **14**, 1419–1425.

42. Breit, T. M., Beishuizen, A., Ludwig, W. D., Mol, E. J., Adriaansen, H. J., van Wering, E. R., and van Dongen, J. J. (1993) tal-1 deletions in T-cell acute lymphoblastic leukemia as PCR target for detection of minimal residual disease. *Leukemia* **7**, 2004–2011.

43. Breit, T. M., Mol, E. J., Wolvers-Tettero, I. L., Ludwig, W. D., van Wering, E. R., and van Dongen, J. J. (1993) Site-specific deletions involving the tal-1 and sil genes are restricted to cells of the T cell receptor alpha/beta lineage: T cell receptor delta gene deletion mechanism affects multiple genes. *The Journal of Experimental Medicine* **177**, 965–977.

44. Szczepanski, T., van der Velden, V. H. J., and van Dongen, J. J. M. (2002) real-time quantitative (RQ)-PCR for the detection of minimal residual disease in childhood acute lymphoblastic leukemia. *Haematologica* **87** (suppl. 1), 183–191.

45. Langerak, A. W., Wolvers-Tettero, I. L., van Gastel-Mol, E. J., Oud, M. E., and van Dongen, J. J. (2001) Basic helix-loop-helix proteins E2A and HEB induce immature T-cell receptor rearrangements in nonlymphoid cells. *Blood* **98**, 2456–2465.

46. van der Velden, V. H., Cazzaniga, G., Schrauder, A., Hancock, J., Bader, P., Panzer-Grumayer, E. R., Flohr, T., Sutton, R., Cave, H., Madsen, H. O., Cayuela, J. M., Trka, J., Eckert, C., Foroni, L., Zur Stadt, U., Beldjord, K., Raff, T., van der Schoot, C. E., and van Dongen, J. J. (2007) Analysis of minimal residual disease by Ig/TCR gene rearrangements: guidelines for interpretation of real-time quantitative PCR data. *Leukemia* **21**, 604–611.

47. Verhagen, O. J., Wijkhuijs, A. J., van der Sluijs-Gelling, A. J., Szczepanski, T., van der Linden-Schrever, B. E., Pongers-Willemse, M. J., van Wering, E. R., van Dongen, J. J. M., and van der Schoot, C. E. (1999) Suitable DNA isolation method for the detection of minimal residual disease by PCR techniques. *Leukemia* **13**, 1298–1299.

48. Pongers-Willemse, M. J., Verhagen, O. J., Tibbe, G. J., Wijkhuijs, A. J., de Haas, V., Roovers, E., van der Schoot, C. E., and van Dongen, J. J. M. (1998) Real-time quantitative PCR for the detection of minimal residual disease in acute lymphoblastic leukemia using junctional region specific TaqMan probes. *Leukemia* **12**, 2006–2014.

49. Beishuizen, A., Verhoeven, M. A., Mol, E. J., Breit, T. M., Wolvers-Tettero, I. L., and van Dongen, J. J. (1993) Detection of immunoglobulin heavy-chain gene rearrangements

by Southern blot analysis: recommendations for optimal results. *Leukemia* 7, 2045–2053.

50. Beishuizen, A., Verhoeven, M. A., Mol, E. J., and van Dongen, J. J. (1994) Detection of immunoglobulin kappa light-chain gene rearrangement patterns by Southern blot analysis. *Leukemia* 8, 2228–2236.

51. Breit, T. M., Wolvers-Tettero, I. L., Beishuizen, A., Verhoeven, M. A., van Wering, E. R., and van Dongen, J. J. (1993) Southern blot patterns, frequencies, and junctional diversity of T-cell receptor-delta gene rearrangements in acute lymphoblastic leukemia. *Blood* 82, 3063–3074.

52. van Wering, E. R., van der Linden-Schrever, B. E., van der Velden, V. H. J., Szczepanski, T., and van Dongen, J. J. M. (2001) T-lymphocytes in bone marrow samples of children with acute lymphoblastic leukemia during and after chemotherapy might hamper PCR-based minimal residual disease studies. *Leukemia* 15, 1301–1303.

53. van Wering, E. R., van der Linden-Schrever, B. E., Szczepanski, T., Willemse, M. J., Baars, E. A., van Wijngaarde-Schmitz, H. M., Kamps, W. A., and van Dongen, J. J. M. (2000) Regenerating normal B-cell precursors during and after treatment of acute lymphoblastic leukaemia: implications for monitoring of minimal residual disease. *British Journal of Haematology* 110, 139–146.

54. van Lochem, E. G., Wiegers, Y. M., van den Beemd, R., Hahlen, K., van Dongen, J. J. M., and Hooijkaas, H. (2000) Regeneration pattern of precursor-B-cells in bone marrow of acute lymphoblastic leukemia patients depends on the type of preceding chemotherapy. *Leukemia* 14, 688–695.

55. Van der Velden, V. H. J., Wijkhuijs, J. M., and Van Dongen, J. J. M. (2008) Non-specific amplification of patient-specific Ig/TCR gene rearrangements depends on the time point during therapy: implications for minimal residual disease monitoring. *Leukemia* 22, 641–644.

56. van der Velden, V. H., Hoogeveen, P. G., Pieters, R., and van Dongen, J. J. (2006) Impact of two independent bone marrow samples on minimal residual disease monitoring in childhood acute lymphoblastic leukaemia. *British Journal of Haematolology* 133, 382–388.

57. van der Velden, V. H. J., Jacobs, D. C., Wijkhuijs, A. J., Comans-Bitter, W. M., Willemse, M. J., Hahlen, K., Kamps, W. A., van Wering, E. R., and van Dongen, J. J. M. (2002) Minimal residual disease levels in bone marrow and peripheral blood are comparable in children with T cell acute lymphoblastic leukemia (ALL), but not in precursor-B-ALL. *Leukemia* 16, 1432–1436.

58. Moppett, J., van der Velden, V. H., Wijkhuijs, A. J., Hancock, J., van Dongen, J. J., and Goulden, N. (2003) Inhibition affecting RQ-PCR-based assessment of minimal residual disease in acute lymphoblastic leukemia: Reversal by addition of bovine serum albumin. *Leukemia* 17, 268–270.

Chapter 8

Array-Based Comparative Genomic Hybridization as a Tool for Analyzing the Leukemia Genome

Jon C. Strefford and Helen Parker

Summary

Comparative genomic hybridization (CGH) is arguably the most significant technical development in the molecular cytogenetics era, and has contributed considerably to our further understanding of the cancer genome. In essence, DNA from a cancer specimen (test DNA) labeled with the fluorescence reporter molecule (or fluorochrome) is hybridized to a target genome in the presence of a differentially labeled control DNA (reference DNA). The two DNA populations compete for hybridization sites on normal metaphase chromosomes, so that the resulting fluorescence ratio is a reflection of the copy number change in the test sample. The copy number changes are mapped to their position on the chromosome template. Over recent years, the chromosomal template has been largely superseded by microarray formats (aCGH), in which changes in copy number can be mapped to the genome sequence at a high resolution. This advance allows the genome to be studied at an unbridled resolution and at a high-throughput, whilst posing several technical, statistical and interpretive challenges. It is the aim of this chapter to introduce the fundamental concepts of aCGH and to provide an overview of the steps involved in a successful aCGH processing. The materials required for BAC and oligonucleotide aCGH are included, with detailed methods and a range of refinements to improve the success rate and quality of aCGH data.

Key words: Comparative genomic hybridization, CGH, Microarray, Copy number changes, Acute lymphoblastic leukemia

1. Introduction

Screening the entire genome in a single reaction with chromosomal comparative genomic hybridization (CGH, **Fig. 1**) offered huge advantages over laborious gene targeted techniques such as

C.W.E. So (ed.), Leukemia, *Methods in Molecular Biology, vol. 538*
© Humana Press, a part of Springer Science + Business Media, LLC 2009
DOI: 10.1007/978-1-59745-418-6_8

Southern analysis, polymerase chain reaction (PCR) and fluorescence in situ hybridization (FISH) *(1)*. However, the metaphase template is made up of highly condensed super-coiled DNA resulting in a limited resolution of 8–10 Mb for a single copy gain or loss. The smallest copy number gains detected by cCGH are in the range of 2 Mb in size, but this is dependent on the level of the copy number gain compared to the reference genome. While capable of highlighting recurrent aberrant chromosomal regions and facilitating positional cloning studies, the resolution of cCGH is unable to precisely localize sequences or genes of interest. In addition, the analysis of cCGH is incompatible with automation, as a skilled cytogeneticist is required to interpret the inverted 4′,6-diamidino-2-phenylindole (DAPI)-stained chromosome banding patterns of the template chromosomes.

cCGH has been largely superseded by DNA microarray formats (array CGH or aCGH) which offers considerable improvements in resolution and provides mapping of the copy number directly onto the genome sequence (**Fig. 1**) *(2)*. This involves the same competitive hybridization of a test and reference genome as cCGH, but the hybridization template comprises of a nucleic acid sequence of known genomic location spotted onto an array slide, used to assess the genomic location of the copy number changes in the test DNA sample. The initial approaches used arrays made from large-insert genomic clones such as bacterial artificial chromosomes (BAC) *(3)*. Producing sufficient BAC DNA and assuring its quality is difficult

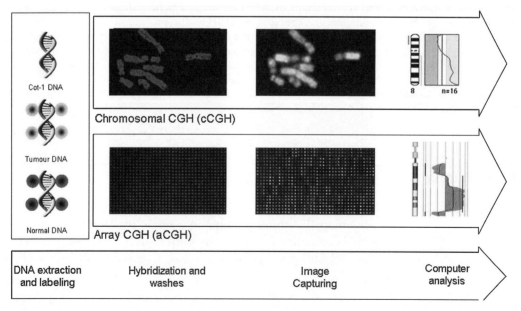

Fig. 1. Comparative genomic hybridization (CGH) at the chromosomal and array level. Nick translation labeling is adequate for cCGH, but random-primer based labeling procedures are required for array platforms. After labeling, DNA samples compete for hybridization sites on the chromosome or array template. After hybridization and washes, the resulting hybridization ratio is a reflection of the copy number changes in the tumor sample.

and time-consuming, so a great deal of effort has been invested into DNA amplification procedures. These techniques include ligation-mediated polymerase chain reaction (PCR) *(4)*, degenerate primer PCR *(5)* and rolling cycle amplification *(6)*. A range of BAC platforms now provide total human genome coverage *(7, 8)*. Arrays fabricated from less complex nucleic acids such as cDNAs *(9)*, selected PCR products *(10)* and oligonucleotides *(11–13)* are now widely available.

Although aCGH platforms vary, sample processing is similar. Firstly, the test and reference DNA samples are assessed for both quality and quantity. Often an enzyme digestion step is included to ensure genomic DNA of the correct fragment size for hybridization onto the array. The fragmented DNA samples are differentially random-primer labeled with fluorescent reporter molecules, before several steps of purification. These purification steps are included to remove unincorporated fluorochromes, which dramatically improve the quality of aCGH data. The test and reference samples are competitively hybridized to the microarray containing sequences representing the target genome where the labeled fragments compete for their complementary sites. This is achieved in the presence of Cot-1 DNA, which suppresses the repetitive regions throughout the genome. After hybridization, incompletely bound DNA molecules are removed with a series of washes and the arrays are dried and scanned. Data is extracted, aligned with the genome sequence and the copy number changes are identified. With certain array platforms a dye-swap experiment may be performed, in which the test DNA labeled with both fluorescent molecules is hybridized with the oppositely labeled reference DNA sample. These duplicate experiments proved more statistically significant data. The multifaceted processes of aCGH are highly complex and it is beyond the scope of this chapter to cover them in their entirety. The purpose of this chapter is to introduce the fundamental concepts of aCGH processing and to highlight those steps critical to the successful completion of the process.

1.1. Current Platforms

A range of aCGH platforms are widely available, which fall into two basic categories. The first is constructed from large-insert DNA clones (hereafter referred as 'BAC aCGH') such as yeast artificial chromosomes (YAC; 0.2–2 Mb in size), bacterial artificial chromosomes (BAC; 50–70 kb), P1 (70–100 kb), PAC (130–150 kb) or cosmids (30–45 kb). BAC aCGH platforms often contain duplicate or triplicate copies of the same feature, allowing hybridization evaluation and providing more robust data. The second comprises of those fabricated with shorter oligonucleotide sequences (of approximately 60 bp in size, hereafter referred as 'Oligo aCGH'). Both systems result in clones that share sequence homology with known regions of the human genome which can be used to construct a high-resolution genomic template for CGH hybridization. BAC platforms have the advantage of high signal intensities and the easy confirmation of results by FISH using the same clones as spotted onto the array. The production of consistently high-quality BAC aCGH arrays can be problematical and laborious. It can be difficult to produce adequate quantities of DNA for array manufacture. Oligonucleotide arrays can be spotted at high-density, resulting in greater resolution and with highly statistically significant data output. Due to the efficient in situ fabrication process, custom arrays targeting specific subsets of the genome are readily available. However, confirmation of the copy number changes may not be possible using traditional molecular cytogenetic techniques as it is often difficult to identify FISH probes close to the breakpoints. This has been largely overcome by the development of alternative molecular approaches such as quantitative genomic PCR, multiplex ligation-dependant probe amplification (MLPA) *(14)* or molecular copy number counting (MCC) *(15)*.

BAC aCGH platforms include the gene-targeted Array300 from Vysis (distributed by Abbott Diagnostics). The Array300 contains features spotted in triplicate which targets 287 loci including telomeres, microdeletions, oncogenes and tumor suppressor genes. In conjunction with the GenoSensor image capture and analysis system, this platform allows abnormal gene amplifications and deletions to be detected at a sensitivity of a single copy number change. Several other commercial companies offer BAC platforms at approximately 1 Mb resolution. In particular, BlueGnome market their 'CytoChip', which contains more than 3,300 DNA clones spotted at 1 Mb genomic resolution as well as a further 400 selected to cover regions associated with 90 known genetic conditions. Spectral Genomics market the Spectral Chip 2600 array which includes 2,600 large-insert DNA clones at a 1 Mb resolution. The use of this platform is included in **Subheading 3**. Oligo aCGH platforms are beginning to dominate the market, with several flexible solutions. Agilent Technologies use inkjet SurePrint array fabrication, which in combination with their eArray software allows complete flexibility in array design. They currently also offer several 'off the shelf' products, including whole genome profiling with 44,000 (44 k) and 244,000 (244 k) oligonucleotides positioned throughout the human genome (the protocols presented in the Oligo aCGH section focus on the use of these arrays). Multiple copies of the 44 k array can be multipacked onto a single slide to reduce cost. NimbleGen market an ultra-high resolution platform with feature densities of 385,000 oligonucleotides with flexibility comparable to the Agilent platform. A comprehensive list of commercial and academic array manufacturers is provided in **Table 1**.

Table 1
Commercial sources of microarrays for CGH, including product name, provider, and web address

Array type	Product name	Provider	Web address
BAC	GenoSensor Array 300	Abbott Diagnostics	https://www.vysis.com/
	Spectral arrays	Perkin Elmer	http://www.spectralgenomics.com/
	1 Mb BAC CGH	Array Genomics	http://www.arraygenomics.com/
	CytoChip	Cambridge BlueGnome	http://www.cytochip.com/
	Hum32 k, Hum Array3.2	UCSF Cancer Centre	http://www.cancer.ucsf.edu/array/
	SMRT Array	BC Cancer Centre	http://www.bccrc.ca/arraycgh/
Oligo	244A CGH array	Agilent	http://www.chem.agilent.com/
	Fine-tiling arrays	NimbleGen	http://www.nimblegen.com/
	OGT CGH arrays	Oxford Gene Technology	http://www.ogt.co.uk/
	GeneChip® Arrays	Affymetrix	http://www.affymetrix.com/

1.2. Applications to Childhood Leukemia

Over recent years, preliminary data has been emerging on the application of aCGH to the study of the acute leukemia genome. In an attempt to unveil recurrent genomic alterations in acute lymphoblastic leukemia (ALL) patients who lack established chromosomal changes of diagnostic or prognostic significance, we have analyzed a series of 58 patients with aCGH *(16)*. Copy number alterations were observed in 83% of the patients and some novel regions of recurrent copy number alterations were revealed. We showed that the genome of these patients was often more complex than seen by conventional cytogenetics. Similar observations were made by Paulsson and co-workers in a small series of patients with high hyperdiploidy *(17)*.

Intrachromosomal amplification of chromosome 21 (iAMP21) is arguably the most important molecular prognostic marker among patients with B-lineage ALL identified in recent years. These patients have a significantly inferior event free survival at 5 years compared with other ALL patients: 29% versus 78% *(18)*. Employing aCGH, we have shown a common region of amplification flanking the *RUNX1* gene, subtelomeric deletions and considerable copy number heterogeneity around the centromere in these iAMP21 patients *(19)*. aCGH has also identified a number of novel genetic abnormalities in T-lineage ALL, worthy of further study. Duplications of 9q34 have recently been highlighted as a recurrent finding in pediatric T-cell ALL with amplification of a common region of approximately 4 Mb including the *NOTCH1* gene *(20)*. Other work from this group highlighted a novel recurrent deletion on the short arm of chromosome 11, del(11)(p12p13) *(21)*, providing evidence of a novel mechanism leading to the activation of the *LMO2* gene in pediatric T-ALL patients. Although amplification of the *ABL1* gene was originally observed in 6% of T-ALL *(22)*, a subsequent study characterized is as an episomal amplification of an in-frame fusion between exon 31 of *NUP214* and exon 2 of *ABL1 (23)*.

2. Materials

2.1. Quantification of DNA and Assessment of Quality

1. UV-VIS spectrophotometer (NanoDrop ND-1000).
2. Qubit™ fluorometer (Invitrogen Cat. no. Q32857).
3. Quant-iT DNA assay kit; Quanti-iT dsDNA Broad Range (contains Quant-iT dsDNA BR reagent, Quant-iT buffer, component C) (Invitrogen Cat. no. Q33130).
4. Qubit assay tubes (Invitrogen Cat. no. Q32856).
5. Gel electrophoresis equipment.

2.2. Genomic DNA Amplification

There are a large number of kits available in the market. Several are listed below and the protocol presented later in this chapter is based on the REPL-g Mini Kit.

1. REPLI-g Mini Kit. Store at –80°C (contains REPLI-g Mini Reaction Buffer, REPLI-g Mini DNA Polymerase) (Qiagen Cat. no. 150025 or 150023).
2. GenomiPhi High Yield DNA Amplification Kit (GE Healthcare Cat. no. 25-6600-20).
3. GenomePlex Complete Whole Genome Amplification (WGA) Kit (Sigma-Aldrich Cat no. WGA2).

2.3. BAC aCGH

2.3.1. Microarray Slides

Spectral Chip™ 2600 BAC Array Kit (5 Pack) (contains Spectral HYB Buffers) (Perkin Elmer Cat. no. 4027-0010).

2.3.2. Restriction Digest of Genomic DNA (See Note 1)

1. *Eco*RI restriction enzyme (10 U/µl). Store at –20°C (Invitrogen Cat. no. 15202-021) (*see* **Note 1**).
2. React 3 10× buffer (supplied with *Eco*RI restriction enzyme).
3. QIAprep Spin Miniprep Kit (contains Buffer PE, Buffer PB, QIAprep Spin Miniprep column, Buffer EB) (Qiagen Cat. no. 27106 or 27104) for clean-up of amplified-digested DNA.

4. Heat block or water bath which allows consistent temperatures of between 37°C and 100°C.

5. Genomic test DNA. Store at 4°C.

6. Reference DNA. Store at 4°C (Promega Cat. no. G1471 (male) Cat no. G1521 (female)).

7. Nuclease free water.

2.3.3. Fluorescent Labeling of Genomic DNA

1. BioPrime® Array CGH Genomic Labelling System (Invitrogen Cat. no. 18095011).

2. Cy3-dCTP & Cy5-dCTP (Perkin Elmer Cat no. NEL 576-577, *see* **Note 2**).

3. Spectral Labelling Buffer. Store at –20°C (Perkin Elmer Cat. no. 4040-0010).

4. 0.5 M EDTA (ethylenediaminetetraacetic acid), pH 8.0.

2.3.4. Microarray Hybridization

1. Spectral HYB Buffer I and II (supplied with the BAC array slides). Store at –20°C.

2. 5 M NaCl (sodium chloride).

3. Isopropanol.

4. 70% Ethanol.

5. 22 × 50 mm cover slips (VWR international 631-0148).

6. Aluminum foil.

7. Kapak Pouches (VWR international 11214-301).

8. Impulse Heat Sealer.

9. Rocking Platform Incubator (Shake 'N' Bake Hybridization Oven Boekel Scientific Cat. no. B6400).

2.3.5. Microarray Washing and Drying

1. Petri dishes.

2. Saline-sodium citrate buffer (SSC).

3. Sodium dodecyl sulphate (SDS).

4. Deionised formamide (*see* **Notes 3** and **4**).

5. Igepal (Sigma I7771).

6. Milli-Q water.

7. Tank of high purity nitrogen gas.

2.4. Oligo aCGH

2.4.1. Microarray Slides

Human genome oligo CGH microarray kit (Agilent Cat. no. G4411B).

2.4.2. Restriction Digest of Genomic DNA (See Note 5)

1. *Alu I* restriction enzyme (10 U/μl). Store at –20°C (Promega Cat. no. R6281) (*see* **Note 5**).

2. *Rsa I* restriction enzyme (10 U/μl). Store at –20°C (Promega Cat. no. R6371).

3. 10× Buffer C (supplied with restriction enzyme *Rsa I*).

4. Acetylated BSA (supplied with restriction enzyme *Rsa I*).

5. Heat block or water bath which allows consistent temperatures of between 37 and 100°C.

6. Genomic test DNA. Store at 4°C.

7. Reference DNA. Store at 4°C (Promega Cat. no. G1471 (male) Cat no. G1521 (female)).

8. Nuclease free water.

2.4.3. Fluorescent Labelling of Genomic DNA

1. Genomic DNA Labelling Kit PLUS (contains random primers, 5× buffer, 10× dNTP, exo-klenow fragment). Store at –20°C (Agilent Cat. no. 5188-5309).

2. Clean-up of labeled genomic DNA.

3. 1× TE (Tris–EDTA) buffer (pH 8.0) (Promega Cat. no. V6231).

4. Microcon YM-30 filter units (Millipore Cat. no. 42410).

2.4.4. Preparation of Labeled DNA for Hybridization

1. Human Cot-1 DNA. Store at –20°C (Invitrogen Cat. no. 15279-011).

2. Agilent oligo aCGH hybridization kit (contains 10× blocking agent, 2× hybridization buffer, *see* **Note 6**). Store at 4°C (Agilent Cat. no. 5188-5220).

2.4.5. Microarray Hybridization

1. Hybridisation chambers (Agilent Cat. no. G2534A).

2. Hybridisation chamber gasket slides (Agilent Cat. no. G2534-60003).

3. Hybridisation oven (Agilent Cat. no. G2545A).

4. Hybridisation oven rotator (Agilent Cat. no. G2530-60029).

2.4.6. Microarray Washing and Drying

1. Agilent oligo aCGH wash buffer 1 and 2 set (Agilent Cat. no. 5188-5226).

2. Stabilization and drying solution (*see* **Note 7**) (Agilent Cat. no. 5185-5979).

3. Acetonitrile (Sigma Cat. no. 271004-1l).

4. 250-ml capacity slide staining dish, with slide rack (×5) (Wheaton Cat. no. 900200).

2.5. Scanning

All scanning procedures in this chapter use the following scanner:

1. Agilent Microarray scanner (Agilent Cat. no. G2565BA).

2.6. Feature Extraction

1. Agilent feature extraction software.

2.7. Data Analysis

Several software platforms are discussed earlier in the chapter, but two are focused upon in **Subheadings 2** and **3**.

1. SpectralWare software (this software performs the feature extraction as well).
2. CGH Analytics software (*see* **Note 8**).

3. Methods

3.1. Quantification of DNA and Assessment of Quality

For optimal performance use high quality, intact genomic DNA (*see* **Notes 9** and **10**).

3.1.1. UV Absorbance-Based Spectrophotometer Quantification of DNA

To quantify and measure the purity of the DNA sample, a Nano-Drop-1000 UV-VIS spectrophotometer is recommended. UV light is absorbed by the DNA at a wavelength of 260 nm, and by proteins at 280 and 230 nm. Other contaminates such as carbohydrates also absorb at 230 nm. NanoDrop-1000 measures absorbance of each of these wavelengths and calculates the concentration of the DNA from the 260 nm absorbance. The 260/280 nm and 260/230 nm ratios indicate the degree of sample contamination by protein or carbohydrates. The ratio should fall between 1.5 and 2. A lower value indicates high level contamination.

3.1.2. Fluorescent Quantification of DNA

Due to the inaccuracy of measuring DNA at low concentrations with spectrophotometer-based systems, it is recommended that a fluorescent method is also used (*see* **Note 11**). Fluorescence assays are potentially several magnitudes more sensitive that the most sensitive UV absorbance measurements particularly for measuring concentrations of between 10 pg/μl and 1,000 ng/μl. One such kit is the Quant-iT DNA broad range assay kit that allows simple and sensitive concentration measurements, even in the presence of RNA and many common contaminants.

1. Label the lids of the assay tubes (*see* **Note 12**) required for the standards and user samples.
2. Prepare control 1 by dilution of the 100 ng/μl λ dsDNA BR standard from the Component C.
3. Prepare control 2 by dilution of the 100 ng/μl λ dsDNA BR standard from the Component C.
4. Make the working solution by diluting the Quant-iT™ dsDNA BR reagent 1:200 in Quant-iT buffer.
5. Vortex all tubes briefly.
6. Incubate the tubes for 2 min at room temperature.

7. Calibrate the Qubit fluorometer using controls 1 and 2.

8. Analyze DNA concentration with the fluorometer.

9. Multiply by the value given by the dilution factor to determine concentration of your original sample (*see* **Note 13**).

3.1.3. Quality Assessment of DNA

To assess DNA quality, gel electrophoresis is recommended. Intact genomic DNA, run through a 1% agarose gel, for approximately 1 h, at 100 V will be visualized as a discrete band. Degraded DNA will appear as a smear.

3.2. Genomic Amplification

Amplification of genomic DNA may be performed if insufficient amounts are available (i.e., 0.1–0.5 µg) (*see* **Note 14**). High quality, intact DNA is required.

1. Equilibrate heat blocks or water baths to 30 and 65°C.

2. Add 0.1 µl of genomic DNA to a 1.5-ml nuclease-free tube. Add nuclease-free water to bring to a final volume of 20 µl.

3. Thaw all components and move to ice.

4. Prepare the master mix by combining 29 µl reaction buffer and 1 µl DNA polymerase, on ice. Quick freeze the remainder of components on dry ice and return to storage at –80°C.

5. In the tubes containing the genomic DNA, add 30 µl of master mix to make a total volume of 50 µl.

6. Transfer the sample tubes to a circulating water bath or heat block at 30°C for 16 h.

7. Transfer the sample tubes to a circulating water bath or heat block at 65°C for 10 min to inactivate the enzymes, move to ice.

3.3. BAC aCGH Methodology

3.3.1. Restriction Digest of Genomic DNA

1. Equilibrate heat blocks or water baths to 37°C and 72°C.

2. Add 1 µg of genomic test DNA to two separate 1.5-ml nuclease-free tubes, repeat with the reference DNA. Add nuclease-free water to bring to a final volume of 43 µl.

3. On ice, add 5 µl of React 3 10× buffer and 2 µl *Eco* R1 to each reaction tube. Mix the reactions by flicking the tube, and pulse spin.

4. Transfer the samples to 37°C for 16 h.

5. Transfer the samples to 72°C for 10 min to inactivate the enzymes (*see* **Note 15**).

3.3.2. Cleanup of Digested DNA

Before using for the first time, prepare Buffer PE from the QIAprep Spin Miniprep Kit by adding 100% ethanol to the Buffer PE bottle (add the correct quantity of ethanol for the correct volume of buffer).

1. Add 500 µl Buffer PB to each 100 µl sample.

2. Apply sample to a Miniprep Column. Spin for 1 min at 17,900 × g and discard the flow-through.

3. Add 750 µl Buffer PE to each Miniprep Column. Spin for 1 min at 17,900 × g and discard the flow-through.

4. Spin for 60 s at 17,900 × g to remove residual wash buffer.

5. Place the Miniprep Column in a clean 1.5-µl tube.

6. To elute the DNA, add 25 µl Buffer EB to the centre of each spin column, and incubate at room temperature for 1 min.

7. Spin for 1 min at 17,900 × g to collect purified DNA.

8. Quantify the DNA using the NanoDrop ND-1000 UV-VIS spectrophotometer. At least 500 ng of digested DNA from each sample should be used for labeling.

3.3.3. Fluorescent Labelling of Genomic DNA

1. Equilibrate heat blocks or water baths to 100°C, 37 and 65°C.

2. Add nuclease-free water to the reaction tubes to bring to a volume of 25 µl, add 20 µl of 2.5× random primers/reaction buffer mix from the BioPrime® Array CGH Genomic Labelling System. Mix the samples well and pulse spin.

3. Transfer the samples to a heat block or circulating water bath at 100°C for 5 min. Place on ice for 5 min and pulse spin again.

4. Prepare a labeling mastermix by combining 2.5 µl Spectral Labelling Buffer, 1.5 µl Cy3-dCTP or Cy5-dCTP and 1 µl klenow fragment per sample.

5. Add 5 µl of Cy3-dCTP mastermix to one test and one reference DNA sample, and 5 µl of Cy5-dCTP mastermix to the remaining test and reference DNA samples. Mix the samples and pulse spin.

6. Transfer the samples to a heat block or water bath at 37°C for 2 h (*see* **Note 16**).

7. Add 5 µl of 0.5 M EDTA pH 8.0 to each sample. Transfer to a heat block or water bath at 72°C for 10 min to inactivate the enzymes, then move to ice.

8. Samples can be stored at –20°C or hybridized directly.

3.3.4. Microarray Hybridisation

1. Add 45 µl Hybridisation Buffer I to each tube containing the combines of differentially labeled test and reference DNA samples from **Subheading 3.3.3.8** (*see* **Note 17**).

2. Precipitate the samples by adding 12.9 µl 5 M NaCl and 130 µl isopropanol. Mix the samples and incubate at room temperature, in the dark for 20 min.

3. Centrifuge at ≥10,000 × g for 20 min. Remove the supernatant and add 500 µl 70% ethanol. Centrifuge at ≥10,000 × g for 3 min, remove the supernatant and air dry the pellet for 10 min at room temperature, in the dark.

4. Add 10 µl nuclease-free water to the pellets. Let stand at room temperature for 10 min. Ensure the pellets are thoroughly resuspended and add 30 µl Spectral hybridization Buffer II. Mix well by pipetting.

5. Denature the DNA by transferring the samples to 72°C for 10 min, then place on ice for 5 min.

6. Transfer the samples to 37°C for 30 min.

7. Pipette each sample in a line down the centre of an array. A diagonal mark on the lower right hand corner indicates the upright bottom of the slide when viewed vertically. Cover with a 22 × 60 mm cover slip (*see* **Note 18**).

8. Place each slide in a hybridization chamber. Add 10 µl of water to the wells on both sides of each chamber (*see* **Note 19**).

9. Close the chambers, individually wrap them with aluminum foil and place inside separate plastic pouches, with wet paper towels to prevent evaporation.

10. Heat seal the pouches and place them in a shaking platform incubator at 37°C for 16 h.

3.3.5. Microarray Washing and Drying

1. Pre-warm 25 ml of the following solutions at 50°C, in individual Petri dishes, for a maximum of 2 h; 2× SSC, 50% deionized formamide 2× SSC, 0.1% Igepal, 0.2× SSC.

2. Briefly soak the slide in 2× SSC, 0.5% SDS (make fresh each time) at room temperature and slide the cover slip off using clean forceps. Avoid peeling off the cover slip by force.

3. Using forceps, transfer the slides to the pre-warmed 2× SSC, 50% formamide. Incubate in a shaking incubator at 50°C for 20 min.

4. Repeat **step 2** using 2× SSC, 0.1% Igepal.

5. Repeat **step 2** using 2× SSC for 10 min.

6. Transfer the slides to a petri dish of Milli-Q water at room temperature. Rock for 5 s.

7. Repeat **step 6** using a fresh Petri dish of water.

8. Immediately dry the slides with a stream of nitrogen gas.

9. Store the slides in a dark box until scanned.

10. Clean the hybridization chambers by soaking for 1 day in distilled water, a second day in Milli-Q water and dry with tissue.

3.4. Oligo aCGH Methodology

3.4.1. Restriction Digest of Genomic DNA

1. *See* **Note 20**: Equilibrate heat blocks or water baths to 37 and 65°C.

2. Thaw reagents. Briefly vortex 10× Buffer C and pulse spin. Store reagents on ice.

3. Add 0.5–3 µg of genomic test DNA and reference DNA to separate 1.5-ml nuclease-free tubes. Add nuclease-free water to bring to a final volume of 20.2 µl.

4. Prepare a digestion mastermix by combining 2.0 µl nuclease-free water, 2.6 µl 10× buffer C, 0.2 µl acetylated BSA, and 0.5 µl of Alu I and Rsa I, on ice, in the order indicated.

5. Add 5.8 µl of digestion mastermix to each reaction tube containing the genomic DNA to make a total volume of 26 µl.

6. Transfer the samples to a heat block or water bath at 37°C for 2 h.

7. Transfer the samples to a heat block or water bath at 65°C for 20 min to inactivate the enzymes, then move to ice (*see* **Note 21**).

3.4.2. Fluorescent Labelling of Genomic DNA (See Note 22)

1. Equilibrate heat blocks or water baths to 95, 37, and 65°C.

2. Add 5 µl of random primers to each reaction tube to make a total volume of 29 µl. Mix by pipetting up and down gently.

3. Transfer the samples to 95°C for 3 min, then place on ice for 5 min.

4. Prepare a labeling mastermix by combining 2 µl nuclease-free water, 10 µl 5× buffer, 5 µl 10× dNTP, 3 µl Cy3-dUTP or Cy5-dUTP and 1 µl exo-klenow, on ice, in the order indicated.

5. Add 21 µl of labeling mastermix to each reaction tube. Test DNA and reference DNA are differentially labeled.

6. Transfer the samples to 37°C for 2 h.

7. Transfer the samples at 65°C for 10 min to inactivate the enzymes, and then move to ice.

8. Reactions can be stored overnight at –20°C, in the dark.

3.4.3. Cleanup of Labeled Genomic DNA

1. Add 430 µl of 1 × TE buffer (pH 8.0) to each reaction tube.

2. Place a Microcon YM-30 filter into a 1.5-ml tube and load each sample into the filter. Centrifuge for 10 min at 8,000 × g (room temperature). Discard the flow-through.

3. Add 480 µl of 1 × TE to each filter. Centrifuge for 10 min at 8,000 × g (room temperature). Discard the flow-through.

4. Invert the filter into a fresh 1.5-ml tube. Centrifuge for 1 min at 8,000 × g (room temperature).

5. Measure the volume of each elute. If the volume exceeds 80.5 µl, return the sample to its filter and centrifuge for 1 min at 8,000 × g (room temperature). Discard the flow-through (*see* **Note 22**).

6. Repeat **steps 4** and **5** until each sample volume is ≤ 80.5 µl.

7. Bring the sample volumes to 80.5 µl with 1 × TE. Remove 2 µl of each sample to determine the yield and specific

activity using the microarray function of the NanoDrop ND-1000 UV-VIS Spectrophotometer.

8. Combine the appropriate cyanine 5-labeled and cyanine 3-labeled samples for a total mixture volume of 158 μl.

9. Reactions can be stored overnight at –20°C, in the dark.

3.4.4. Preparation of Labeled DNA for Hybridisation

1. Add 1,350 μl nuclease-free water to the lyophilized 10× Blocking Agent. Leave at room temperature for 60 min to reconstitute sample. Store at –20°C when reconstituted.

2. Equilibrate heat blocks or water baths to 95 and 37°C.

3. Add 50 μl human Cot-1 DNA, 52 μl 10× blocking agent and 260 μl 2× hybridization buffer to each sample. Mix by pipetting up and down gently and pulse spin.

4. Transfer the samples to 95°C for 3 min. Immediately transfer the samples to 37°C for 3 min.

5. Centrifuge the sample for 1 min at $17,900 \times g$.

3.4.5. Microarray Hybridisation

1. Load a clean gasket slide into the SureHyb hybridization chamber base with the label facing up and aligned with the rectangular section of the chamber base.

2. Slowly dispense 490 μl of hybridization sample mixture into the gasket well. This should be done by slowly dispensing the solution as you move the pipette along the length of the glass slide. Do not allow the sample to touch the rubber seal (*see* **Note 23**).

3. Place a microarray onto the gasket slide, so the numeric barcode side is facing up and the labeled barcode is facing down (*see* **Note 24**). Assure that the sandwich-pair is properly aligned (*see* **Note 25**).

4. Place the chamber cover onto the sandwiched slides and slide the clamp assembly onto both pieces. Hand-tighten the clamp onto the chamber.

5. Vertically rotate the assembled chamber to wet the slides and assess the mobility of the bubbles (*see* **Note 26**). Tap the assembly on a hard surface to move stationary bubbles.

6. Place the chamber in the rotator rack in a hybridization oven set at 65°C. Ensure the rotator rack is correctly balanced. Rotate at 20 rpm for 40 h (*see* **Note 27**).

3.4.6. Wash Preparation

1. Always use clean equipment when conducting the wash procedures. Use only dishes that are dedicated for use in aCGH experiments.

2. The temperature of Oligo aCGH wash buffer 2 must be at 37°C for optimal performance.

3. Dispense an appropriate volume of wash buffer 2 into a disposable plastic bottle and warm overnight at 37°C.

4. If the stabilization and drying solution shows visible precipitation, warming of the solution will be necessary to redissolve the compound.

5. Warm the solution overnight at 37°C in a closed container with sufficient head space to allow for expansion.

6. Gently shake the container to obtain a homologous solution.

7. After the precipitate is completely dissolved, allow the solution to equilibrate to room temperature prior to use.

3.4.7. Microarray Washing and Drying

1. Always use fresh oligo aCGH wash buffer 1 and 2 for each wash of up to five slides.

2. The acetonitrile and stabilization and drying solution may be used for washing a total of 20 slides (*see* **Note 28**).

3. Completely fill slide-staining dish 1 with wash buffer 1 at room temperature.

4. Place a slide rack into slide-staining dish 2 and add a magnetic stir bar. Fill with enough wash buffer 1, at room temperature, to cover the slide rack. Place on a magnetic stir plate.

5. Place slide-staining dish 3, and a magnetic stir bar on a magnetic stir plate.

6. In the fume hood, fill slide-staining dish 4 approximately ¾ full with acetonitrile. Add a magnetic stir bar and place the dish on a magnetic stir plate.

7. In the fume hood, fill slide-staining dish 5 approximately ¾ full with stabilization and drying Solution. Add a magnetic stir bar and place the dish on a magnetic stir plate.

8. Remove one hybridization chamber from the incubator. Place it on a flat surface, loosen and slide off the clamp assembly before removing the cover.

9. Remove the array-gasket sandwich from the chamber base by lifting the slides from their ends. Without letting go of the slides, quickly transfer them to slide-staining dish 1, and completely submerge them in Wash Buffer 1.

10. Pry the sandwich open from the barcode end using the blunt ends of the provided forceps. Drop the gasket slide to the bottom of the staining dish. Remove the microarray slide and place it into the slide rack in slide-staining dish 2, with minimum exposure to air (*see* **Note 29**).

11. Repeat **steps 8** and **9** for up to four additional slides. Washing of a maximum of five slides at 1 time is advised to facilitate uniform washing.

12. When all slides in the batch are placed in slide-staining dish 2, stir for 5 min.

13. To prevent wash buffer 2 from cooling down leave it in the incubator or water bath until there are approximately 30 s of wash 1 left, then pour it into slide-staining dish 3. Transfer the slide rack into slide-staining dish 3 and stir for 1 min (*see* **Note** 30).

14. Remove the slide rack from slide-staining dish 3 and tilt it slightly to minimize wash buffer carry-over. Immediately transfer the slide rack to slide-staining dish 4 containing acetonitrile, and stir using setting 4 for 1 min.

15. Transfer the slide rack to slide-staining dish 5 filled with stabilization and drying solution and stir using setting 4 for 30 s. Slowly remove the slide rack over 5–10 s to minimize droplets on the slides (*see* **Notes 31** and **32**).

3.4.8. Cleaning the Equipment

1. Do not use detergent to wash the staining dishes as some detergents may leave fluorescent residue on the dishes.

2. Clean with acetonitrile. Acetonitrile wash removes any residue of stabilization and drying solution from the slide-staining dishes, racks and stir bars.

3. Place the slide rack and stir bar into the slide-staining dish and transfer to a magnetic stir plate.

4. Fill the dish with acetonitrile.

5. Turn on the stir plate and wash at room temperature for 5 min using setting 4.

6. Discard the acetonitrile appropriately.

7. Repeat **steps 1–4**.

8. Air dry everything in the vented fume hood.

9. Run copious amounts of Milli-Q water through the slide-staining dishes, racks and stir bars. Empty out the water collected in the dishes at least 5 times, until all traces of contaminating material are removed.

3.5. Array Scanning

Scan the slides immediately after washing to minimize the impact of environmental oxidants on the signal intensities.

1. Assemble the slides into the slide holders for the scanner such that the active side of the array is facing up and will be covered when the slide holder is closed. The lasers scan through the glass slide rather than across the surface.

2. Place the assembled slide holders into the array carousel.

3. Use the scan control software to indicate the following; which slots the arrays are located in, the scan area (provided with the microarrays), the dye channels to red and green and

the PMT to 100%. The scan resolution should be set to 10 and 5 μm for low and high density arrays respectively.

3.6. Image Capture and Analysis

Image capture and analysis is a critical step in the production of high quality aCGH data and can have considerable impact on subsequent analysis such as copy number identification. Analysis of the array image seeks to extract the fluorescent intensity of each spot or feature on the array, where the independent fluorescent wavelengths are specific for the tumor and normal hybridized DNA.

3.6.1. Image Acquisition

Prior to data analysis, all features on the microarray slide must be captured electronically at high resolution. This step is typically performed with laser-based scanning systems that acquire two differential wavelengths, either sequentially or simultaneously. The speed, throughput and resolution of the scanning equipment are variable, although scanning resolutions of between 5 and 10 μm are required for high-resolution oligo aCGH experiments. **Table 2** shows a range of commercially available scanners.

3.6.2. Image Analysis

There are now many commercial and academic providers of image analysis software (hereafter referred as 'feature extraction software'), Today, these types of analysis are rather complex and can not be completely explained here. However, in simplified terms they follow the processes shown in **Fig. 2**. The steps are divided into gridding, segmentation, intensity extraction and background correction. Regardless of the array platform, each spot or feature will need to be identified. This is accomplished with a 'gridding' protocol that aligns a predefined grid to the features on the array image. This is most often performed automatically, but sometimes requires review and refinement by the user, particularly for BAC arrays than can exhibit variability in fabrication. This 'grid template' file will generally be supplied with

Table 2
Commercially available scanner systems

Scanner	Supplier	Website
DNA microarray scanner	Agilent Technologies	http://www.chem.agilent.com/
GenePix	Axon Instruments	http://www.axon.com/
Revolution 4200	Vidar Systems Corporation	http://www.microarrayscanner.com/
ProScanArray HT	Perkin Elmer	http://www.perkinelmer.com/
NovaRay Detection Platform	Alpha Innotech Corporation	http://www.alphainnotech.com/
LS Reloaded	Tecan	http://www.tecan.com/

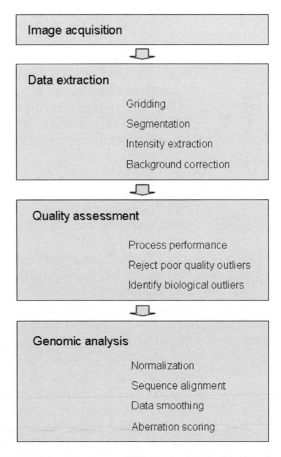

Fig. 2. The steps required to process aCGH data for the identification of copy number changes. After scanning (image acquisition), data is extracted and its quality is assessed. Genomic analysis allows regions of copy number changes to be identified and mapped onto the human genome.

the microarrays and installed in the feature extraction software. Once the features have been identified, they need to be separated from the background. The shape of each spot is identified, where the simplest assumption is that everything within a circle is a feature and everything outside is considered to be the background. More sophisticated models are also used, such as adaptive shape segmentation which imposes a 'best fit' shape to the feature and does not assume a circular structure. In addition, the pixel intensity profile of the feature can be used to more accurately identify signal verses background. Feature intensities are then extracted from both the background and feature followed by background correction. This is necessary as array images often contain signal in the areas between the features that represent non-specific/background fluorescence. This background can be accounted for by subtraction from the feature intensity to achieve a more accurate estimate of the biologically relevant feature signal. This type of background correction is often performed locally to the feature in question as levels of background can vary across the microarray.

Once the data has been extracted and corrected, software packages generally assess the data quality to allow efficient monitoring of microarray processing performance, reject any outlier features exhibiting poor characteristics, flag biologically relevant outliers and calculate statistical confidences. With sub-optimal data quality, these software packages identify key metrics to help pinpoint certain steps in the methodology where conditions may have been compromised. The most important quality measurement is derived from the standard deviation (SD) of the fluorescence ratio of all features on the array, where an increased SD indicates high levels of background and poor data quality. Typically, this entire process is coordinated by the 'feature extraction protocol' generally provided with the microarrays.

Table 3
Commercial and academic providers of analysis software

Software title	Provider	Web address
CGH Analytics	Agilent Technologies	http://www.chem.agilent.com/
BlueFuse	Cambridge BlueGnome	http://www.cambridgebluegnome.com/
SignalMap	NimbleGen	http://www.nimblegen.com/
SpectralWare	Spectral Genomics	http://www.spectralgenomics.com/
ImaGene-CGH	Biodiscovery	http://www.biodiscovery.com
LSPHMM	University of British Columbia	http://www.cs.ubc.ca/~sshah/acgh/
CGHPRO	Max Plank Institute	http://www.molgen.mpg.de/~abt_rop/molecular_cytogenetics/ArrayCGH/CGHPRO/
VAMP	InsitutCurie	http://bioinfo-out.curie.fr/actudb/
ArrayCyGHt	Catholic University of Korea	http://genomics.catholic.ac.kr/arrayCGH/
CGH-Explorer	Norwegian Radium Hospital	http://www.ifi.uio.no/forskning/grupper/bioinf/Papers/CGH/
CGH-Miner	University of Stanford	http://www-stat.stanford.edu/~wp57/CGH-Miner/
Normalise Suite	Ontario Cancer Institute	http://www.utoronto.ca/cancyto/software
CGHAnalyzer	Penn Genomic Institute	http://www.genomics.upenn.edu/
SeeGH	University of British Columbia	http://www.bccrc.ca/ArrayCGH/software.html

3.7. Genomic Analysis   Once the feature data has been extracted from the array, further
analysis is required to identify regions of copy number change.
There are now a large number of commercial and academic software providers, each with their own strengths and weaknesses.
A comprehensive list of current software packages is provided
in **Table 3**. An example of the application of different aCGH
platforms is shown in **Fig. 3**. Initially, both fluorescent channels
are combined to give ratio values for each unique feature (i.e.,
fluorescence ratios). All non-control features are aligned onto the
human genome sequence by assigning each feature to its correct
location. The data is normalized to a ratio value of 1.0 or a log
ratio of 0.0, so that copy number changes can be identified as
deviations of the fluorescence ratios away from these values
at any given genomic location. Cut-off values for this process
can be defined in several ways, but are often derived from the

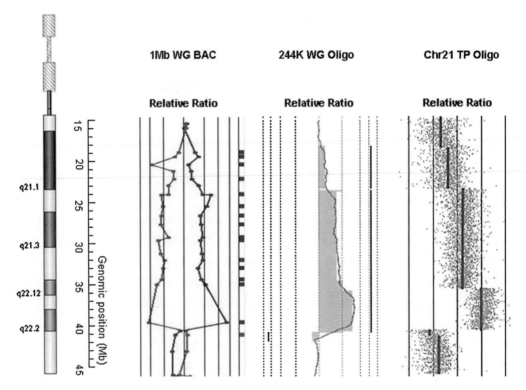

Fig. 3. Chromosome 21 copy number changes identified in patients with acute lymphoblastic leukaemia with varying
aCGH platforms and software packages. Chromosome 21 is positioned vertically on the left with genomic distances in
megabases. To the right of the chromosome 21 idiogram is a profile using a 1 Mb BAC from Spectral Genomics analyzed
with the SpectralWare software. Each dye-swap experiment is shown by the *light* and *dark lines*, and double deviation
from a central ratio of 1.0 showed a copy number gain when the dark profile deviates to the right. The same patient is
then shown using the 244 k whole genome array from Agilent. Deviation of the profile to the right shows copy number
gain. It can be clearly seen that using this increased resolution allows the region of amplification to be further refined.
Finally, to the right is a profile of the same patient with a high resolution chromosome 21 tiling path array from Nimble-
Gen. In essence, this array tiles through chromosome 21 with 60-bp oligonucleotides positioned every 50 bp along 21q,
resulting in entire sequence coverage.

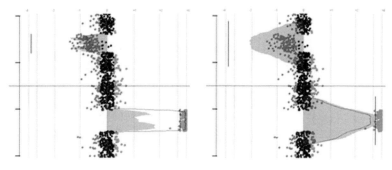

Data smoothing at 0.5Mb
genomic window

Data smoothing at 2.0Mb
genomic window

Fig. 4. *C-MYC* amplification in a patient with acute leukaemia profiled with the 244 k oligo aCGH platform. The spots represent lost, normal and gained copy number respectively for a single data points from the ratio values at a given genomic location. The extent of the shift to the right or left shows the degree of copy number gain or loss respectively relative to the normal control DNA sample. The *shaded area* shows the regions defined as abnormal by the Z-score-based aberration identification algorithm. Both *right* and *left* images show profiling data from the 8q24 region, where the data smoothing has been performed at 0.5- and 2.0-Mb window sizes. At larger window sizes, it can be seen that Z-score analysis can lose sensitivity at breakpoint identification.

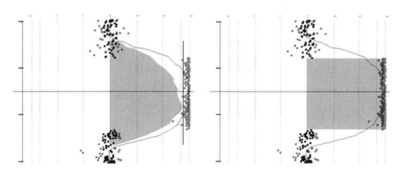

Z-score aberration scoring

ADM1 aberration scoring

Based on standard
deviation

Based on mathematical
prediction

Fig. 5. *C-MYC* amplicon mapping with oligo aCGH. Data is show as in **Fig. 4**. Both images show copy number data on the C-MYC region at 8q24, where the *left* and *right* images show breakpoint delineation with Z-scoring and ADM1 (aberration detection method 1) mathematical modeling respectively. Z-score analysis allows rapid identification of global copy number changes, but can often incorrectly score the extent of copy number changes, while ADM1 scoring can precisely identify breakpoint regions but risks the identification of false positive regions of copy number changes.

standard deviation of all the features on an array. For example, many investigators use cut-off values that are greater than 3 times the SD of the array. With BAC aCGH where the features are large sequences and exhibit intense signals, analysis can be performed on a feature by feature basis, particularly if a dye-swap experiment is included to improve statistical significance. With oligo aCGH, data is generated from a number of consecutive oligonucleotide features rather than a single feature, to vastly improve the significance of the data, a process often described as 'data smoothing' *(24–26)*. Data smoothing can be performed at fixed genomic distances or with a pre-defined number of features. Using relatively large genomic regions to determine copy number changes results in highly significant data, but resolution can be lost **(Fig. 4)**. Copy number changes can be identified using SD-based cut-offs, as in the case of Z-score analysis, or with more complex aberrations scoring algorithms that mathematically predict the most likely regions of copy number change **(Fig. 5)**.

4. Notes

1. As an alternative to enzyme digestion, the genomic DNA can be fragmented using a sonicator, at 100 amplitude for 1 min.

2. Cyanine 3-dUTP and Cyanine 5-dUTP are light sensitive and are subject to degradation by multiple freeze–thaw cycles. Aliquot appropriate volumes and minimize light exposure throughout the labeling procedure. These reagents are hazardous. Avoid inhalation, swallowing, and contact with skin.

3. Formamide is hazardous and may cause harm to unborn babies. Irritating to eyes, harmful by inhalation, by contact with skin and if swallowed.

4. Formamide can be deionized with mixed bead resin (Bio-Rad Cat. no. 143-6425). Briefly, 100 ml of formamide is treated with 5.0 g of resin and left to stir. The pH of the solution should be 7.0. Filter through 0.2-μm nylon filter (Nalgene Cat. no. 153-0020) and store at 4°C until required.

5. Several other enzymes can be used to fragment the DNA. The choice is important for labeling efficiency. A balance needs to be maintained between decreasing the average fragment size (which can improve labeling efficiency) and retaining sufficient sequence length to ensure complementary binding during hybridization.

6. Lithium chloride (LiCl) is a component of Agilent's 2× hybridization buffer. It is hazardous and may cause harm to breast-fed babies. There is a possible risk of impaired fertility. It targets central nervous system and is harmful by inhalation, by contact with skin and if swallowed. Lithium dodecyl sulphate (LDS) is a component of Agilent's 2× hybridization buffer. It is harmful by inhalation and irritating to eyes, respiratory system and skin. Triton is a component of Agilent's 2× hybridization buffer. It is harmful if swallowed and can cause serious damage to the eyes. Wear suitable PPE.

7. Stabilization and drying solution is designed to protect against ozone-induced degradation of cyanine dyes. If you are washing slides in an ozone-controlled environment and the ozone level is less then 5 ppb follow the wash instructions up to **step 11**. Remove the slides slowly from wash buffer 2, taking 5–10 s.

8. The PC requirements depend on the type and resolution of the array platform. A standard desktop PC will be perfectly adequate for low resolution arrays, such as a 1 Mb whole genome BAC or the 44 k oligo arrays. The array TIFF images themselves are scanned at low resolution and are therefore relatively small. The data files themselves contain quantities of data easily handled by, for example a 1.5 GHz Pentium III processor with 1GB RAM. However, when a high resolution array such as a 244 k oligonucleotide array is used the resulting scanned TIFF images and data files can be more than 200 Mb in size. This would be incredibly slow on a standard PC. We currently have a Quad-core Xeon processor with 2GB of RAM, which performs the analysis of this type of data quickly and efficiently.

9. The DNeasy tissue kit (Qiagen Cat. no. 69504) and PURE-GENE cell and tissue kit (Gentra Cat. no. D-5500A) are recommended for high quality genomic DNA isolation from cell lines and tissue samples.

10. Data produced with aCGH platforms is a representation of the total DNA in a sample. If the sample is heterogeneous or contains high levels of normal cell contamination, the ability of the experiment to detect any copy number changes could be severally compromised. This is particularly apparent when poor quality data is obtained which can compound the problem. It is recommended that only leukemia samples with more than 70% blast cells are used for aCGH analysis.

11. Samples exhibiting similar DNA concentrations by both UV and fluorescent techniques are suitable for aCGH analysis. This will avoid errors in the quantity of DNA added to the array and improve data quality.

12. Use only thin-wall, clear 0.5-ml PCR tubes. There are several other manufacturers such as VWR who produce the Axygen PCR-05-C tubes (Cat. no. 10011-830).

13. Several fluorometers including the Qubit can perform the calculations automatically. Refer to the manufacturer's documentation for instructions.

14. Amplification of less than 0.05 μg of genomic DNA is not recommended, and the signal to noise ratio may be decreased.

15. At this stage 2 μl of digested genomic DNA may be run on a 0.8% agarose gel to assess the completeness of the digestion. The majority of the digested products should be between 200 and 500 bp in length.

16. Alternately prepare double the volume of labeling mastermix, add 5 μl to each sample and transfer the samples to a heat block or water bath at 37°C for 1 h. Transfer the samples to a heat block at 100°C for 5 min, then move to ice for 5 min. Add an additional 5 μl master mix to each reaction tube and transfer to a heat block or water bath at 37°C for 1 h.

17. The color of the combined labeled DNA samples should be violet/purple, indicating successful labeling of both the test and reference DNA samples. If the sample is pink or blue, this could suggest that one of the labeling reactions was suboptimal.

18. It is essential that the entire array is covered, that air bubbles are avoided and that the cover slip is mobile. Keep the slides horizontal at all times from this point on.

19. It is vital that the microarray does not dry during hybridization. Ensure the array remains humidified and check the status of the chambers several times during hybridization. If the microarray does dry, the results are invariably unusable.

20. DNA clean-up is required when small volumes of genomic DNA have been amplified according to **Subheading 3.1.2**. Perform clean-up according to **Subheading 3.2.2**.

21. Instead of labeling, samples can be stored at –20°C until required.

22. It is recommended that instead of only cleaning up the labeled sample twice if the sample volume is too large, all samples should be passed through the column twice as this removes more unincorporated fluorochromes and dramatically improves the results.

23. Ensure that the majority of the sample is dispensed at the barcoded end of the gasket slide.

24. The microarray slide can be positioned so that the two corners furthest from the barcode are touching the correspond-

ing corners of the gasket slide. The remaining corners of the slide can then be lowered to a distance of a few millimeters above the gasket slide. It can then be gently dropped to ensure that no hybridization solution escapes from the gasket which may compromise the seal between the microarray and gasket.

25. When the microarray and gasket slides are sandwiched together the barcodes should be aligned. Place the non-barcoded end of the microarray into the chamber base, at a 45° angle. Assure that it is aligned with the gasket slide. Balance the barcoded end on the tip of the forceps and lower into place. If most of the sample is dispensed at the barcoded end of the gasket slide, the array will not make contact with it until it is almost in place. Therefore surface tension will not cause the sample to breach the rubber seal.

26. It is critical that bubbles do not remain fixed in position as the array is rotated. This will result in no hybridization at those positions on the array. In addition, it is worth checking the level of hybridization solution in the chamber which should be well above half way. Low levels of hybridization solution may result in sub-optimal signal intensities in the centre of the array.

27. The arrays should be checked after 1 day of hybridization to ensure that all the bubbles are still moving and no leaking has occurred. If any problems can be detected here, the array can be salvaged by moving bubbles or by adding more hybridization solution.

28. Agilent Stabilization and drying solution contains acetonitrile. It is toxic and flammable. Acetonitrile wash and stabilization and drying solution must be used in a vented fume hood. Use gloves and eye/face protection.

29. With practice, this can be done quickly and efficiently. Be careful to avoid any contact between the gasket slide and the active side of the array.

30. Alternately, to maintain the wash buffer 2 at 37°C, place a slide staining dish into a 1.5-L dish three-fourths filled with water and warm to 37°C overnight in an incubator. Place the pre-warmed 1.5-L glass dish filled with water and containing slide-staining dish 3 on a magnetic stir plate with a heating element. Fill slide-staining dish 3 approximately ¾ full with wash buffer 2 (pre-warmed to 37°C). Add a magnetic stir bar. Turn on the heating element and maintain the temperature of Wash Buffer 2 at 37°C.

31. If droplets of stabilization and drying solution form on the bottom edge of the slides, they can be re-submerged and slowly lifted out. Check the slides for precipitates, particularly around

the edges and the barcode. They will affect the focusing of the lasers during scanning, so should be carefully wiped off. Do not touch the active surface of the arrays.

32. Do not air dry or spin dry the slides. This can cause water-marks to appear on the glass slide surface, which can interfere with the scanning process.

Acknowledgements

The authors are grateful to Professor Christine Harrison for critical reading of the manuscript. This work was funded by Leukaemia Research, United Kingdom.

References

1. Kallioniemi, A., et al. (1992). Comparative genomic hybridisation for molecular genetic analysis of solid tumours. *Science* **258**(5083),818–821.

2. Solinas-Toldo, S., et al. (1997). Matrix-based comparative genomic hybridization: biochips to screen for genomic imbalances. *Genes Chromosomes Cancer* 20, **399**–407.

3. Pinkel, D., et al. (1998). High resolution analysis of DNA copy number variation using comparative genomic hybridization to microarrays. *Nat Genet* **20**, 207–211.

4. Snijders, A.M., et al. (2001). Assembly of microarrays for genome-wide measurement of DNA copy number. *Nat Genet* **29**, 263–264.

5. Fiegler, H., et al. (2003). DNA microarrays for comparative genomic hybridization based on DOP-PCR amplification of BAC and PAC clones. *Genes Chromosomes Cancer* **37**, 223.

6. Smirnov, D.A., Burdick, J.T., Morley, M. & Cheung, V.G. (2004). Method for manufacturing whole-genome microarrays by rolling circle amplification. *Genes Chromosomes Cancer* **40**, 72–77.

7. Ishkanian, A.S., et al. (2004). A tiling resolution DNA microarray with complete coverage of the human genome. *Nat Genet* **36**, 299–303.

8. Krzywinski, M., et al. (2004). A set of BAC clones spanning the human genome. *Nucleic Acids Res* **32**, 3651–3660.

9. Pollack, J.R., et al. (1999). Genome-wide analysis of DNA copy-number changes using cDNA microarrays. *Nat Genet* **23**, 41–46.

10. Dhami, P., et al. (2005). Exon array CGH: detection of copy-number changes at the resolution of individual exons in the human genome. *Am J Hum Genet* **76**, 750–762.

11. Brennan, C., et al. (2004). High-resolution global profiling of genomic alterations with long oligonucleotide microarray. *Cancer Res* **64**, 4744–4748.

12. Callagy, G., et al. (2005). Identification and validation of prognostic markers in breast cancer with the complementary use of array-CGH and tissue microarrays. *J Pathol* **205**, 388–396.

13. Barrett, M.T., et al. (2004). Comparative genomic hybridization using oligonucleotide microarrays and total genomic DNA. *Proc Natl Acad Sci USA* **101**, 17765–17770.

14. Schouten, J.P., et al. (2002). Relative quantification of 40 nucleic acid sequences by multiplex ligation-dependent probe amplification. *Nucleic Acids Res* **30**, e57.

15. Daser, A., et al. (2006). Interrogation of genomes by molecular copy-number counting (MCC). *Nat Methods* **3**, 447–453.

16. Strefford, J.C., et al. (2007). Genome complexity in acute lymphoblastic leukaemia is revealed by array-based comparative genomic hybridization. *Oncogene* **26**, 4306–4318.

17. Paulsson, K., et al. (2006). Identification of cryptic aberrations and characterization of translocation breakpoints using array CGH in high hyperdiploid childhood acute lymphoblastic leukemia. *Leukemia* **20**, 2002–2007.

18. Moorman, A.V., et al. (2007). Prognosis of children with acute lymphoblastic leukaemia (ALL) and intrachromosomal amplification of chromosome 21 (iAMP21). *Blood* **109**, 2327–2330.

19. Strefford, J.C., et al. (2006). Complex genomic alterations and gene expression in acute lymphoblastic leukemia with intra-chromosomal amplification of chromosome 21. *Proc Natl Acad Sci USA* **103**, 8167–8172.

20. van Vlierberghe, P., et al. (2006). A new recurrent 9q34 duplication in pediatric T-cell acute lymphoblastic leukemia. *Leukemia* **20**, 1245–1253.

21. van Vlierberghe, P., et al. (2006) The cryptic chromosomal deletion, del(11)(p12p13), as a new activation mechanism of LMO2 in pediatric T-cell acute lymphoblastic leukemia. *Blood* **108**, 3520–3529.

22. Barber, K.E., et al. (2004). Amplification of the ABL gene in T-cell acute lymphoblastic leukemia. *Leukemia* **18**, 1153–1156.

23. Graux, C., et al. (2004). Fusion of NUP214 to ABL1 on amplified episomes in T-cell acute lymphoblastic leukemia. *Nat Genet* **36**, 1084–1089.

24. Jong, K., Marchiori, E., Meijer, G., Vaart, A.V. & Ylstra, B. (2004). Breakpoint identification and smoothing of array comparative genomic hybridization data. *Bioinformatics* **20**, 3636–3637.

25. Hupe, P., Stransky, N., Thiery, J.P., Radvanyi, F. & Barillot, E. (2004). Analysis of array CGH data: from signal ratio to gain and loss of DNA regions. *Bioinformatics* **20**, 3413–3422.

26. Eilers, P.H. & de Menezes, R.X. (2005) Quantile smoothing of array CGH data. *Bioinformatics* **21**, 1146–1153.

Chapter 9

Application of SNP Genotype Arrays to Determine Somatic Changes in Cancer

Manu Gupta and Bryan D. Young

Summary

Genetic abnormalities in leukaemia range from single gene defects to chromosomal translocations, inversions, losses and gains. While conventional technologies can detect macroscopic abnormalities, finding smaller regions remained a challenge until the recent introduction of high-resolution genomic platforms. Microarrays based on single nucleotide polymorphisms is one such technology. It has made possible genome-wide allelic association studies of predisposition to common clinical problems. This approach is also being used to identify somatic changes in cancer, such as loss, gain and copy-neutral loss of heterozygosity (CN-LOH), which are below the level of detection by conventional systems. Such arrays have been used to identify key genes involved in paediatric acute lymphoblastic leukaemia. We have used these arrays to identify regions of CN-LOH on a genome-wide scale in a large series of acute myeloid leukaemia samples, which so far has not been possible through any other technology.

Key words: SNP microarrays, DNA copy-number change, Loss of heterozygosity, Uniparental disomy, Acquired homozygosity

1. Introduction

1.1. Background

Comparison of genomic DNA sequences between individuals reveals some base positions at which two, or in some cases more than two, bases can occur. Such a variation is called single nucleotide polymorphism (SNP). To date, more than 11 million SNPs have been reported in the human population in public databases like dbSNP. The frequency of individual SNPs may vary in different ethnic groups.

The sequence variation due to a SNP, depending on its location in the genome, may have different phenotypic consequences. The non-synonymous SNPs in the coding region of the genome

C.W.E. So (ed.), Leukemia, *Methods in Molecular Biology, vol. 538*
© Humana Press, a part of Springer Science + Business Media, LLC 2009
DOI: 10.1007/978-1-59745-418-6_9

may affect the structure or the function of the encoded protein by coding for a different amino acid. Even the synonymous SNPs may affect the stability or folding of the mRNA. The SNPs in the non-coding region may affect transcriptional regulation, mRNA processing efficiency, mRNA isoform expression or induce epigenetic changes. Hence, SNPs may directly lead to phenotypic variations in humans.

Some SNPs are in linkage with other SNPs on the same haplotype and are inherited together more frequently then expected. This phenomenon is known as linkage disequilibrium (LD). Because of LD, a SNP may serve as a marker for other SNPs. The widespread occurrence of SNPs in the genome makes them useful as markers for population genetics, evolutionary studies and also for disease genetics through genome-wide allelic association studies.

Currently, there is considerable interest in the use of SNPs as they can serve as markers to identify genes that predispose individuals to common multifactorial diseases including cancer. Many low, medium and high-throughput technologies that can genotype a few SNPs in multiple samples or genotype about one million SNPs per sample have been developed and have been reviewed (1–3). High-throughput platforms like GeneChip® Mapping arrays (Affymetrix Inc.), and lately BeadChip® arrays (Illumina Inc.), have been used in several large-scale studies. These arrays were originally designed for linkage and association studies (4–8), however, in recent years they have found various other applications.

Such arrays are normally used to genotype DNA prepared from specimens under standard conditions. However it is possible to extend their application to other sources of nucleic acids. For example, they have been applied to genotype formalin-fixed paraffin-embedded (FFPE) samples (9–11), to genotype whole genome amplified DNA (12, 13), to the analysis of DNA methylation (14, 15) and also to the analysis of allelic expression (16, 17). We have conducted a study on a large number of acute myeloid leukaemia (AML) samples to determine loss of heterozygosity (LOH), gains and losses of DNA through the use of GeneChip® Mapping arrays.

1.2. GeneChip® Mapping Arrays

These arrays are based on the principle of reverse dot blot where the oligonucleotides are attached to a solid surface to form an array and the DNA to be analysed is hybridized to these arrays. The DNA that is hybridized has reduced genomic complexity as a result of fragmentation with restriction enzymes and selective PCR amplification of the resulting fragments (18).

Different arrays that can genotype 10,000 (10 k), 50,000 (50 k), and 250,000 (250 k) SNPs were made available a few years ago. There exists only one array for 10 k SNPs while there are two arrays each for 50 and 250 k, each querying a different set of

Color Plates

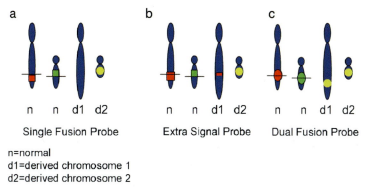

n=normal
d1=derived chromosome 1
d2=derived chromosome 2

Chapter 3, Fig. 3. Diagrammatic representation of (**a**) single fusion, (**b**) extra signal, and (**c**) dual fusion probes. Different sizes and positioning of probes on normal chromosomes produces a range of signal patterns for the same cytogenetic rearrangement. Probes which span a chromosomal breakpoint will produce a split signal between both derivative chromosomes. Normal chromosomes (n) show a single *red* or *green* signal, the derived chromosomes 1 and 2 (d1 and d2) show the patterns expected for each probe type.

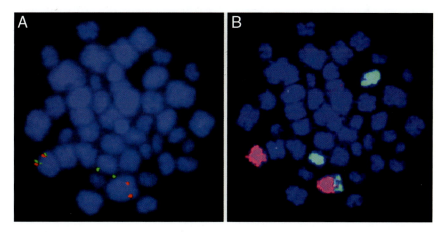

Chapter 3, Fig. 6. Sequential metaphase FISH to identify a chromosomal partner. (**a**) A breakapart locus-specific probe to *TLX3* shows a split signal pattern. The intact fusion hybridises to 5q35, the red signal remains on the derived chromosome 5, der(5), and the green signal has translocated to an unknown partner chromosome. (**b**) After washing and re-hybridising with whole chromosome paint 5 (*red*) and 7 (*green*), the partner chromosome is identified as chromosome 7. Further FISH may be carried out to identify the partner gene involved, using published data on known genes, or by breakpoint mapping (*see* **Subheading 3.7**).

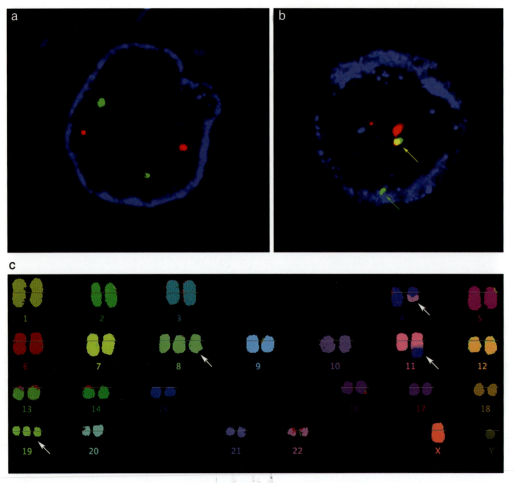

Chapter 4, Fig. 1. Examples of combined immunophenotyping and FISH and M-FISH. (*For complete caption go to Page 59*)

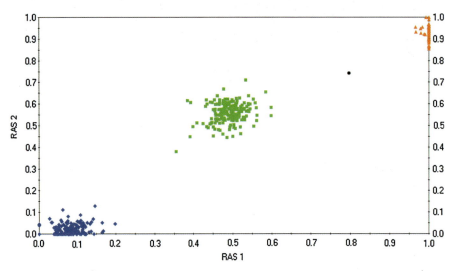

Chapter 9, Fig. 3. Three well separated clusters represent three genotypes for SNP rs717366 tested on GeneChip® 10 k 2.0 arrays. Each *dot* represents genotype for one sample. Spots in *diamond shape* (*bottom left*) represent homozygous alleles, in *triangles* (*top right*) the alternate allele in homozygous state and, in *squares* (*middle*) samples having heterozygous state for the alleles. One sample marked as *black circle* represents sample for which the algorithm could not call any genotype and was given a "no call".

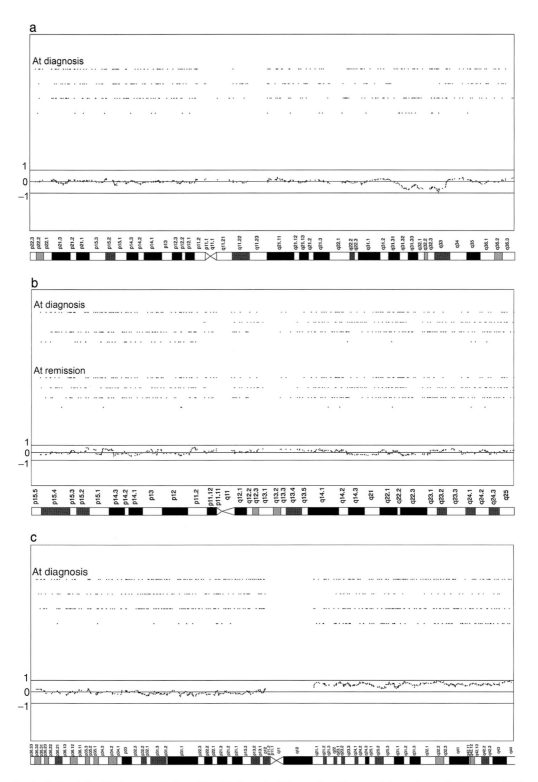

Chapter 9, Fig. 4. Graphical representation of the data from six AML samples. (*For complete caption go to Page 193–195*)

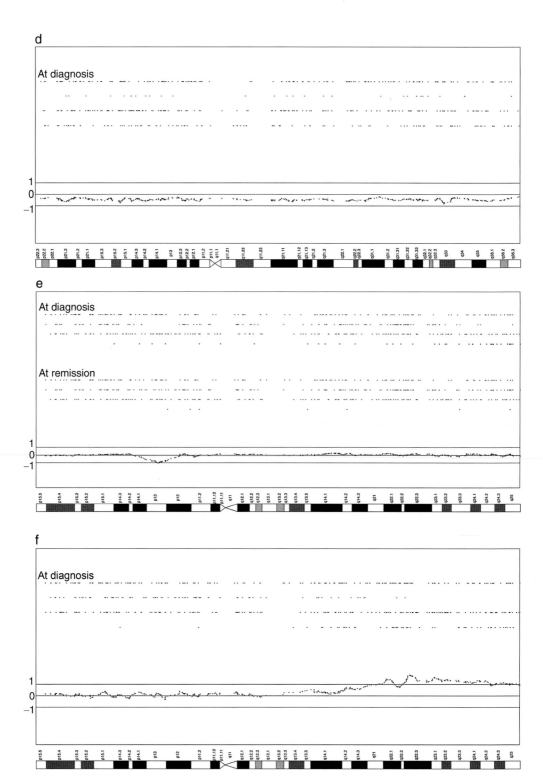

Chapter 9, Fig. 4. (continued)

SNPs depending on the restriction enzyme (Xba I, Hind III, Nsp I, or Sty I) used in the experiment. The two 50 k arrays (50 k Xba I and 50 k Hind III) together have usually been referred to as 100 k in the literature while the two 250 k arrays (250 k Nsp I and 250 k Sty I) as 500 k. The array design consists of 25-mer long oligonucleotides complementary to a perfect match of the A allele sequence (PM_A) and to the perfect match of the B allele sequence (PM_B) synthesized on the array. To determine the specificity in binding, a single base mismatch is introduced at the centre position of each 25mer for each allele (MM_A and MM_B). The PM and MM probe pairs allow estimation of signal versus noise. For each of the above four types of oligonucleotides, there are in total five oligonucleotides with a slight variation in the sequence flan-king the SNP giving 20 oligonucleotides per SNP on the sense strand. The same number of oligonucleotides are designed for the anti-sense strand giving in total 40 oligonucleotides per SNP on 10 and 50 k arrays. The 250 k arrays consist of between 24 and 40 oligonucleotides per SNP represented by PM_A, PM_B, MM_A, and MM_B.

Recently, new SNP 5.0 and 6.0 arrays have been introduced that have oligonucleotides encoding about 440,000 and 906,000 SNPs, respectively, plus almost an equal number of non-SNP loci for DNA copy-number analysis yielding information on 800,000 and 1.8 million loci, respectively. Both 5.0 and 6.0 arrays use Nsp I and Sty I restriction enzymes. The 6.0 arrays include 424,000 tag SNP markers from the international HapMap project, mitochondrial SNPs and SNPs in recombination hotspots. These arrays contain perfect match oligonucleotides and no mismatch oligonucleotides for most of the SNPs; SNP 5.0 has four replicate oligonucleotides each for PM_A and PM_B while SNP 6.0 has three replicate oligonucleotides each for PM_A and PM_B thus making in total eight and six oligonucleotides per SNP per array, respectively. However, for quality control purposes, both arrays have PM_A, PM_B, MM_A, and MM_B oligonucleotides for 3,000 SNPs similar to 10 and 50 k arrays. The median inter-marker distance on 6.0 arrays over all the 1.8 million loci combined is less than 700 bases.

The initial selection of SNPs on GeneChip arrays was based on the computational prediction of restriction fragments likely to be amplified by the assay. Further selection was based on SNP call rate, quality of genotype clusters, accuracy and reproducibility of genotype calls, heterozygosity, genome-wide coverage, distance from repeat regions, Mendelian inheritance pattern and Hardy-Weinberg equilibrium.

1.3. BeadChip® Arrays

These genotyping platforms are available from Illumina Inc. The arrays based on their proprietary Infinium II® assay (19) can genotype 109,000 (exon centric), 240,000, 317,000, 550,000,

650,000, or 1 million SNP loci. The SNPs on these arrays are tag SNPs derived from the HapMap data. Arrays based on their GoldenGate assay® can genotype 384–1,536 SNPs in 16 samples (slide format) or 96 samples (plate format). The later assay has also been adapted to study up to 1,536 methylation sites across the genome. These platforms are more amenable to custom-designed arrays.

2. Materials

The materials and methods described in this chapter are for GeneChip® Mapping 10 k 2.0 array platform. The methods for other higher resolution GeneChip® arrays are very similar and readers are advised to refer the company manual for them.

2.1. Restriction Digestion

1. High quality test genomic DNA: 250 ng.
2. Xba I (20,000 U/ml): New England Biolab (NEB). This is supplied together with NE buffer 2 and Bovine serum albumin (BSA; 100×, i.e. 10 mg/ml).
3. Molecular biology grade H_2O.
4. 200-μl tubes with caps (MJ Research). For multiple samples, use of PCR plates and plate covers is recommended.
5. Thermal cycler (for pre-PCR purposes).

2.2. Ligation

1. T4 DNA ligase (400,000 cohesive end U/ml): New England Biolab (NEB). This is supplied together with T4 DNA ligase buffer.
2. 5 μM adaptor Xba (Box 1 in GeneChip® Mapping 10 k Xba Assay kit; Part no. 900441).
3. Molecular biology grade H_2O.
4. 200-μl tubes with caps (MJ Research).
5. Thermal cycler (for pre-PCR purposes).

2.3. Polymerase Chain Reaction

1. Molecular biology grade H_2O.
2. dNTP (2.5 mM each).
3. 10 μM PCR primer (Box 1 in GeneChip® Mapping 10 k Xba Assay kit; Part no. 900441).
4. AmpliTaq Gold DNA polymerase 5 U/μl (Applied Biosystems). This is supplied with $MgCl_2$ (25 mM) and PCR Buffer II (10×).
5. 1.5-ml Microfuge tubes (Eppendorf).
6. Thermal cycler (for post-PCR purposes).

2.4. Gel Electrophoresis	1. Gel running apparatus.
	2. 2% TBE agarose gel.
	3. DNA marker 50–10,000 bp.
	4. 1% TBE for loading gel apparatus.
	5. 6× gel loading dye.

2.5. Purification

1. Manifold – QIAvac multiwell unit (Qiagen).
2. MinElute 96 UF PCR purification kit (Qiagen).
3. EB buffer (Qiagen).
4. Biomek seal and sample aluminium foil lids (Beckman).
5. Plate shaker.
6. Vacuum regulator that can create ~800 mbar vacuum.

2.6. Quantification

1. Spectrophotometer (NanoDrop Technologies).
2. EB buffer (Qiagen).

2.7. Fragmentation

1. Fragmentation reagent (DNase I) (Box 3 in GeneChip® Mapping 10 k Xba Assay kit; Part no. 900441).
2. 10× fragmentation buffer (Box 3 in GeneChip® Mapping 10 k Xba Assay kit; Part no. 900441).
3. Molecular biology grade H_2O.
4. Thermal cycler (for post-PCR purposes).

2.8. Labelling

1. GeneChip DNA labelling reagent (Box 3 in GeneChip® Mapping 10 k Xba Assay kit; Part no. 900441).
2. Terminal deoxynucleotidyl Transferase (TdT, 30 U/µl) (Box 3 in GeneChip® Mapping 10 k Xba Assay kit; Part no. 900441).
3. 5× Terminal deoxynucleotidyl transferase buffer (Box 3 in GeneChip® Mapping 10 k Xba Assay kit; Part no. 900441).

2.9. Hybridization

1. MES hydrate (Sigma).
2. MES Sodium salt (Sigma).
3. Molecular biology grade H_2O.
4. DMSO 100% (Sigma).
5. EDTA, 500 mM (Ambion).
6. Denhardt's solution, 50× concentrate (Sigma).
7. Herring sperm DNA (10 mg/ml) (Promega).
8. Human Cot-1 (1 mg/ml) (Invitrogen).
9. Oligonucleotide control reagent (Box 3 in GeneChip® Mapping 10 k Xba Assay kit; Part no. 900441).

10. 5 M Tetramethyl Ammonium Chloride (TMACL) (Sigma).

11. 10% surface-Amps20 (Tween-20) (Pierce Chemical): diluted to 3% in molecular biology grade H_2O.

12. Prepare 1,000 ml of 12× MES stock solution by mixing 70.4 g MES hydrate and 193.3 g MES Sodium salt in 800 ml of molecular biology grade H_2O. Adjust the volume to 1,000 ml. The pH should be between 6.5 and 6.7. Filter the solution through a 0.2-μM filter (for storage *see* **Note 1**).

2.10. Washing

1. 20× SSPE (3 M NaCl, 0.2 M NaH_2PO_4, 0.02 M EDTA) (BioWhittaker Molecular Applications/Cambrex).

2. 10% Surfact-Amps20 (Tween-20) (Pierce Chemical).

3. Molecular biology grade H_2O.

4. 0.5 mg Biotinylated anti-streptavidin antibody (goat) (Vector Laboratories).

5. R-Phycoerythrin Streptavidin (SAPE) (Molecular Probes).

6. Denhardt's solution, 50× concentrate (Sigma).

7. MES hydrate (Sigma-Aldrich).

8. MES sodium salt (Sigma-Aldrich).

9. 5 M NaCl, RNase-free, DNase-free (Ambion).

10. Wash buffer A, non-stringent: Make a 1,000 ml stock solution by mixing 300 ml of 20× SSPE, 1.0 ml of 10% Tween-20 and 699 ml of H_2O. Filter the solution through a 0.2-μm filter. This will give final concentrations as 6× SSPE and 0.01% Tween-20. It should be stored at room temperature.

11. Wash buffer B, stringent: Make a 1,000 ml stock solution by mixing 30 ml of 20× SSPE, 1.0 ml of 10% Tween-20 and 969 ml of H_2O. Filter the solution through a 0.2-μm filter. This will give final concentrations as 0.6× SSPE and 0.01% Tween-20. It should be stored at room temperature.

12. Antibody stock solution: Resuspend 0.5 mg of anti-streptavidin antibody in 1 ml of H_2O.

13. Prepare 1,000 ml of 12× MES stock solution (the stock prepared during hybridization can be used).

14. 1× Array holding buffer: 8.3 ml of 12× MES stock buffer, 18.5 ml of 5 M NaCl, 0.1 ml of 10% Tween-20 and 73.1 ml of H_2O. Store at 2–8°C and protect from light. The final 1× concentration will be 100 mM MES, 1 M [Na^+] and 0.01% Tween-20.

15. Prepare stain buffer by mixing 666.7 μl of H_2O, 300 μl of 20× SSPE, 3.3 μl of 3% Tween-20 and 20 μl of 50× Denhardt's. This will give the final concentration as 6× SSPE, 0.01% Tween-20 and 1× Denhardt's in a total volume of 990 μl.

16. Prepare SAPE stain solution by mixing 5.0 µl of 1 mg/ml SAPE with 495 µl of stain buffer made above. This will give 10 µg/ml as the final concentration of SAPE. This solution should be made immediately before use (*see* **Note 2**).

17. Prepare antibody stain solution by mixing 5.0 µl of 0.5 mg/ml biotinylated antibody to the remaining 495 µl of stain buffer. This will give 5 µg/ml as the final concentration of the antibody.

3. Methods

The volumes given here are for one sample only. For multiple samples, the volumes should be calculated accordingly. In general, it is a good laboratory practice when dealing with multiple samples to make master-mix volumes in excess of 5%. All the mixes should preferably be made on ice unless indicated otherwise. If not proceeding to the subsequent step, the products should be stored at −20°C. The various steps involved in the method are shown in **Fig. 1**.

3.1. In Pre-PCR Room

3.1.1. Restriction Digestion

In this step, the genomic DNA is broken into smaller fragments. The restriction enzyme used recognizes a specific sequence of nucleotides on the double-stranded DNA and cleaves it. This generates fragments, each with two overhanging ends that have a complementary base sequence and have a tendency to associate with each other or with any other similar complementary overhang by forming base-pairs. It is recommended that a positive control reaction with a known good quality DNA be run with each batch of test DNAs being processed.

1. Set a program in the pre-PCR thermal cycler: 37°C for 120 min, 70°C for 20 min and 4–12°C to hold the products at a low temperature.

2. Dilute the 100× BSA (10 mg/ml) ten times, i.e. to a concentration of 10× (1 mg/ml).

3. Mix in a 200-µl tube the following: 10.5 µl molecular biology grade H_2O, 2 µl of 10× NEB buffer 2, 2 µl of 10× BSA prepared above, 0.5 µl of 20 U/µl Xba I and 5 µl of 50 ng/µl Genomic DNA (*see* **Notes 3–5**).

4. Close the tube tightly with tube cap, mix the contents by vortex and spin down briefly.

5. Place the tube in a thermal cycler and run the program set in **step 1**. Temperature of 37°C is optimal for Xba I enzyme activity, 70°C is used to inactivate the enzyme and 4–12°C is used to hold the products at low temperature.

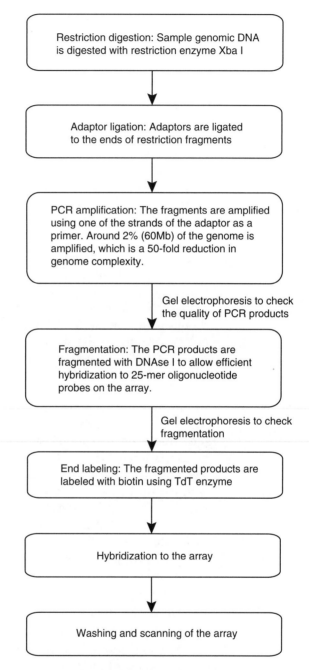

Fig. 1. Steps involved in GeneChip® Mapping 10 k Xba assay.

3.1.2. Ligation

Here, double-stranded oligonucleotides (T4 adaptors) that have overhangs with sequence complementary to the overhanging ends of the fragments generated above are ligated to the fragments using a ligase enzyme. All resulting products will have the sequence derived from the adaptors on both the ends of each fragment and a unique sequence derived from genomic DNA in the middle.

1. Set a program in the pre-PCR thermal cycler: 16°C for 120 min, 70°C for 20 min and 4–12°C to hold.

2. Make a mix for ligation in 200-μl tubes: 1.25 μl of 5 μM adaptor Xba, 2.5 μl of 10× T4 DNA ligase buffer (*see* **Note 6**) and 1.25 μl of T4 DNA ligase.

3. Add the above mix to 20 μl of digested DNA.

4. Close the tube tightly with tube cap, mix the contents by vortex and spin down briefly.

5. Place the tube in pre-PCR thermal cycler and run the program set in **step 1**: 16°C is used for ligation (*see* **Note 7**), 70°C to inactivate the enzyme and 4–12°C to hold the products at low temperature.

6. Dilute each ligation product fourfold to 100 μl with molecular biology grade H_2O.

3.1.3. PCR

PCR is required to reduce the complexity of the genome and to increase the number of the DNA templates to levels required for specific and sensitive detection of single-base changes. In the protocol for 10 k arrays, around 2% of the genome is amplified during the PCR reaction thus reducing the genome complexity 50-folds (*see* **Note 8**). Four PCR reactions (each = 100 μl) per sample are needed to produce sufficient amount (~20 μg) of product for hybridization to one array. For each batch of sample being processed, one negative control reaction (without DNA) can be included at this step to assess the presence of contamination.

1. Set a program in the post-PCR thermal cycler using "Calculated Temperature" option: 95°C for 3 min (1 cycle), 95°C for 30 s, 59°C for 30 s, and 72°C for 30 s (35 cycles for **steps 2–4**), 72°C for 7 min (1 cycle) and 4–12°C to hold.

2. Make the following master mix in a 1.5-ml tube: 10 μl of 10× PCR buffer, 10 μl of 2.5 mM dNTPs, 10 μl of 25 mM $MgCl_2$, 7.5 μl of 10 μM PCR primer Xba, 2 μl of 5 U/μl AmpliTaq Gold and 50.5 μl molecular biology grade H_2O. The volumes above are for one reaction only and as four reactions per sample need to be run, the volumes should be calculated accordingly.

3. Add 90 μl of PCR mix to the 10 μl of ligated and diluted DNA. This will give a total volume of 100 μl per reaction.

4. Close the tube tightly with tube cap, mix the contents by vortex and spin down briefly.

5. Place the tube in the post-PCR thermal cycler and run the program set in **step 1** using the "Heated Lid" option.

3.2. In Post-PCR Room

3.2.1. Gel Electrophoresis

Visualize the PCR products on a 2% TBE gel by running 3 μl of one reaction per sample mixed with 1 μl of 6× gel loading dye at 120 V for 40–60 min. The fragment's sizes should range between 250 and 1,000 bp.

3.2.2. Purification

The purification method retains the required double-stranded DNA fragments bigger than 100 bp and allows the removal of primers (smaller than 20mers), unincorporated nucleotides, and salts through the filter membrane (for an alternative method, *see* **Note 9**).

1. Connect the vacuum manifold to the source of vacuum.

2. Place a tray inside the base of the manifold to collect the waste. Place a PCR purification plate on the top of the manifold and cover the wells of the plate that are not needed with plate cover.

3. Pool the four PCR reactions for each sample into one well of the purification plate. It is important not to pierce the filter membrane at the base of the plate.

4. Apply the vacuum (~800 mbar) and wait until the wells are completely dry.

5. Add 50 μl molecular biology grade H_2O while the vacuum is on. Allow the wells to dry completely. Repeat this washing step two more times.

6. Release the vacuum and remove the plate from the manifold. Remove any liquid from the bottom of the plate by gently tapping the plate on a stack of clean absorbent paper.

7. Add 47 μl EB buffer to each well, cover the plate with adhesive plate cover and moderately shake the plate on a plate shaker for 5 min.

8. Recover the purified PCR product by pipetting the eluate out of each well. It is easier to recover the products by holding the plate at a slight angle.

3.2.3. Quantification

Read the yield of 1.5–2 μl product on Nanodrop® using EB buffer as blank. Adjust the concentration of the product to 20 μg of PCR product per 45 μl solution by adding EB buffer. Move 45 μl of the product to a new 200-μl tube (for multiple samples, *see* **Note 10–11**).

3.2.4. Fragmentation

To allow efficient hybridization to 25-mer oligonucleotides on the array, the PCR products are randomly fragmented to <100 bp with fragmentation reagent deoxyribonuclease I (DNase I, for short) that catalyzes the hydrolytic cleavage of phosphodiester linkages in the DNA backbone. This step is critical in obtaining optimal assay performance.

1. Set a program in the post-PCR thermal cycler: 37°C for 30 min, 95°C for 15 min and 4–12°C to hold.

2. Add 5 μl of 10× fragmentation buffer to each 45 μl purified product and mix by pipetting.

3. Dilute the fragmentation reagent to 0.048 U/μl with fragmentation buffer and molecular biology grade H_2O. Since

the fragmentation reagent is viscous, it is advisable to make a minimum of 125 µl stock solution to avoid any pipetting errors and ensure proper mixing. Do not scale down the volumes even if you are working with a small number of samples. The final concentration of fragmentation buffer should be 1×, e.g. if fragmentation reagent has an initial concentration of 3 U/µl, then mix 2 µl of fragmentation reagent, 12.5 µl of 10× fragmentation buffer and 110.5 µl of H_2O.

4. Add 5 µl of diluted fragmentation reagent (0.048 U/µl) to each 50 µl diluted PCR product. The total volume at this stage would be 55 µl.

5. Gently pipette up and down several times to mix (*see* **Note 12**).

6. Close the tube tightly with a cap and spin briefly.

7. Place the tube in a thermal cycler pre-heated at 37°C and run the program set in **step 1**.

8. Spin the tube briefly after fragmentation reaction.

9. Run 4 µl of the fragmented products on a 2% TBE agarose gel. Most of the products should appear below 100 bp (*see* **Note 13**).

3.2.5. Labelling

In these steps, biotin is added as a label to the ends of fragmented DNA using TdT enzyme. The GeneChip DNA labelling reagent contains biotin.

1. Set a program in the post-PCR thermal cycler: 37°C for 2 h, 95°C for 15 min and 4–12°C to hold.

2. Prepare master mix for labelling: 14 µl of 5× TdT buffer, 2 µl of 5 mM GeneChip DNA labelling reagent and 3.4 µl of 30 U/µl TdT. This will give a total volume of 19.4 µl. Mix by pipetting.

3. Add 19.4 µl of labelling master mix to the sample containing 50.6 µl of fragmented DNA.

4. Close the tube tightly with a cap and spin briefly.

5. Place the tube in a thermal cycler and run the program set in **step 1**.

6. Spin briefly again after the reaction is complete.

3.2.6. Hybridization

In these steps, the labelled products (probes) are mixed with reagents that assist the hybridization of probes to the array. A number of reagents like Human Cot-1, Denhardt's solution and herring sperm DNA are used to minimize non-specific binding of the probes to the arrays. Human Cot-1 DNA is predominantly 50–300 bp in size and enriched for repetitive DNA sequences such as the *Alu* and *Kpn* family members. Denhardt's solution is a mixture of high-molecular weight polymers capable of saturating non-specific binding sites. DMSO is used to reduce the formation of secondary structures by the probes.

1. Prepare hybridization mix as: 12 μl of 12× MES buffer, 13 μl of 100% DMSO, 13 μl of 50× Denhardt's solution, 3 μl of 500 mM EDTA, 3 μl of 10 mg/ml Herring sperm DNA, 2 μl oligonucleotide control, 3 μl of 1 mg/ml Human Cot-1, 1 μl of 3% Tween-20 and 140 μl of 5 M TMACL in a final volume of 260 μl.

2. Add 70 μl of the probes to the above mix.

3. Heat the mix at 95°C for 10 min to denature the probes. Place on ice for 10 s.

4. Spin down briefly to collect any condensate. Mix again by pipetting.

5. Inject 80 μl of the above mix into the 10 k array cartridge (*see* **Note 14**). The remaining mix can be stored at –20°C for future use.

6. Allow hybridization in a hybridization oven rotating at 60 rpm at 48°C for 16–18 h.

3.2.7. Washing

In these steps, the arrays are washed and stained to generate signals from the probes hybridized to the arrays. Staining is carried out in three steps consisting of Streptavidin Phycoerythrin (SAPE) stain (streptavidin binds very strongly to biotin used as label), followed by an amplification step in which a biotinylated goat anti-streptavidin antibody binds to SAPE to increase the effective number of biotin molecules on the target and the final step of staining with SAPE again. Phycoerythrin is a fluorophore and gives a quantifiable signal that corresponds to the input of genomic DNA in the first step of the experiment, i.e. restriction digestion.

1. After hybridization for 16 h, remove the array from the oven and remove the hybridization cocktail from it using a pipette. The cocktail can be stored at –80°C for repeating hybridization, if needed.

2. Load the array with 80 μl of holding buffer (*see* **Note 15**).

3. The subsequent washing and staining procedures listed below are carried out using Affymetrix fluidics station and GCOS software.

   (a) Wash with non-stringent wash buffer A for six cycles at 25°C.

   (b) Wash with stringent wash buffer B for six cycles at 45°C.

   (c) Stain the probe array with SAPE for 10 min at 25°C.

(d) Wash post stain with non-stringent wash buffer A for six cycles at 25°C.

(e) Stain for 10 min in antibody solution at 25°C.

(f) Stain for 10 min in SAPE solution at 25°C.

(g) Wash extensively with non-stringent wash buffer A for ten cycles at 30°C. The holding temperature is 25°C.

(h) Following the final wash, the arrays are kept filled with the holding buffer.

3.2.8. Scanning

The arrays are scanned to record the signal intensity at each locus. This step needs GeneChip scanner GCS30007G with autoloader and GCOS software.

3.2.9. Data Analysis

To check the quality of the data and call the genotypes GTYPE software is used. The manufacturer's instructions should be followed.

To understand the basic principle behind genotype calling *see* **Note 16–19, Figs. 2** and **3** and **Table 1**. For analysis on DNA copy-number changes and LOH, that has been the major application of SNP arrays in cancer research, *see* **Note 20–27**, and **Figs. 4** and **5**. Limitations of SNP arrays are discussed in **Note 28**.

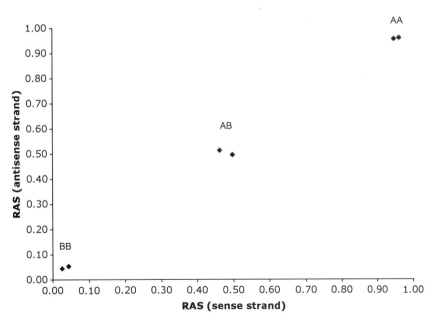

Fig. 2. Plot of hypothetical data from **Table 1** to visualize genotype calls for six samples. The three clusters with *two dots* each represent the genotypes for six samples. The *bottom left* cluster represent two samples with genotype BB, the *top right* cluster represent two samples with genotype AA and the *middle* cluster represent two samples with genotype AB.

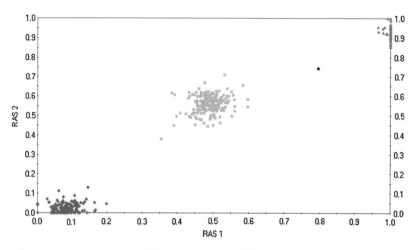

Fig. 3. Three well separated clusters represent three genotypes for SNP rs717366 tested on GeneChip® 10 k 2.0 arrays. Each *dot* represents genotype for one sample. Spots in *diamond shape* (*bottom left*) represent homozygous alleles, in *triangles* (*top right*) the alternate allele in homozygous state and, in *squares* (*middle*) samples having heterozygous state for the alleles. One sample marked as *black circle* represents sample for which the algorithm could not call any genotype and was given a "no call". (*see* Color Plates)

Table 1
Hypothetical signal values for a SNP on a microarray in six different samples

Sample ID	A_{si}	B_{si}	A_{asi}	B_{asi}	$A_{si}/(A_{si} + B_{si})$ (X axis)	$A_{asi}/(A_{asi} + B_{asi})$ (Y axis)
1	3,562	200	3,326	159	0.95	0.95
2	100	3,605	151	3,359	0.03	0.04
3	1,694	1,965	1,568	1,496	0.46	0.51
4	3,698	149	3,569	152	0.96	0.96
5	156	3,359	202	3,671	0.04	0.05
6	1,955	1,966	1,698	1,739	0.50	0.49

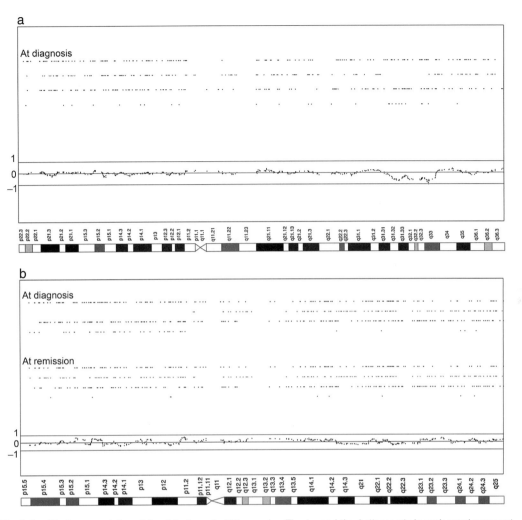

Fig. 4. Graphical representation of the data from six AML samples. The *top* and the *bottom* parts in each panel represent genotype calls from a tumor DNA and the copy-number estimation as $\log_2$ ratio, respectively. For two of the six cases, paired remission control samples were available and their genotype is shown in the middle part of (**b**) and (**e**). Each *dot* represents a SNP locus according to its physical location on the chromosome. The *blue* genotype calls depict homozygous alleles (AA or BB), the *red dots* represent heterozygous alleles (AB), and the *black dots* represent "no calls." In the copy number plot the *middle solid line* represents $\log_2$ ratio of zero equivalent to two copies of DNA; the *upper solid line* represents $\log_2$ ratio of 1 equivalent to four copies of DNA and *lower solid line* represents $\log_2$ ratio of −1 equivalent of 1 DNA copy. The $\log_2$ ratio data for each sample is shown by *black dots*, each representing a SNP. The *dots* represent average of $\log_2$ ratios of signal intensity in a running window of 3–10 SNPs. (**a**) Deletion between 7q31.31-7q33 in AML sample 1 is shown by loss of heterozygous calls (absence of *red dots*) in the tumor DNA and decrease in $\log_2$ ratio. (**b**) UPD between 11pter-11p11.2 in sample 2 is shown by loss of heterozygous calls in the tumor DNA and diploid DNA copy-number but retention of heterozygous calls in the remission control. (**c**) Gain of 1q in sample 3 is shown by $\log_2$ ratios of about 0.6 in this region. (**d**) Sample 4, monosomy 7 is indicated by all the $\log_2$ ratios below zero and loss of heterozygous calls. Retention of some heterozygous calls and many "no calls" implies contamination from normal DNA. (**e**) The diagnostic sample from patient 5 has UPD between 11q23-11qter interrupted by heterozygous calls and "no calls" while remission control was normal and retained heterozygous calls. (**f**) Amplification at 11q in sample 6 is represented by $\log_2$ ratios well above 1 in this region and LOH. (*see* Color Plates)

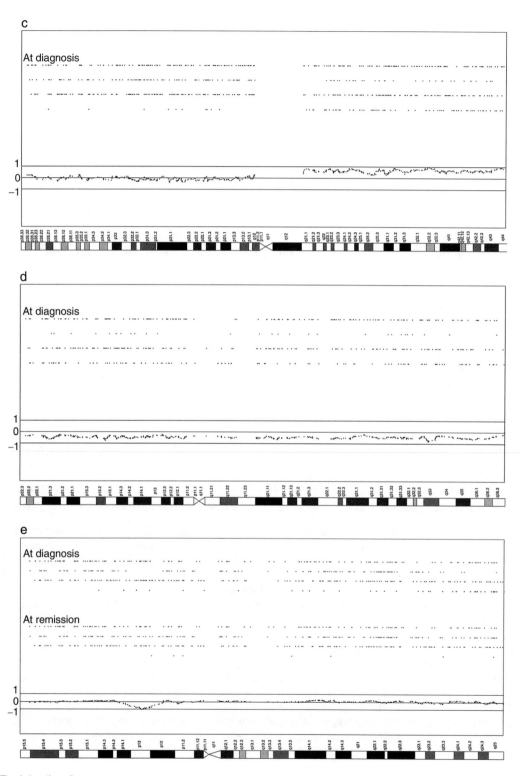

Fig. 4. (continued)

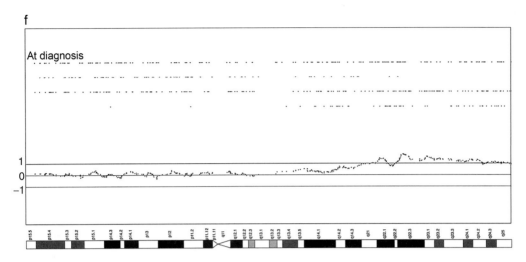

Fig. 4. (continued)

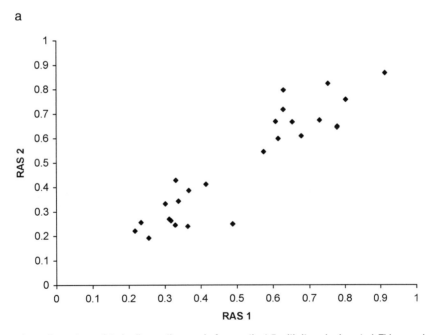

Fig. 5. Comparison of genotype plots in diagnostic sample from patient 5 with its paired control. This case had UPD on 11q at diagnosis but not in its paired control (also *see* **Fig. 4e**). SNPs with "no call" in the region of UPD at diagnosis (**a**) and the corresponding SNPs in remission sample (**b**) are shown. The SNPs that were originally heterozygous in the control have moved in the direction of homozygous clusters in the diagnostic sample suggesting LOH in a proportion of cell in the diagnostic sample.

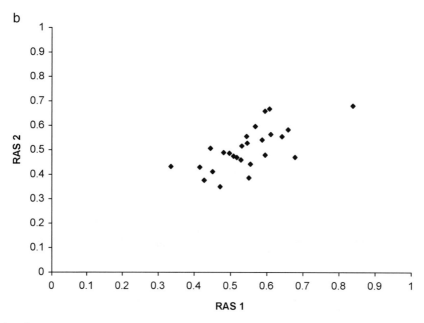

Fig. 5. (continued)

---

4. Notes

1. Store the MES stock at 2–8°C and protect from light. Discard if solution is yellow.

2. SAPE should be stored protected from light at 4°C and should never be frozen.

3. Good quality DNA free of PCR inhibitors is required. Quality can be checked by running DNA on 1% agarose gel and by checking the ratio of absorptions at 260 nm versus 280 nm and 260 nm versus 230 nm.

4. A concentration of 50 ng/μl is recommended. However, if the sample is already more dilute, higher volumes of DNA can be used to get 250 ng and volume should be adjusted by reducing the volume of H_2O in the digestion mix.

5. Too little or excess of DNA could affect the results. Lower quantity may not give the required 20 μg PCR amplified products while if excess DNA is used, the restriction enzyme may not be enough to cleave all the strands.

6. ATP is an essential co-factor for the reaction. To prevent breakdown of ATP in the buffer, multiple freeze thaw cycles should be avoided. It should be thawed gradually on the bench or in the palm of hand. Once thawed, it should be placed on ice.

7. T4 DNA ligase is most active at 25°C. However in order to perform successful ligations, the optimal enzyme temperature needs to be balanced with the melting temperature T_m (also the

annealing temperature) of the DNA fragments being ligated. If the ambient temperature exceeds T_m, homologous pairing of the overhanging ends will not occur because the high temperature disrupts hydrogen bonding. The shorter the DNA fragments, the lower the T_m. Thus for overhanging ends (overlaps) less than ten base pairs long, ligation experiments are performed at low temperatures for a long period of time (often overnight).

8. In case of the 250 k array, ~10% of the genome is amplified and hybridized to the arrays while in case of SNP 6.0 arrays, it is ~30%.

9. For dealing with few samples at a time, we use an alternative method for PCR purification in our lab. It requires Ultrafree-MC centrifugal filter devices (Millipore, Cat. No. UFC3LTKNB), a centrifuge, molecular biology grade H_2O and buffer EB (Qiagen). Pool all the four PCR reactions (400 µl) into one clean-up filter column. Spin at $2,000 \times g$ at room temp until the column is dry. Discard the liquid in the bottom of the tube. Wash the products by adding 250 µl molecular biology grade H_2O to the column and spin at $2,000 \times g$ until the column is dry. Repeat the washing step twice. Add 47 µl of EB buffer and leave for 1 min. Gently mix by pipetting and remove eluate from top of the filter to a clean 200-µl tube.

10. If there are many samples, quantification can be done using a spectrophotometeric plate reader. Dilute 4 µl of PCR product 40-folds up to 160 µl and read absorbance at 260 nm using EB buffer as blank. Calculate the amount of product as per the information in the spectrophotometer handbook. Adjust the concentration of the product to 20 µg of PCR product per 45 µl solution by adding EB buffer.

11. If the total yield is less than 20 µg, it may be worth running additional PCR reactions with the unused ligation products. All the PCR products can later be combined by using original eluate for collection.

12. Never vortex DNase I as it is especially sensitive to physical denaturation. It must be prepared fresh before use and should not be stored.

13. If the majority of the products are not below 100 bp, it indicates incomplete fragmentation and it may be necessary to re-fragment. In such a case, we add an additional 5 µl of the fragmentation mix to the products and run the program in the thermal cycler: 37°C for 5 min, 95°C for 15 min and 12°C to hold. Check again by running the products on agarose gel.

14. Arrays are loaded through the bottom septa while another pipette tip is inserted into the top septa. This allows air to vacate the chamber.

15. If needed, the arrays can be held in holding buffer at 4°C for up to 3 h. It should be equilibrated to room temperature before proceeding to the next step.

16. *Genotype calling*: The data generated in terms of signal intensity from either platform (GeneChip or BeadChip) can be transformed using different algorithms to derive the genotypes. The end point for all the algorithms is however the same; to get three distinct clusters per SNP locus across the tested samples as shown in **Fig. 2**. The cluster on the bottom left represents samples with homozygous alleles and cluster on the top right represents samples with homozygous alternate alleles while the cluster in the middle represents samples with heterozygous alleles. Each dot represents a genotype for a sample. If good quality DNA is used in the experiment, the call rate, i.e. "percent of SNPs on the array successfully genotyped" is generally above 95%. The call rate also gives an idea of the quality of the whole experiment. SNP loci for which genotype cannot be called successfully are given a "no call."

Here, we demonstrate the concept of genotype calling through an example. Consider the two possible alleles at a SNP locus as A and B, and their derived signal intensities on the microarrays as A_{si} and B_{si} respectively on the sense strand, and A_{asi} and B_{asi} respectively on the antisense strand. Consider six samples with arbitrary signal intensities for both the alleles on the microarrays as shown in columns 2–5 of **Table 1** (*see* **Note 17**). Plotting the signal intensity of allele A from the sense strand as a fraction of the total signal intensity for both the alleles on the sense strand, i.e. $A_{si}/(A_{si} + B_{si})$ as in column 6 of **Table 1** [henceforth called as relative allele signal (RAS)] on the X-axis and the corresponding value for the antisense strand, i.e. $A_{asi}/(A_{asi} + B_{asi})$ as in column 7 of **Table 1** on the y-axis would give three clusters, each representing a genotype as in **Fig. 2**. The cluster at the bottom left (consisting of samples 2 and 5) corresponds to BB homozygous genotype, the cluster on the top right corresponds to AA genotype (samples 1 and 4) and the one in the middle corresponds to AB genotype (samples 3 and 6). Ideally, both the RAS values tend to be 1 for AA homozygous genotype, 0 for BB homozygous genotype and 0.5 for AB heterozygous genotype. If, for a given SNP, the dots form a tight cluster and if the clusters are well separated, it indicates a good experimental design for that SNP. For a given sample the quantity or the number of copies of each allele present at the first step of the experiment would affect its signal intensity on the arrays. This intensity would determine where the dot would fall on the plot of the RAS values and hence the genotype that will be derived. If the alleles are not present in perfect 1:1 ratio (heterozygous state), 2:0 ratio (homozygous state) or 1:0 ratio (as in the case of deletion) either due to amplification of one allele, e.g. presence of three or more copies of one allele as opposed to one copy of the other, or due to contamination from DNA of normal cells or tumour sub-clone, the dots would appear to be shifted towards the space between the heterozygous and homozygous cluster, and moved away from the cluster to which it would otherwise belong. In such a case, the dot may not belong to any cluster and will be given a "no call" (*see* **Note 18–19**). Please note that the above is a simplified explanation to help the readers understand how clustering to derive genotypes work and the actual algorithms may be more complex.

The figures shown further in this chapter are from our large study on 454 AML samples that were hybridized to 10 k 2.0 arrays. To derive genotypes from 10 k 2.0 arrays, Affymetrix uses an algorithm called Modified Partitioning Around Medoids (MPAM). Firstly, from the DNA probes hybridized to 40 different oligonucleotides per SNP on the array, two RAS values are derived, one for the forward and one for the reverse strand. The MPAM algorithm uses these values to call genotypes *(18)*. **Figure 3** shows the data output from the 10 k 2.0 platform for SNP rs717366. For this SNP, genotype was successfully called for all but one of the 454 samples. The samples successfully called are represented by three well-separated clusters (blue, green and red) while the failed sample for this SNP (represented by black dot that does not belong to any cluster) was given a "no call."

Newer genotype calling algorithms: A large number of the studies published on whole genome genotyping so far have used the GeneChip® platform, as these platforms were introduced into the market earlier than others. As the technology has matured, better algorithms have been developed to improve genotype calling. These include SNiPER (for 10 k) and BRLMM (for 500 k) and the recently developed ones that use data only from matched probes include SNiPER-HD (for 500 k), BRLMM-P (for SNP 5.0) and BirdSeed (for 6.0 arrays). Algorithm CHIAMO was developed by the Wellcome Trust Case-Control Consortium *(4)* and was used in large scale association studies.

17. The signal for allele B in samples homozygous for allele A and vice versa represents the noise due to background or non-specific hybridization.

18. If a sample has gained two additional copies of DNA for the allele B, the two alleles will be present in the ratio of 1:3 and the genotype will be ABBB. To see how the number of copies of an allele affects derivation of genotype, try to plot the RAS values for a sample with $A_{si} = 1,000$, $B_{si} = 3,000$, $A_{asi} = 1,100$, and $B_{asi} = 3,300$ on **Fig. 2**. This would also help the readers to understand the **Notes 21**, **23–26** better.

19. "No calls" generally occur in the regions of aberration (copy number changes or LOH), but, the regions of aberration do not necessarily have "no calls."

20. *Determining copy-number changes and loss of heterozygosity (LOH) on a genome-wide basis:* The hybridization signal intensities at each SNP locus can be used to estimate relative DNA copy numbers in human tissues. This has been the major application of SNP arrays, so far, in cancer research. Ideally, signal value from DNA of tumour sample at a SNP locus on the array is compared with the corresponding value from non-tumour (germ line) sample from the same individual (called as paired control). Log_2 ratios of signal values are generally used to estimate the copy numbers. A log_2 ratio of zero indicates normal (diploid) copies of DNA, a log_2 ratio of –1 indicates one copy of DNA, 0.585 indicates three copies of DNA and 1 indicates four copies of DNA. These are theoretical estimates; practically the values fluctuate around these values because of the noise in the data. A number of software programs are available to analyze the copy number changes and LOH through the data generated by SNP arrays, e.g. Copy Number Analysis Tool (CNAT) from Affymetrix for GeneChip® arrays and BeadStudio from Illumina for Bead-Chips. Other softwares for GeneChip® arrays such as Copy Number Analyser for GeneChip® (CNAG), DChip and Genome Oriented Laboratory File (GOLF) are freely available. All the plots in this chapter with copy-number ratios are an output from GOLF. Most of the above programs use "Hidden Markov Model" to automatically identify regions of copy-number change and/or LOH.

Deletion – LOH due to loss of genetic material: **Fig. 4a** shows the data on chromosome 7 for an AML sample. The deletion between 7q31.31-7q33 is shown by loss of heterozygous calls (absence of red dots) in this region and a corresponding decrease in log_2 ratio of the hybridisation signals. The significance of identifying chromosomal aberrations through arrays is highlighted by increasing number of studies discovering the underlying target genes. Identification of deletions on 9p in 30% of B-progenitor acute lymphoblastic leukaemia (ALL) cases helped uncover PAX5 as the target gene *(20)*; in Wilm's tumour, deletions identified in 15 of 51 cases on chromosome X helped identification of WTX gene as the target *(21)*; CTNNA1 was identified as target gene in AML cases with deletion on 5q *(22)*; PTPRD was identified as a candidate tumour suppressor gene in cutaneous squamous cell carcinoma *(23)*.

Uniparental disomy (UPD) – LOH without loss of genetic material: Copy-neutral LOH, also known as uniparental disomy, can be detected by SNP arrays but cannot be detected by conventional karyotype analysis, fluorescent in situ hybridization (FISH) or array-CGH. UPD can arise by mitotic recombination, chromosomal non-disjunction followed by deletion or duplication or by trisomy rescue. **Figure 4b** shows the data on chromosome 11 for an AML sample. The UPD between 11pter-11p11.2 in the tumour DNA is shown by the loss of heterozygous calls (absence of red dots) and the normal diploid DNA copy number while heterozygosity is retained in the remission (paired control) sample. UPD is frequently observed in myeloproliferative disorders at 9p and *JAK2* gene underlying the UPD region was found to be the target frequently mutated *(24)*. In AML, UPD is observed most frequently at 13q, 11p, and 11q *(25)*

Gains: **Fig. 4c** shows the data on chromosome 1 for an AML sample. The gain on entire q-arm is shown by $\log_2$ ratio consistently above zero (*see* **Note 21**).

In many cases, paired controls are not available; however, it may still be possible to analyze DNA copy numbers and LOH (*see* **Note 22**). Furthermore, there are many issues to be kept in mind to correctly interpret the data for DNA copy number and LOH (*see* **Note 23–26**). Understanding of the concept of genotype calling depicted in **Figs. 2–3** is critical to understand these notes.

21. Studies have shown that in case of high-level amplification, SNP arrays can correctly identify regions of amplification but may underestimate the level of amplification *(26, 27)*. This situation arises due to saturation effects that are well known for oligonucleotide arrays. If it is important to know the level of amplification, it is advisable to confirm the results with an alternative method, e.g. real-time PCR.

22. A pool of DNA samples from unaffected controls or bioinformatically pooled signal intensities from SNP array data of individual controls can be used as reference to calculate $\log_2$ ratios in the test samples. Deletions are easier to identify as decrease in $\log_2$ ratio is accompanied by LOH while gains can be identified by increase in $\log_2$ ratios of consecutive SNPs. However, it may be difficult to identify UPDs as the $\log_2$ ratio would not be affected and the apparent region of LOH could really be an acquired UPD or could be observed due to various germ-line events like consanguinity, markers within a long-haplotype in strong linkage disequilibrium, extended haplotypes, areas of low SNP coverage or minor alleles with a low frequency. One way to identify UPDs in such a situation is to use additional large number of unaffected unrelated controls. Using data from such controls, a limit for the minimum number of consecutive homozygous

SNPs can be set at which no or only a few regions of homozygosity are observed. Majority of the regions under this limit would represent regions of homozygosity due to germline events listed above. In the test samples, regions with a number of consecutive homozygous SNPs above the set limit would reflect regions of UPD. The number of regions observed in controls at the set limit would reflect false positive rate. It may be necessary to allow few heterozygous calls and/or "no calls" within the limit to account for genotyping errors resulting due to contamination with the normal DNA or the presence of DNA from the subclones that do not contain the aberration. Since, the density of SNPs on the arrays varies across the genome, this criteria would have a reduced sensitivity in certain regions of the genome. Also, regions of UPD smaller than the defined limit may not be detectable. Alternatively, instead of using a limit as defined above, using the heterozygosity estimates for each SNP it has been made possible by algorithm DChip to predict regions of UPD *(28)*. If a string of consecutive SNPs have high rate of heterozygosity in the general population but show up as homozygous in the test sample, it might indicate a region of UPD. This criteria would have reduced sensitivity than the analysis against a paired control; it would however be better than using a limit for the minimum number of consecutive homozygous SNPs.

23. *Contamination:* If the aberrant DNA from leukaemic cells is contaminated with non-aberrant DNA (from non-leukaemic cells or leukaemic subclone), it may result in the arrays reflecting a lower level of loss or gain than actual. Experiments mixing tumour and normal cells in differing proportions have defined approximately 70% tumour content as a lower limit for detection of an aberration on both the platforms, GeneChip® and BeadChips® *(29–31)*. Such a contamination may also lead to observation of many heterozygous calls (or "no calls") in the regions of LOH (as shown in **Fig. 4d**).

24. *No calls:* As described in note 20 and 22, in our AML study we defined the criterion of UPD as at least 48 homozygous SNPs out of 50 consecutive SNPs (i.e. two heterozygous calls allowed among 50 consecutive homozygous SNPs). Using this criteria, the region of UPD between 11q23-11qter could not be detected in one of the samples and it could only be discovered by comparing SNP calls in the diagnostic tumour sample with its paired control (**Fig. 4e**). Between 11q23-11qter, the number of heterozygous calls and "no calls" in the control sample were 36 and 2, respectively. The corresponding SNPs in the diagnostic sample were AA (3 SNPs), BB (4 SNPs), AB (5 SNPs), and "no calls" (26 SNPs).

With so many "no calls" and a normal DNA copy number, it would be difficult to infer an aberration. In this case, even the "no calls" helped to infer the aberration as UPD. We compared the 26 "no calls" in the diagnostic sample (**Fig. 5a**) with the corresponding calls in the remission control sample (**Fig. 5b**) by plotting the RAS values on XY-scatter plot. The values for heterozygous SNPs in the control were present in the middle of the graph while in the diagnostic sample the corresponding values had drifted apart in the direction of the homozygous clusters. This non-random drift suggested that some of the cells actually acquired homozygosity (LOH) in this genomic region but it was not acquired in enough cells at the time of sample collection to make the dots reach the homozygous clusters and hence "no calls."

25. *Regions of gain with LOH:* The higher contribution in signal intensity due to the amplification of a single allele may dwarf the signal intensity from the non-amplified allele, pulling the dot on the plot of RAS values towards the homozygous cluster corresponding to the amplified allele. If signal due to amplification is enough, it will pull the dot into the homozygous cluster and will be called as a homozygous allele; if not enough, it may fall between the heterozygous and homozygous allele clusters and given a "no call." If many SNPs in tandem within a region appear homozygous, the region would appear to have gain and apparent LOH (**Fig. 4f**). In such a case, it is advisable to test multiple genotype calling algorithms or confirm the results with an alternative method like real-time PCR.

26. *Copy number reduction without LOH:* Such a case can arise when a sample has a karyotype with an average ploidy of four. If only two copies of certain chromosomes are present (either these chromosomes are not duplicated with the rest of the genome or two copies, one from each parent, are subsequently lost), then a 50% drop in fluorescence intensity would be observed, and each chromosome would be derived from a different parent.

27. *Improvements in copy-number and LOH analysis using newer algorithms:* Novel applications of SNP arrays may depend a lot on the development of new computational algorithms. Algorithm Probe level allele-specific quantification (PLASQ) can analyse allelic composition of aberrant regions, giving information about the haplotype of the region being amplified or deleted *(27)*. A new feature in the DChip program can infer LOH from tumours without paired controls by taking into account SNP intermarker distance, SNP-specific heterozygosity rates and haplotype structure of the human genome *(28)*. A new feature in CNAG can allow allele-specific estimation of

copy-numbers and LOH analysis in tumour samples without paired controls, even in the presence of 70–80% normal cell contamination *(32)*. Some of the above algorithms also take into consideration the experimental conditions such as the length of fragments containing the SNP that are generated after restriction digestion and the GC content, etc.

28. *Limitations of SNP arrays:*

(a) If the SNP of interest is not on the arrays, it may not always be possible for every platform to develop custom designed arrays and conventional or non-commercial methods may be needed.

(b) In rare cases, if there is a SNP under the restriction site (in case of GeneChip arrays) or under the primer (in case of BeadChips), it can give erroneous results.

(c) The SNP arrays until recently were not ideal to investigate copy number polymorphism in normal individuals as many SNPs in these regions were not represented on the arrays and were dropped during various selection criteria. However, in the new SNP 5.0 and 6.0 arrays and BeadChip 1 million chip, inclusion of probes specifically for copy number analysis should alleviate this problem.

(d) In GeneChip arrays, only the SNPs within the restriction fragments are represented on the arrays. Considering that only around 30% of the genome is amplified and hybridized in the SNP 6.0 array protocol, the SNPs on the rest of the genome cannot be queried. In contrast, in the BeadChip protocol, the whole genome is amplified and hence any SNP can be queried.

(e) Copy number changes in samples with ploidy of three or above may not always be easy to interpret.

Acknowledgements

The work described in this chapter was supported by the grants from the Leukaemia Research Fund (05054 to Bryan D. Young) and Cancer Research UK (C6277/A6789 to Bryan D. Young).

References

1. Fan JB, Chee MS, Gunderson KL. (2006) Highly parallel genomic assays. *Nat Rev Genet.* 7, 632–44.

2. Syvanen AC. (2001) Accessing genetic variation: genotyping single nucleotide polymorphisms. *Nat Rev Genet.* **2**, 930–42.

3. Syvanen AC. (2005) Toward genome-wide SNP genotyping. *Nat Genet.* 37 Suppl, S5–10.

4. Wellcome Trust Case Control Consortium. (2007) Genome-wide association study of 14,000 cases of seven common diseases and 3,000 shared controls. *Nature.* **447**, 661–78.

5. Easton DF, Pooley KA, Dunning AM, Pharoah PD, Thompson D, Ballinger DG, et al.

(2007) Genome-wide association study identifies novel breast cancer susceptibility loci. *Nature.* **447**, 1087–93.

6. Kemp Z, Carvajal-Carmona L, Spain S, Barclay E, Gorman M, Martin L, et al. (2006) Evidence for a colorectal cancer susceptibility locus on chromosome 3q21-q24 from a high-density SNP genome-wide linkage scan. *Hum Mol Genet.* **15**, 2903–10.

7. Sellick GS, Longman C, Brockington M, Mahjneh I, Sagi L, Bushby K, et al. (2005) Localisation of merosin-positive congenital muscular dystrophy to chromosome 4p16.3. *Hum Genet.* **117**, 207–12.

8. Tomlinson I, Webb E, Carvajal-Carmona L, Broderick P, Kemp Z, Spain S, et al. (2007) A genome-wide association scan of tag SNPs identifies a susceptibility variant for colorectal cancer at 8q24.21. *Nat Genet.* **39**, 984–8.

9. Jacobs S, Thompson ER, Nannya Y, Yamamoto G, Pillai R, Ogawa S, et al. (2007) Genome-wide, high-resolution detection of copy number, loss of heterozygosity, and genotypes from formalin-fixed, paraffin-embedded tumor tissue using microarrays. *Cancer Res.* **67**, 2544–51.

10. Lips EH, Dierssen JW, van Eijk R, Oosting J, Eilers PH, Tollenaar RA, et al. (2005) Reliable high-throughput genotyping and loss-of-heterozygosity detection in formalin-fixed, paraffin-embedded tumors using single nucleotide polymorphism arrays. *Cancer Res.* **65**, 10188–91.

11. Oosting J, Lips EH, van Eijk R, Eilers PH, Szuhai K, Wijmenga C, et al. (2007) High-resolution copy number analysis of paraffin-embedded archival tissue using SNP BeadArrays. *Genome Res.* **17**, 368–76.

12. Berthier-Schaad Y, Kao WH, Coresh J, Zhang L, Ingersoll RG, Stephens R, et al. (2007) Reliability of high-throughput genotyping of whole genome amplified DNA in SNP genotyping studies. *Electrophoresis.* **28**, 2812–7.

13. Zhou X, Temam S, Chen Z, Ye H, Mao L, Wong DT. (2005) Allelic imbalance analysis of oral tongue squamous cell carcinoma by high-density single nucleotide polymorphism arrays using whole-genome amplified DNA. *Hum Genet.* **118**, 504–7.

14. Bibikova M, Lin Z, Zhou L, Chudin E, Garcia EW, Wu B, et al. (2006) High-throughput DNA methylation profiling using universal bead arrays. *Genome Res.* **16**, 383–93.

15. Yuan E, Haghighi F, White S, Costa R, McMinn J, Chun K, et al. (2006) A single nucleotide polymorphism chip-based method for combined genetic and epigenetic profiling: validation in decitabine therapy and tumor/normal comparisons. *Cancer Res.* **66**, 3443–51.

16. Milani L, Gupta M, Andersen M, Dhar S, Fryknas M, Isaksson A, et al. (2007) Allelic imbalance in gene expression as a guide to cis-acting regulatory single nucleotide polymorphisms in cancer cells. *Nucleic Acids Res.* **35**, e34.

17. Pant PV, Tao H, Beilharz EJ, Ballinger DG, Cox DR, Frazer KA. (2006) Analysis of allelic differential expression in human white blood cells. *Genome Res.* **16**, 331–9.

18. Matsuzaki H, Loi H, Dong S, Tsai YY, Fang J, Law J, et al. (2004) Parallel genotyping of over 10,000 SNPs using a one-primer assay on a high-density oligonucleotide array. *Genome Res.* **14**, 414–25.

19. Steemers FJ, Chang W, Lee G, Barker DL, Shen R, Gunderson KL. (2006) Whole-genome genotyping with the single-base extension assay. *Nat Methods.* **3**, 31–3.

20. Mullighan CG, Goorha S, Radtke I, Miller CB, Coustan-Smith E, Dalton JD, et al. (2007) Genome-wide analysis of genetic alterations in acute lymphoblastic leukaemia. *Nature.* **446**, 758–64.

21. Rivera MN, Kim WJ, Wells J, Driscoll DR, Brannigan BW, Han M, et al. (2007) An X chromosome gene, WTX, is commonly inactivated in Wilms tumor. *Science.* **315**, 642–5.

22. Liu TX, Becker MW, Jelinek J, Wu WS, Deng M, Mikhalkevich N, et al. (2007) Chromosome 5q deletion and epigenetic suppression of the gene encoding alpha-catenin (CTNNA1) in myeloid cell transformation. *Nat Med.* **13**, 78–83.

23. Purdie KJ, Lambert SR, Teh MT, Chaplin T, Molloy G, Raghavan M, et al. (2007) Allelic imbalances and microdeletions affecting the PTPRD gene in cutaneous squamous cell carcinomas detected using single nucleotide polymorphism microarray analysis. *Genes Chromosomes Cancer.* **46**, 661–9.

24. James C, Ugo V, Le Couedic JP, Staerk J, Delhommeau F, Lacout C, et al. (2005) A unique clonal JAK2 mutation leading to constitutive signalling causes polycythaemia vera. *Nature.* **434**, 1144–8.

25. Raghavan M, Lillington DM, Skoulakis S, Debernardi S, Chaplin T, Foot NJ, et al. (2005) Genome-wide single nucleotide polymorphism analysis reveals frequent partial uniparental disomy due to somatic recombination in acute myeloid leukemias. *Cancer Res.* **65**, 375–8.

26. Bignell GR, Huang J, Greshock J, Watt S, Butler A, West S, et al. (2004) High-resolution analysis of DNA copy number using oligonucleotide microarrays. *Genome Res.* **14**, 287–95.

27. LaFramboise T, Weir BA, Zhao X, Beroukhim R, Li C, Harrington D, et al. (2005) Allele-specific amplification in cancer revealed by SNP array analysis. *PLoS Comput Biol.* 1, e65.

28. Beroukhim R, Lin M, Park Y, Hao K, Zhao X, Garraway LA, et al. (2006) Inferring loss-of-heterozygosity from unpaired tumors using high-density oligonucleotide SNP arrays. *PLoS Comput Biol.* 2, e41.

29. Lindblad-Toh K, Tanenbaum DM, Daly MJ, Winchester E, Lui WO, Villapakkam A, et al. (2000) Loss-of-heterozygosity analysis of small-cell lung carcinomas using single-nucleotide polymorphism arrays. *Nat Biotechnol.* 18, 1001–5.

30. Peiffer DA, Le JM, Steemers FJ, Chang W, Jenniges T, Garcia F, et al. (2006) High-resolution genomic profiling of chromosomal aberrations using Infinium whole-genome genotyping. *Genome Res.* 16, 1136–48.

31. Zhao X, Li C, Paez JG, Chin K, Janne PA, Chen TH, et al. (2004) An integrated view of copy number and allelic alterations in the cancer genome using single nucleotide polymorphism arrays. *Cancer Res.* 64, 3060–71.

32. Yamamoto G, Nannya Y, Kato M, Sanada M, Levine RL, Kawamata N, et al. (2007) Highly sensitive method for genomewide detection of allelic composition in nonpaired, primary tumor specimens by use of affymetrix single-nucleotide-polymorphism genotyping microarrays. *Am J Hum Genet.* 81, 114–26.

Chapter 10

Retroviral/Lentiviral Transduction and Transformation Assay

Bernd B. Zeisig and Chi Wai Eric So

Summary

Non-random chromosomal translocations can be found in about half of acute leukaemia patients and mostly lead to either over-expression of proto-oncogenes or creation of novel fusion genes. To assess the oncogenic potential and characterize the underlying mechanisms mediated by these candidate oncoproteins, a retroviral transduction/transformation assay (RTTA) has been successfully employed to study the biological impacts of a number of proto-oncoproteins and novel fusion proteins in primary hematopoietic cells both in vitro and in vivo. To further widen the application of the RTTA, a lentiviral transduction/transformation assay (LTTA) has also been developed to target the most quiescent hematopoietic stem cells (HSCs). This chapter will cover both the RTTA and LTTA for studying candidate oncogenes involved in human leukaemia.

Key words: Acute leukaemia, AML, oncogene, fusion gene, serial replating assay, transformation of primary cells, self-renewal, retrovirus, lentivirus

1. Introduction

Recurring chromosomal translocations are frequently found in acute leukaemias and specifically associate with distinctive sub-types of the diseases *(1)*. At a molecular level, gene rearrangements mostly result in either over-expression of proto-oncogenes or generation of novel fusion genes. It is clear from pre-natal back-tracking data *(2)* that these illegitimate gene rearrangements occur at a very early stage and probably represent the first initiating event for the overt leukaemia (*see* Chapter "Backtracking of Leukemic Clones to Birth"). In order to define the roles and study the underlying transformation mechanisms mediated by these candidate oncoproteins, the establishment of proper disease

C.W.E. So (ed.), Leukemia, *Methods in Molecular Biology, vol. 538*
© Humana Press, a part of Springer Science + Business Media, LLC 2009
DOI: 10.1007/978-1-59745-418-6_10

models is the first and essential step towards the understanding of the diseases.

Growth-factor-dependent cell lines have been historically the most commonly used systems for exploring the properties of candidate oncoproteins. However, they suffer from the accumulation of pre-existing and irrelevant mutations as a result of long-term passages. To this end, transgenic approaches have been used to develop in vivo models for a number of candidate oncoproteins. While these were a breakthrough for in vivo disease modelling, which minimize the pitfalls due to pre-existing irrelevant mutations, the expression of transgenic constructs are dependent on a combination of the choices of promoters and their integration sites. The lack of specific enhancers/promoters and their random integration have significantly limited the usefulness of the transgenic approaches to a small number of oncogenes. To overcome these issues, knock-in models have been developed to accurately mimic the temporal and spatial expression of the candidate oncoproteins under their endogenous promoters *(3)*. Although embryonic lethality has been a major issue associated with this approach, the second-generation and much improved conditional knock-in and translocator models using tissue-specific Cre mice have conferred an additional level of control on the spatial and temporal expression of the candidate genes *(4)*. These knock-in approaches have, no doubt, made revolutionary progress in disease modelling. However, the limitations of these knock-in approaches are (1) the lack of tissue- and/or temporal-specific Cre mice, which limits their practical use to only when appropriate Cre mice are available; (2) the simultaneous expression of candidate genes in a large number of cells, which is different from clonal development of leukaemia from a single or few initiating cells; and (3) the extremely time-consuming and costly methods, which are therefore almost impracticable for structure/function analysis. In contrast to the knock-in approaches, the retroviral transduction/transformation assay (RTTA) using purified hematopoietic stem cells and/or progenitor cells has offered an alternative solution to study both the in vivo and in vitro functions of any given oncoproteins involved in leukaemic transformation in a much shorter time and more cost-effective manner.

In a classical RTTA, murine primary hematopoietic precursor/stem cells enriched by 5′ fluorouracil (5-FU) treatment *(5)* or positively selected for expression of the progenitor marker c-Kit *(6)* are transduced with a retrovirus carrying a proto-oncogene or a fusion gene of interest (**Fig. 1**). The retroviral transduction is assisted by a brief incubation in conditions that stimulate cell division, which allow the insertion of retroviral DNA into the host's genome. To assess the leukaemogenic potential of the proto-oncogene or the fusion gene in vivo, transduced cells are injected into lethally irradiated syngeneic mice. Alternatively,

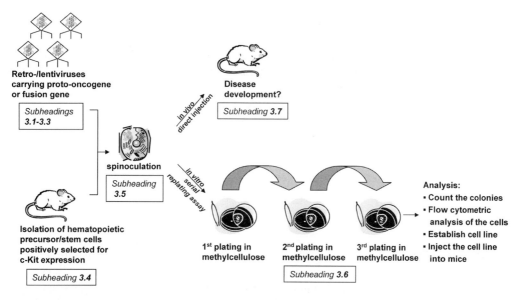

Fig. 1. Schematic overview of the retroviral/lentiviral transduction and transformation assay. In this assay, retro- or lentiviral supernatant (described in **Subheadings 3.1–3.3**) is incubated with c-Kit-enriched hematopoietic stem and progenitor cells (described in **Subheading 3.4**). Viral transduction is carried out and assisted with centrifugation, a process called spinoculation (described in **Subheading 3.5**). Transduced bone marrow cells can be used in a serial replating assay to assess the transforming potential of the gene of interest in vitro (described in **Subheading 3.6**). Alternatively, transduced bone marrow cells can be injected into lethally irradiated mice to assess leukemogenic potential of the gene of interest in vivo (described in **Subheading 3.7**).

transduced cells can be plated into a methylcellulose medium supplemented with cytokines supporting cell growth towards the myeloid lineage. They will then be serially re-plated every 6–7 days to investigate the cellular transformation potential in vitro. In this serial re-plating assay, non-transformed cells form colonies only in the initial plating but then rapidly exhaust their self-renewal potential and are not able to form colonies by the third round of plating. In contrast, transformed cells that have acquired enhanced self-renewal properties can form compact colonies in the third plating. These cells may also be expanded in liquid culture to establish cell lines. Transformed cells can then be injected into sub-lethally irradiated syngeneic mice to determine their leukaemogenic potential in vivo (**Fig. 1**).

The RTTA can be further modified (1) to target distinctive subpopulations of hematopoietic cells highly purified by fluorescence activated cell sorting (FACS) *(7, 8)* (*see* Chapters "Gene Expression Profiling of Leukemia Stem Cells" and "Identification and Characterization of Hematopoietic Stem and Progenitor Cell Populations in Mouse Bone Marrow by Flow Cytometry"); (2) to target quiescent cells such as HSCs using a lentiviral gene transfer vector. Here we describe in detail the procedures for both the RTTA and its variant, the lentiviral transduction/transformation assay (LTTA), in which gene delivery is mediated by lentivirus instead of retrovirus. In both cases, replication-deficient viruses are produced, i.e., all the proteins necessary for generating the viruses are provided *in trans* by either the packaging cell line or co-transfection of helper plasmids. The cells infected with the replication-defective virus are unable to produce new virus, thereby increasing the targeting specificity and at the same time the biosafety for researchers.

2. Materials

2.1. General Materials

1. D10 cell culture medium: Dulbecco's Modified Eagle Medium (DMEM), with 10% fetal calf serum (FCS), 100 IU/ml penicillin and 100 μg/ml streptomycin; store at 4°C.

2. R10 cell culture medium: RPMI 1640 with 10% FCS, 100 IU/ml penicillin and 100 μg/ml streptomycin; store at 4°C.

3. Suspension medium (SM): Phosphate buffered saline (PBS) with 0.2% FCS, 100 IU/ml penicillin and 100 μg/ml streptomycin; store at 4°C.

4. Plastic ware: 10-cm plates; 10- and 50-ml conical-base test tubes; 10-ml pipettes; 1.5- and 2-ml Eppendorf tubes; 6-, 24-, and 96-well (U- or V-shaped bottom) plates; T25 tissue culture flasks; FACS tubes (12 × 75 mm 5-ml round-bottom polystyrene tubes); 1- and 10-ml syringes; 27G½ Tuberculin syringe (injection syringe) (Becton Dickinson); 18G blunt-end needles; 25G needles; 40-μm cell strainers; 0.45-μm syringe filters.

5. Dissection tools: Micro-dissecting scissors and forceps (Sigma).

6. Haematocytometer, trypan blue.

7. Tissue culture incubator (37°C and 5% CO_2).

8. Biological safety cabinet.

9. Centrifuges: Sorvall Legend RT, swinging bucket rotor (75006445) or equivalent; Eppendorf 5415R microcentrifuge or equivalent.

10. Vortex: Genie 2 (Scientific Industries) or equivalent.

11. Waterbath.

2.2. Virus Production

1. GP2-293 packaging cell line (Clontech) for retroviral production; HEK 293 cell line (ATCC, CRL-1573) for lentiviral production.

2. 250 ml 2 × HBS: 4.0 g NaCl, 0.18 g KCl, 0.05 g Na_2HPO_4, 2.5 g HEPES, 0.5 g glucose, 230 ml water. Adjust to pH

7.05, fill up to 250 ml with water, and check pH again. Filter-sterilize and aliquot into 50-ml conical-base test tubes and store at −80°C. Store the working solution at 4°C (*see* **Notes 1** and **2**).

3. 100 ml 2 M CaCl$_2$: 29.4 g CaCl$_2$·2H$_2$O (FW=147.02) fill to 100 ml with water, filter-sterilize, and aliquot into 15-ml conical base test tubes. Store at 4°C.

4. Plasmids (Clontech) for retrovirus production: Retroviral plasmid-DNA (e.g., pMSCV), viral helper plasmid-DNA (Vesicular Stomatitis Virus Glycoprotein Epitope, pVSV-G).

5. Plasmids *(9, 10)* for lentivirus production (see **Note 3**): Lentiviral plasmid-DNA (e.g., pRRLsin), lentiviral helper plasmid-DNA (e.g., pCMVΔR8.74), viral helper plasmid-DNA (Vesicular Stomatitis Virus Glycoprotein Epitope, pVSV-G).

6. Solution to inactivate virus: 1% Virkon solution (*see* **Note 4**).

2.3. Viral Titration

1. Antibiotics: Geneticin, puromycin, hygromycin; store at 4°C.

2. Polybrene (1,5-dimethyl-1,5-diazaundecamethylene polymethobromide). Prepare a 10 mg/ml stock solution (2,000×) in water. Filter-sterilize and store at 4°C.

3. May–Grünwald solution.

4. Giemsa solution.

2.4. c-Kit Selection of Primary Bone Marrow Cells

1. A 6- to 10-week-old syngeneic mouse (*see* **Note 5**).

2. Erythrocyte lysis buffer: 10 mM KHCO$_3$, 150 mM NH$_4$Cl, 0.1 mM EDTA in water. Filter-sterilize and store at 4°C.

3. c-Kit (CD117) magnetic beads (Miltenyi Biotec); store at 4°C.

4. MACS MultiStand (Miltenyi Biotec).

5. MiniMACS separation unit (Miltenyi Biotec).

6. MS column (Miltenyi Biotec).

7. Cytokines (Peprotech):

   – Recombinant murine stem cell factor, SCF (1,000× stock solution: 20 μg/ml).

   – Recombinant murine interleukin-3, IL-3 (1,000× stock solution: 10 μg/ml).

   – Recombinant murine interleukin-6, IL-6 (1,000× stock solution: 10 μg/ml).

Dilute cytokines in PBS + 0.1% BSA, and store at −80°C. Once thawed, store at 4°C. Alternatively, dilute and store cytokines according to the manufacturer's instructions.

2.5. Spinoculation (Viral Transduction with Centrifugation)

1. Polybrene as described in **Subheading 2.3**.

2. Cytokines as described in **Subheading 2.4**.

2.6. Methylcellulose Replating Assay (In Vitro)

1. Methylcellulose M3231 (Stem Cell Technologies); long-term storage at –20°C, store working bottle at 4°C (*see* **Note 6**).

2. Cytokines (Peprotech) as described in **Subheading 2.4**, plus recombinant murine granulocyte/macrophage-colony stimulating factor, GM-CSF (1,000× stock solution: 10 μg/ml).

3. Antibiotics as described in **Subheading 2.3**.

4. FACS antibodies (Biolegend): CD11b (Mac-1, clone M1/70), Gr-1 (clone RB6-8C5), CD117 (c-Kit, clone 2B8), B220 (clone RA3-6B2), CD4 (RM4-5), CD8 (clone 53-6.7), CD45.1 (clone A20), CD45.2 (clone 104). These antibodies have mouse IgG2a, rat IgG2a, or rat IgG2b isotypes. Depending on the configuration of the flow cytometer, different combinations of fluorochromes will be used in conjugation with the antibodies. In general, antibody dilution for FACS analysis is 1:200.

5. Propidium iodide (Sigma). Prepare a 1 mg/ml stock solution (1,000×) in water. Store protected from light at 4°C.

6. Flow cytometer: (e.g. LSRII, BD Biosciences) or equivalent.

7. INT (*p*-Iodonitrotetrazolium Violet, Sigma). Prepare a 1 mg/ml stock solution (10×) in water. Filter-sterilize and store protected from light at 4°C.

2.7. Transplantation and Disease Analysis (In Vivo Transformation Assay)

1. ^{137}Cs γ-irradiator (e.g., GammaCell 40, Nordion; or IBL 637 irradiator, GammaService Ltd).

2. Perspex irradiation chamber (Ellard Instrumentation Ltd, Cat.No.MIC-6).

3. Cylindrical mouse restrainer (Ellard Instrumentation Ltd).

4. PBS.

5. Erythrocyte lysis buffer as described in **Subheading 2.4**.

6. Recipient mice (at least 6 weeks old) (*see* **Note 5**).

7. FACS antibodies as described in **Subheading 2.6**.

8. Propidium iodide as described in **Subheading 2.6**.

9. Cytokines as described in **Subheading 2.4**.

10. 100 ml 10% formaline: 0.5 g NaCl, 1.5 g Na_2SO_4, 10 ml 40% formaldehyde. Fill up to 100 ml with water. Store at 4°C.

11. Flow cytometer (e.g., LSRII, BD Biosciences, or similar).

3. Methods

3.1. General Precautions

The method described in this chapter employs viruses that are capable of targeting both murine and human cells. Although replication defective retro- and lentiviral systems are used, i.e., genes for replication are absent in the viral genomes, virus must still be handled with caution. All handling, storage, and disposal of biohazard waste must be in accordance with institutional rules and regulations. Viruses generated by the described method can be inactivated by overnight incubation in 1% Virkon solution. All consumables that get in contact with viruses should be decontaminated, e.g., using Virkon solution before disposal.

3.2. Virus Production

3.2.1. Production of Replication-Deficient Retroviruses

1. For each transfection (testing construct), seed 4–5 × 10⁶ GP2-293 cells onto a 10-cm plate with 8 ml of pre-warmed D10. Incubate overnight (o/n) in an incubator (*see* **Note 7**).

2. Sixteen hours later, replace the old medium with 8 ml of pre-warmed D10 (*see* **Note 8**). Put the plates back in the incubator.

3. Place 2×HBS at room temperature (RT) to warm up. Invert several times before use. For each transfection take a 10-ml conical base test tube and add 500 μl of 2×HBS (RT).

4. Label one Eppendorf tube for each construct and add reagents in the following order: 415 μl of H_2O, 15 μl of retroviral DNA construct (1 μg/μl), 9 μl of VSV-G envelope DNA (1 μg/μl), 61 μl of 2 M $CaCl_2$. Mix 2–3 times by pipetting up and down, and vortex briefly (*see* **Note 9**).

5. Add the H_2O/DNA/$CaCl_2$ solution drop wise to 2×HBS using a P1000 pipette while vortexing the 2×HBS.

6. Immediately add the HBS/H_2O/DNA/$CaCl_2$ mixture onto a labelled plate with GP2-293 cells in a drop-wise fashion. Swirl the plate and put it back in the incubator.

7. Repeat **steps 5** and **6** for other samples.

8. Twenty-four hours after transfection, replace the old medium with 10 ml of pre-warmed D10 (*see* **Note 8**), and put the plate back in the incubator. Repeat for other samples.

9. Forty-eight hours after transfection, collect viral supernatant (48-h virus) by aspirating the old medium with a 10-ml syringe (*see* **Note 10**). Attach a 0.45-μm filter to a syringe and filter the viral supernatant into a 10-ml conical test tube (*see* **Note 4**).

10. Aliquot the viral supernatant into Eppendorf tubes and store the virus at –80°C until required (*see* **Note 4**). Alternatively, viral supernatant can be concentrated (*see* **Note 11**).

11. Add 10 ml of pre-warmed D10 (*see* **Note 8**) and put the plate back in the incubator.

12. Repeat **steps 9–11** for other samples.

13. Seventy-two hours after transfection, collect viral and filter the viral supernatant (72-h virus) as previously described for the 48-h virus (*see* **Note 4**).

14. Aliquot the viral supernatant into Eppendorf tubes and store the virus at –80°C until required (*see* **Note 4**).

15. Repeat **steps 13** and **14** for other samples.

3.2.2. Production of Repli-cation Deficient Lentivirus

1. For each transfection (testing construct), seed 4–5 × 10⁶ HEK 293 cells onto a 10-cm plate with 8 ml of pre-warmed D10 and culture o/n in an incubator (*see* **Note 7**).

2. Sixteen hours later, replace the old medium with 8 ml of pre-warmed D10 (*see* **Note 8**). Put the plates back in the incubator.

3. Place 2×HBS at RT to warm up. Invert several times before use. For each transfection take a 10-ml conical base test tube and add 500 μl of 2×HBS (RT).

4. Label one Eppendorf tube for each construct and add reagents in the following order: 406 μl of H_2O, 15 μl of lentiviral DNA construct (1 μg/μl), 9 μl of VSV-G envelope DNA (1 μg/μl), 9 μl of pCMVΔR8.74 DNA (1 μg/μl), 61 μl of 2 M $CaCl_2$. Mix 2–3 times by pipetting up and down, and vortex briefly (*see* **Note 9**).

5. Add the H_2O/DNA/$CaCl_2$ solution drop wise to 2×HBS using a P1000 pipette while vortexing the 2×HBS.

6. Immediately add the HBS/H_2O/DNA/$CaCl_2$ mixture onto a labelled plate with HEK 293 cells in a drop-wise fashion. Swirl the plate and place it back in the incubator.

7. Repeat **steps 5** and **6** for other samples.

8. Harvest the virus (*see* **Note 3**) by following **steps 8–15** as described in **Subheading 3.2.1**.

3.3. Viral Titration

1. Seed 4 × 10³ NIH3T3 cells into each well of a 6-well plate. Label the wells as follows: undiluted, 10^{-2}, 10^{-3}, 10^{-4}, 10^{-5}, and none. Put the plate back in the incubator.

2. Sixteen hours later, pre-warm the centrifuge to 32°C. If the frozen virus is to be titred, warm up the virus in a waterbath at 37°C immediately before use.

3. Prepare virus dilutions, e.g., 10^{-2}, by mixing 20 μl of virus stock with 1,980 μl of D10 (*see* **Note 4**). Prepare 10^{-3}, 10^{-4}, and 10^{-5} dilutions similarly.

4. Aspirate the medium from the NIH3T3 cells and pipette 2 ml of undiluted or diluted virus into the respectively labelled well (*see* **Note 4**). Pipette 2 ml of D10 into the well labelled "none".

5. Add 0.8 μl of polybrene (*see* **Note 12**) and swirl the plate.

6. Place the 6-well plate into the centrifuge and spin for 2 h at 800g at 32°C.

7. After centrifugation, aspirate supernatant and add 2 ml of D10 (*see* **Note 4**). Put the plate back into the incubator.

8. Twenty-four hours later, start selection where appropriate (including well labelled "none"), e.g., using geneticin, puromycin, or hygromycin. The optimal concentration of antibiotics used for selection needs to be determined empirically (e.g., 0.5 mg/ml geneticin for neomycin-resistant NIH3T3 cells) *before* the viral transduction. If GFP is used as a marker, do not add any antibiotics but count the GFP-positive NIH3T3 cells 48 h after viral transduction using either a UV-fluorescent microscope or a flow cytometer. For example, if you count 12 GFP-positive cells (or cell clumps) in the 10^{-5} dilution, the titre in 2 ml of viral supernatant will be approximately 12×10^5 colony forming units (CFUs).

9. Depending on the effectiveness of the chemical selection, we usually select the cells for 6 days. If the medium turns yellowish, replace it with a fresh selection medium.

10. After 6 days, stain remaining cells with May–Grünwald–Giemsa directly in the 6-well plate. To do so, aspirate the medium and carefully put 1 ml of May–Grünwald solution in each well. Incubate for 3 min at RT. Remove the medium and wash the cells once with water. Add 2 ml of Giemsa solution (1:20 dilution with water, freshly prepared) and incubate for 20 min at RT. Afterwards, remove medium and wash the cells once with water. Air-dry the stained cells before counting.

11. Count the number of colonies in the lower dilutions using a microscope with a 5× magnification objective. After selection, only the transduced cells will remain in the plate that have formed colonies (or cell patches). If the selection was complete, no colonies would remain in the control well labelled "none". For example, if you count 12 colonies in the 10^{-5} dilution, then the titre in 2 ml of the virus supernatant will be approximately 12×10^5 CFUs.

3.4. c-Kit Selection of Primary Bone Marrow Cells

1. Sacrifice a mouse (*see* **Note 5**), e.g., by CO_2 inhalation. Prepare femurs and tibias from both hind legs by removing as much flesh as possible. Make sure that both ends of the bones are opened. Otherwise, cut them open using a pair of scissors. Place the bones in PBS. The following steps are then carried out in biological safety cabinet.

2. Aspirate SM using a 10-ml syringe attached to a 25G needle. Label a 10-ml conical base test tube for bone marrow collection.

3. Hold the femur with forceps and puncture it with the needle at one end of the bone. Flush the bone marrow using 2–3 ml of SM until the femur/tibia turns white. Repeat this step for the remaining femur and tibia.

4. Spin down the bone marrow cells ($350g$, 5 min, RT) and aspirate the supernatant. Resuspend the cells in 1 ml of erythrocyte lysis buffer and incubate for 10 min at RT.

5. After lysis, slowly add 10 ml of SM to the lysis buffer/cells and mix gently (*see* **Note 13**).

6. Fit a cell strainer onto a 50-ml conical base test tube and filter the cell suspension.

7. Remove the cell strainer and spin down the cells ($350g$, 5 min, RT). Aspirate the supernatant and wash once with 10 ml of SM.

8. Resuspend the cells in 500 µl of SM and add 15 µl of c-Kit magnetic beads. Mix well and incubate at 4°C for 30 min in the dark.

9. After incubation, add 30 ml of SM to the cells and spin them down ($350g$, 5 min, RT).

10. Place an MS column into a MiniMACS separation unit attached to a MACS MultiStand. Add 500 µl of SM to the MS column for equilibration via gravity.

11. After the centrifugation in **step 9**, aspirate the supernatant and resuspend the cells in 500 µl of SM.

12. Add the cells to the equilibrated MS column. After the cell suspension has passed through the MS column via gravity, wash the column with 500 µl of SM.

13. Repeat the wash step twice with 500 µl of SM each time.

14. After the final drop of medium drains from the MS column, remove the MS column from the MiniMACS separation unit and place it into an Eppendorf tube. Add 1 ml of SM to the MS column and use the plunger to flush out the magnetically labelled cells (*see* **Note 14**).

15. Count the number of viable cells using a hematocytometer together with trypan blue. Usually $1.2–2 \times 10^6$ c-Kit-positive cells can be isolated from one mouse.

16. For each spinoculation (one methylcellulose replating assay), resuspend 20,000 c-Kit-positive cells in 200 µl of R10 supplemented with 20 ng/ml SCF and 10 ng/ml each IL-3 and IL-6 (*see* **Note 15**). Seed the cells into a 96-well plate.

17. For the direct injection experiment, 200,000 c-Kit-positive cells are required for each recipient mouse. Therefore, plate 10 wells with 20,000 cells each for spinoculations (*see* **Note 16**).

18. Leave cells overnight in the incubator. If these cells are to be transduced with lentivirus, this overnight incubation step is optional and spinoculation can be performed directly.

**3.5. Spinoculation
(Viral Transduction
with Centrifugation)**

1. Pre-warm the centrifuge to 32°C. If frozen virus is to be used, thaw the 48-h virus harvested in a waterbath at 37°C.

2. Transfer the c-Kit-positive cells (primary haematopoietic precursor/stem cells) from one well (200 µl) of the 96-well plate into a labelled 10-ml conical base test tube. Add 1.8 ml of the 48-h virus to the cells (*see* **Notes 4** and **17**). Repeat for other samples.

3. Add 0.8 µl of polybrene (*see* **Note 12**) to the cells and mix well (*see* **Note 4**). Repeat for other samples.

4. Place the conical base test tubes into the centrifuge, and spin for 2 h at 800*g* at 32°C (*see* **Note 18**).

5. After spinoculation, aspirate the supernatant and leave approximately 100 µl medium in the conical base test tube.

6. Resuspend the cells with 100 µl of R10 supplemented with double the amounts of SCF (40 ng/ml), IL-3 (20 ng/ml), and IL-6 (20 ng/ml). Transfer the cells from the conical base test tube into a labelled well of a 96-well plate (*see* **Note 4**).

7. Repeat **steps 5** and **6** for other samples.

8. Leave cells overnight in the incubator (*see* **Notes 15** and **19**).

**3.6. Methylcellulose
Replating Assay (In
Vitro Transformation
Assay)**

*3.6.1. First Plating of
Primary Hematopoietic
Precursor/Stem Cells After
Spinoculation*

1. Place a methylcellulose bottle into a waterbath at 37°C. Supplement the methylcellulose with 20 ng/ml SCF, 10 ng/ml IL-3, 10 ng/ml IL-6, 10 ng/ml GM-CSF, 100 IU/ml penicillin, and 100 µg/ml streptomycin.

2. Mix well by shaking the bottle vigorously for 1–2 min. Place the bottle in the centrifuge and briefly spin for 30 s so that all bubbles move to the surface.

3. Attach a 18G blunt-end needle to a 10-ml syringe. Aspirate the methylcellulose and aliquot 0.9 ml methylcellulose into labelled Eppendorf tubes using the marks on the side of the tubes.

4. Add an appropriate amount of antibiotics (e.g., 1 mg/ml geneticin, 1.5 µg/ml puromycin, or 1 mg/ml hygromycin) for selection (*see* **Note 20**). Vortex the Eppendorf tubes in both upside down and upright positions.

5. Take out the 96-well plate with spinoculated cells from the incubator. Most of the cells will form a pellet at the bottom of the plate.

6. Carefully aspirate 120 µl of the medium using a P200 pipette. Use a new pipette tip for every well (*see* **Note 4**).

7. Resuspend cells 2–3 times in the remaining medium and transfer them to an Eppendorf tube containing methylcellulose with appropriate antibiotics (*see* **Note 4**).

8. Vortex the Eppendorf tube in both upside down and upright positions. Briefly spin in a microcentrifuge for 5 s (*see* **Note 21**).

9. Attach a 18G blunt-end needle to a 1-ml syringe. Use it to aspirate and dispense the methylcellulose/cell mix from the Eppendorf tube into a labelled well of a 24-well plate.

10. Since some methylcellulose remains on the walls of the Eppendorf tube, briefly centrifuge the tube to collect the remains at the bottom. Use the same syringe to transfer these into the same well.

11. Repeat **steps 7–10** for other samples.

12. Only use the middle two rows of the 24-well plate for cells, and fill the first and last row of the 24-well plate with water (*see* **Note 22**).

13. Put the plate into the incubator and leave it for the next 6–7 days (*see* **Note 23**).

3.6.2. Re-plating into Second and Third Rounds

1. Pre-warm the SM and methylcellulose (supplemented with cytokines) in a waterbath at 37°C.

2. Take the 24-well plate from the incubator, mark the bottom of the plate with several horizontal lines (best done using a pair of scissors or forceps) to assist colony counting. Write down the numbers (**Fig. 2a**) and type of colonies in each well (*see* **Note 24**). Typical examples of different types of colonies are shown in **Fig. 2b**, upper right panel.

3. For each well, use 8 ml of SM to elute the methylcellulose/cell mix from the 24-well plate and transfer this to a labelled 10-ml conical base test tube.

4. Use the same pipette to further homogenize the medium by pipetting up and down several times. After homogenization, only tiny methylcellulose clumps, if any at all, should be visible.

5. Repeat **steps 3** and **4** for other samples.

6. Spin down the cells (350g, 5 min, RT) and aspirate the supernatant. Resuspend the cells in 500 µl to 1 ml of SM, depending on the initial colony number (e.g., 1 ml for more than 100 colonies, 500 µl for less than 100 colonies). Count the number of cells using a hematocytometer.

7. Attach a 18G blunt-end needle to a 10-ml syringe, aspirate cytokine-supplemented methylcellulose, and dispense 0.9 ml into each labelled Eppendorf tube.

8. Add 20,000 cells in a volume no larger than 100 µl into the 0.9 ml methylcellulose (*see* **Note 25**). Vortex the Eppendorf tube in both upside down and upright positions. Briefly spin in a microcentrifuge for 5 s (*see* **Note 21**).

9. Dispense the methylcellulose/cell mix into 24-well plate as described in **steps 9** and **10** in **Subheading 3.6.1**.

10. Repeat **steps 8** and **9** for other samples.

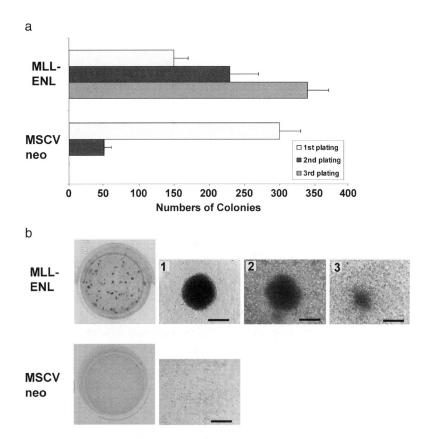

Fig. 2. Typical result of RTTA or LTTA. (**A**) The *bar chart* shows the numbers of colonies after each round of plating of c-Kit-positive cells transduced with retroviruses carrying either MLL-ENL or an empty vector (MSCVneo). The *error bars* indicate standard deviations (SD) of three independent experiments. (**B**) Typical colony morphology. Third-round colonies from c-Kit-positive cells transduced with retroviruses carrying either MLL-ENL or empty vector (MSCVneo) were stained with INT (*left*). The pictures were taken by scanning the whole 24-well plate. Close-ups of single *unstained* third round colonies are shown on the *right*. *Upper panel:* (1) compact colony (frequency > 80%), (2) compact colony with a corona of migrating cells (frequency < 10%), and (3) small and diffuse colony with large corona of migrating cells (frequency < 10%). Only compact colonies as seen in pictures 1 and 2 are counted when the colony numbers are determined. Note that the frequency of different colony types is dependent on the transduced gene. The *lower right panel* shows a typical negative result obtained with the empty vector (MSCVneo) where no colony is formed in the third round of plating. The pictures were taken under a microscope using an objective with 10× magnification. Scale bars indicate 100 μm.

3.6.3. Evaluation and Analysis After Three Rounds of Plating

Counting the Colonies

1. Six to seven days after the third plating, count the number of compact colonies by following **step 2** as described in **Subheading 3.6.2**. In this round, only transformed cells with enhanced self-renewal properties will form compact colonies. The number as well as the morphology of the colonies (**Fig. 2a** and **b**, upper right panel) is dependent on the transduced gene. Non-transformed cells do not form colonies in the third round of plating (**Fig. 2a** and **b**, bottom panel).

Staining Colonies

1. If cells were plated in duplicates, one of them can be used for staining the colonies. Once stained, the cells will not grow any more.

2. For staining, add 100 µl of INT (final concentration 100 µg/ml) directly into the well containing the third-round colonies. In living cells, the colourless INT will be reduced to yield a purple formazan dye. Return the plate into the incubator.

3. Twenty-four hours later, the colonies should be visible as violet dots (**Fig. 2b**, upper left panel).

4. Directly scan the plate with the stained colonies using an ordinary A4 size flatbed scanner or store the plate at 4°C for several days.

Immunophenotyping Using FACS

1. Elute the cells by following **steps 1**, **3**, and **4** as described in **Subheading 3.6.2**. Spin down the cells ($350g$, 5 min, RT) and aspirate the supernatant. Re-suspend the cells in 1 ml of SM.

2. Label the FACS tubes including one for an unstained control and one for an isotype control.

3. Prepare a master mix of FACS antibodies (e.g., c-Kit, Mac-1, Gr-1, etc.) by adding 1 µl of each antibody per sample into an Eppendorf tube. It is advised to include an additional 10% surplus if you have multiple samples.

4. Pipette the antibody master mix into the labelled FACS tubes (e.g., for four different antibodies, pipette 4 µl of the antibody master mix into each FACS tube). Do not add any antibodies into the unstained control tube.

5. Pipette 1 µl of each of the appropriate fluorochrome-labelled isotype control antibodies into the isotype control tube.

6. Pipette 200 µl of the cell suspension containing around 10^4–10^5 cells (*see* **Note 26**) from each sample into its homonymous labelled FACS tube.

7. Pipette 200 µl of cells from one sample into the FACS tube labelled "unstained control" and "isotype control."

8. Gently vortex the FACS tubes, and incubate the samples in the dark for 15–30 min at 4°C.

9. Add 4.5 ml of SM to each FACS tube and centrifuge the cells ($350g$, 5 min, RT). Aspirate the supernatant and resuspend the cells in 400 µl of freshly prepared SM with 1 µg/ml propidium iodide.

10. Analyse the surface marker expression using a flow cytometer (e.g. LSRII, BD Bioscience, or equivalent) following the manufacturer's instructions.

11. Since cells were cultured under myeloid conditions, cells forming the third-round colonies should only express progenitor (e.g., c-Kit) and/or myeloid lineage surface markers (e.g., Mac-1, Gr-1), but not B- (e.g., B220) and T-cell markers (e.g., CD4, CD8a). Typical phenotypes of transformed cells are shown in **Fig. 3a**.

12. In some cases, particularly when transduced cells are not transformed, mast cells expressing high level of c-Kit (and sometime even Sca-1), but not myeloid markers (e.g., Mac-1, Gr-1), appear in the culture and are frequently mistaken for early stem/progenitor cells by less experienced investigators (*see* **Note 27**). Typical FACS plots of mast cells are shown in **Fig. 3b**.

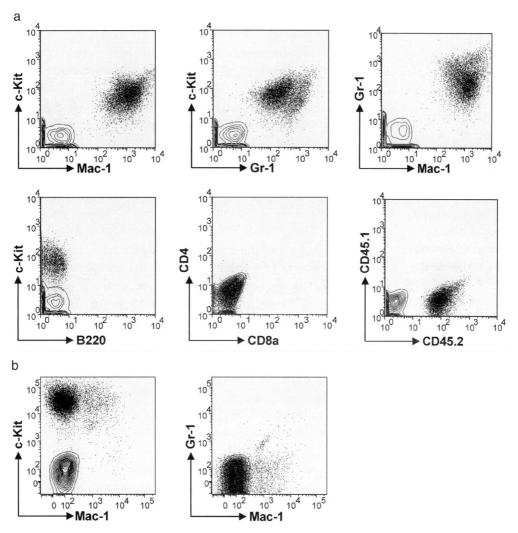

Fig. 3. FACS analysis of cells grown in the third round of plating. (**a**) Phenotypic analysis of cells transformed by MLL-ENL after third round of plating. *Dot plots* represent staining obtained with antibodies specific for the indicated cell surface antigens. *Contour plots* indicate unstained controls. Consistent with the myeloid culture conditions, cells transformed by MLL-ENL express the hematopoietic progenitor marker c-Kit as well as the myeloid markers Mac-1 and Gr-1 (*upper panel*). These cells are negative for B- (B220) and T-cell (CD4, CD8a) markers (*bottom panel, left,* and *middle*). Note that cells expressing CD45.1 or CD45.2 can be easily distinguished by FACS analysis, as shown here by the use of cells that exclusively express CD45.2 (*bottom panel, right*). (**b**) Phenotypical analysis of mast cells. *Dot plots* represent staining obtained with antibodies specific for the indicated cell surface antigens. *Contour plots* indicate unstained controls. Mast cells highly express c-Kit (*left*) but not Mac-1 and Gr-1 (*right*).

Establishment of Cell Lines from the Third-Round Colonies

1. For each sample, spin down the remaining cells ($350g$, 5 min, RT) from **step 1** in **Subheading Immunophenotyping Using FACS**. Aspirate the supernatant and resuspend in 5 ml of R10 supplemented with the same cytokine mix (SCF, IL-3, IL-6, and GM-CSF) used in the methylcellulose replating assay.

2. Transfer the cells into a T25 tissue culture flask and put the flask into the incubator.

3. Monitor cell proliferation by checking the culture daily under the microscope. If the medium turns slightly yellow, add more fresh medium or replace with new medium.

4. Assess the immunophenotype of the cells weekly by FACS analysis as described in **Subheading** "Immunophenotyping Using FACS".

5. In some cases, mast cells emerge and take over the culture. If this occurs, discard the culture and repeat the experiment.

3.7. Transplantation (In Vivo Transformation Assay)

3.7.1. Direct Injection of Primary c-Kit-Positive Hematopoietic Precursor/Stem Cells After Spinoculation into Recipient Mouse

1. Place 5–10 recipient mice into a Perspex irradiation chamber (*see* **Note 5**).

2. Place the irradiation chamber containing the mice inside the irradiator. Following the manufacturer's instructions, lethally irradiate the mice at 950 rad (*see* **Notes 28** and **29**).

3. After irradiation, these mice are ready for transplantation, but we usually wait for few hours before the injection.

4. Prepare the rescue bone marrow cells with the same CD45 marker as the recipient mouse (*see* **Note 30**) by following **steps 1–7** as described in **Subheading 3.4** (*see* **Note 31**).

5. For each recipient mouse, a total of 200,000 spinoculated cells from **step 8** in **Subheading 3.5** is required and pipetted into a 1.5-ml Eppendorf tube.

6. Add 200,000 rescue bone marrow cells prepared in **step 4** into the same tube. Spin cells down for 5 s (*see* **Note 21**) and aspirate the supernatant. Resuspend the cells in no more than 150 µl of PBS.

7. Repeat **steps 5** and **6** for other samples.

8. Place one irradiated mouse in a cylindrical mouse restrainer within a biological safety cabinet by holding its tail and pulling it backwards into the restrainer. Block the entrance using a moveable Perspex lid, which prevents the movement of the mouse.

9. Aspirate 150 µl of the cell suspension using an injection syringe. Use one hand to pull the tail taut. With the other hand, hold the injection syringe, with the bevel of the syringe facing upwards, and inject the cells into the tail vein, which is visible as a dark line on each side of the tail (*see* **Note 32**).

10. After injection, return the mouse to its cage.

11. Repeat **steps 8–10** for other samples.

3.7.2. Injection of In Vitro Transformed Primary Bone Marrow Cells

1. Place 5–10 recipient mice into a Perspex irradiation chamber (*see* **Note 5**).

2. Place the chamber inside the irradiator. Following the manufacturer's instructions, sub-lethally irradiate the mice at 475 rad (*see* **Note 29**).

3. After irradiation, these mice are ready for transplantation.

4. For each injection, 1,000,000 cells from the in vitro transformed cell line in **Subheading** "Establishment of Cell Lines from the Third Round Colonies" will be resuspended in 150 μl of PBS and injected into mice following the **steps 8–9** in **Subheading 3.7.1**.

5. Repeat **step 4** for other samples and cell lines.

3.7.3. Disease Analysis

1. When the mice display signs of sickness (*see* **Note 33**), sacrifice them for autopsy study. If the mice develop leukaemia, they usually have an enlarged spleen and pale bone marrow. Leukemic infiltration to other organs such as the liver is also commonly observed.

2. Prepare bone marrow cells by following **steps 1–7** as described in **Subheading 3.4**.

3. Remove the spleen and the liver under sterile conditions and put them in a 10-ml conical base test tube containing SM.

4. Hold the spleen with forceps and cut it into two pieces. Put one piece into a labelled tube containing 10% formaline for histology.

5. Place a cell strainer in a 10-cm plate filled with 10 ml of SM. Put the other half of the spleen into the cell strainer.

6. Take the plunger from a 10-ml syringe, and use it to prepare a single cell suspension by grinding the spleen against the cell strainer. Discard the cell strainer after the spleen has been homogenized.

7. Transfer the single cell suspension of the spleen to a 10-ml conical base test tube and spin it down (350g, 5 min, RT). Aspirate the supernatant.

8. Resuspend the cells with 1 ml of erythrocyte lysis buffer and incubate for 10 min at RT. Follow **steps 5–7** as described in **Subheading 3.4**.

9. Aspirate the supernatant and resuspend the cell pellet with 5 ml of R10 supplemented with SCF, IL-3, IL-6, and GM-CSF.

10. Take 200 μl and analyse the surface marker expression of these cells by FACS, as described in **Subheading** "Immunophenotyping Using FACS."

11. Transfer the other 4.8 ml into a T25 tissue culture flask and put it into the incubator. Try to establish a cell line.

12. Repeat **steps 5–12** for the liver.

13. Depending on the gene or fusion gene used in the transduction of primary bone marrow cells, the transplanted mice may develop lymphoid, myeloid, or mixed lineaged leukaemias. For detailed diagnosis and classification of the diseases, please refer to the Bethesda proposals *(11, 12)*.

4. Notes

1. "Water" or "H_2O" refers to purified water that has a resistivity of 18.2 MΩ cm and total organic content of less than five parts per billion.

2. The pH of 2×HBS is very important to obtain good transfection efficiencies. It is therefore recommended to double check the pH with a second pH meter. Also, do not warm up 2×HBS in a waterbath at 37°C but do so rather at RT for 20–30 min and shake it vigorously before use.

3. Most lentivirus used for gene transfer are modified human immunodeficiency virus (HIV). The most recent generation of lentiviral packing system lacks all HIV accessory genes as well as regulatory genes *tat* and *rev (10)*, which further increases the biosafety when compared to the previous generation lentivirus.

4. All tips, syringes, filters, tubes, etc. that come in contact with viruses must be sterilized, e.g., overnight in 1% Virkon solution, to inactivate the virus.

5. Syngeneic mice that differ only in one surface marker (e.g., CD45.1 and CD45.2) are valuable tools. They allow researchers to distinguish the donor (e.g., CD45.1) from the recipient (e.g., CD45.2) cells by a simple flow cytometric analysis using antibodies specifically detecting one of these antigens. SJL mice (CD45.1, strain code 277) and C57BL/6 mice (CD45.2, strain code 027) can be purchased from Charles River Laboratories (http://www.criver.com). Take this into consideration when choosing a mouse strain for preparation of bone marrow cells.

6. Methylcellulose is a semi-solid medium. Cells are not freely movable in this medium and therefore the growth of individual cells will result in colony formation.

7. It is important that GP2-293 cells or HEK 293 cells are never more than 70% confluent. Also, do not culture GP2-293 cells

or HEK 293 cells longer than 6–8 weeks. If you do so, cells may become resistant to transfection and/or produce low viral titre. If a drop in transfection efficiency is observed, discard the culture and thaw a new frozen vial of early passage GP2-293 cells or HEK 293 cells.

8. Both GP2-293 and HEK 293 cells tend to detach from the surface of the plate. Therefore add fresh medium very slowly (ideally the pipette-aid is set to "gravity only") and do not aim directly at the cells but rather at the sidewall of the plate.

9. The addition of 1 µg of a non-viral GFP plasmid (e.g., pEGFP-N1, Clontech) to the H_2O/DNA/$CaCl_2$ solution allows you to monitor the transfection efficiency without altering your viral production or generating a GFP virus. In this case, it will allow you to check the transfection efficiency under a UV fluorescent microscope. In the case of good transfection efficiency, more than 80% of cells should be GFP positive 24 h after transfection. This number, as well as the intensity of green fluorescence, may further increase 48 h after transfection. Alternatively, cells can be analysed by FACS after the last batch of virus has been harvested.

10. This procedure usually produces high viral titres (>10^6 CFUs/ml) (**Subheading 3.3**). However, viral titre is dependent on the size of the gene of interest. Larger genes (6–7 kb) yield lower viral titres whereas smaller genes (up to 3 kb) usually yield higher viral titres.

11. Use of VSVG envelope DNA allows not only transduction of all mammalian cells (e.g., human, mouse, and rat) but also the concentration of viral particles. To do so, transfect three plates, instead of one plate, per viral construct. Forty-eight hours after transfection, filter the viral supernatant into an ultracentrifuge tube (Beckman). Spin down the viral particles at ≥ 50,000g for 3 h at 4°C (e.g., a Beckman Ultracentrifuge, SW28 rotor). After centrifugation, aspirate the supernatant and leave approximately 2–3 ml medium in the tube. Resuspend and aliquot the concentrated virus into Eppendorf tubes and store at –80°C until required.

12. Polybrene is a polycation that reduces charge repulsion between the virus and the cellular membrane; i.e., addition of polybrene facilitates the binding of virus to its cellular receptor. However, do not use much higher concentrations of polybrene as this may be toxic to primary cells.

13. If cells are left for longer than 10 min in erythrocyte lysis buffer, some white blood cells may also be lysed. Slow addition of 10 ml of SM will stop the lysis process.

14. As long as the MS column is attached to the MiniMACS separation unit, c-Kit-positive cells are retained in the magnetic

field. Once the MS column is removed from the magnetic field, c-Kit-positive cells can be simply flushed out.

15. Culturing c-Kit-positive primary cells in the presence of SCF, IL-3, and IL-6 promotes cell division. This is of particular importance, because successful integration of the retroviral DNA into the genome of the target cell is dependent on the disappearance of the nuclear membrane that is associated with cell divisions.

16. Between 100,000 and 1,000,000 transduced cells are recommended for direct injection experiments. Within this range, the biological readout is similar, although the latency for developing leukaemia may be shorter with 1,000,000 transduced cells compared to 100,000.

17. If concentrated virus is used, carry out the spinoculation in a 96-well plate. To do so, thaw the concentrated virus, aspirate 100 µl of medium from the primary bone marrow cells, and add back 200 µl of concentrated virus. Add 0.2 µl each of SCF, IL-3, and IL-6 as well as 0.1 µl of polybrene to each well. Since all the cytokines are already added to the cells, the plate can be put directly back in the incubator after the spinoculation.

18. To perform double transduction of two different viruses, use 0.9 ml of each virus. For concentrated virus, add 100 µl of each virus to the cells. If the two viruses used for double transductions encode two different antibiotic resistances, one can simultaneously select for the presence of both proviruses later.

19. To increase transduction efficiency (and numbers of first round colonies), 2–3 consecutive spinoculations are recommended. Usually, 16–24 h after the first spinoculation, perform additional spinoculations using both the 48- and 72-h viruses.

20. The optimal antibiotic concentration needs to be determined for each mouse strain. Concentration given here are for the C57BL/6 mice. After addition of geneticin to methylcellulose, the colour changes from light red to light yellow because of the acidic nature of geneticin. Care must be taken to avoid direct contact of geneticin with cytokines or other antibiotics, which may reduce their activities. Vortex the Eppendorf tube vigorously after the addition of antibiotics before adding the spinoculated cells.

21. Within this 5 s spin, the micro-centrifuge is normally still accelerating and will not yet have reached its full speed. Do not centrifuge the Eppendorf tube containing cells longer than 5 s, as this may crush the cells.

22. Filling up the first and last row of the 24-well plate with water reduces the evaporation of liquid from the wells containing methylcellulose. This protects the samples from drying out.

23. Selection with geneticin and hygromycin usually takes up to 5 days compared to 2 days required for puromycin. Therefore cells should be left in methylcellulose for at least these indicated amounts of time for proper selection. However, if the pH of the methylcellulose dramatically decreases because of high cell density (colour turns from light red to light yellow), re-plate the cells immediately to avoid starvation and cell death.

24. After the first plating, similar numbers of colonies indicate similar viral titres and transduction efficiencies among the viruses used (numbers may range from less than 50 to several hundreds, depending on the size of the gene of interest). If no colonies are obtained after the first plating, either the viral titre is poor (*see* **Notes 7** and **19**) or the gene of interest may be toxic to the cells.

25. Keep the volume of 20,000 cells smaller than 100 μl. Addition of more than 100 μl to 0.9 ml of methylcellulose may dilute the methylcellulose such that cells are not stationed at a fixed position and do not form nice colonies. If the volume of 20,000 cells is larger than 100 μl, spin down the cells (5 min, 350g, RT) and aspirate the supernatant. Resuspend the cells in 50 μl SM for plating.

26. Usually, 1×10^4 to 3×10^5 cells are used for FACS analysis. However, the amount of antibody used is sufficient for FACS staining of up to 5×10^6 cells.

27. Mast cells typically express very high levels of the progenitor surface marker c-Kit (and even Sca-1) but lack expression of myeloid differentiation markers Gr-1 and Mac-1 (an example is shown in **Fig. 3b**). Furthermore, mast cells grow more slowly in culture compared to transformed myeloid cells. In addition, transduced mast cells do not induce leukaemia when injected into mice. If all or most of the cells that formed third-round colonies are mast cells, the transforming potential of the gene of interest is in question. The experiment has to be repeated.

28. Lethal irradiation is carried out to kill all hematopoietic cells in the bone marrow of the mouse. This makes "space" for the injected transduced stem/progenitor cells to home into the bone marrow and reconstitute the hematopoietic system of the recipient mouse. Without proper transplantation, the irradiated mouse will die within days.

29. These are only rough guidelines for lethal (950 rad) or sublethal (475 rad) irradiation. Since several companies offer different irradiation machines, it is vital to perform optimization studies to ensure that the correct dose is given to the mice. Also, different irradiation regimes can be used, i.e.,

a single dose versus split dose irradiation. It is worth noting that different mouse strains require discrete irradiation doses, highlighting again the need for individual optimization.

30. The rescue bone marrow cells should express the same CD45 surface marker as the recipient mouse, which is different from the donor's.

31. After lethal irradiation of a mouse, rescue bone marrow cells are also injected to assist long-term reconstitution of the hematopoietic system of the recipient mouse. This ensures that the mouse will not die because of irradiation side-effects (e.g., anaemia).

32. It is usually easy to tell whether the needle is in the vein correctly, depending on the pressure required to inject the cells. High back-pressure indicates a wrong position. In this case, try to puncture the vein at another position. The maximum volume that can be injected is 200 μl per mouse.

33. Check the transplanted mice daily for signs of sickness/disease. The most typical signs include rough fur, reduced movement, loss of weight, signs of a tumour, hunched posture, and paralysis of the hind legs.

Acknowledgment

The authors would like to thank Amanda Wilson, Jenny Yeung, and other members of the So's lab for constructive advice. This work was supported by the Association for International Cancer Research (AICR), Cancer Research UK, the Kay Kendall Leukaemia Fund, Medical Research Council, Wellcome Trust, and Leukaemia Research Fund. Eric So is an AICR fellow and an EMBO young investigator.

References

1. Look, A. T. (1997) Oncogenic transcription factors in the human acute leukemias. *Science* **278**(5340), 1059–64.

2. Greaves, M. (2003) Pre-natal origins of childhood leukemia. *Rev. Clin. Exp. Hematol.* **7**(3), 233–45.

3. Rabbitts, T. H., Appert, A., Chung, G., et al. (2001) Mouse models of human chromosomal translocations and approaches to cancer therapy. *Blood Cells Mol. Dis.* **27**(1), 249–59.

4. Forster, A., Pannell, R., Drynan, L. F., et al. (2003) Engineering de novo reciprocal chromosomal translocations associated with Mll to replicate primary events of human cancer. *Cancer Cell* **3**(5), 449–58.

5. Lavau, C., Szilvassy. S. J., Slany. R., and Cleary. M. L. (1997) Immortalization and leukemic transformation of a myelomonocytic precursor by retrovirally transduced HRX-ENL. *EMBO J.* **16**(14), 4226–37.

6. So, C. W., and Cleary, M. L. (2002) MLL-AFX requires the transcriptional effector domains of AFX to transform myeloid progenitors and transdominantly interfere with forkhead protein function. *Mol. Cell. Biol.* **22**(18), 6542–52.

7. Cozzio, A., Passegue, E., Ayton, P. M., Karsunky, H., Cleary, M. L., and Weissman, I. L. (2003) Similar MLL-associated leukemias arising from self-renewing stem cells and

short-lived myeloid progenitors. *Genes Dev.* **17**(24), 3029–35.

8. So, C. W., Karsunky, H., Passegue, E., Cozzio, A., Weissman, I. L., and Cleary, M. L. (2003) MLL-GAS7 transforms multipotent hematopoietic progenitors and induces mixed lineage leukemias in mice. *Cancer Cell* **3**(2), 161–71.

9. Zufferey, R., Dull, T., Mandel, R. J., et al. (1998) Self-inactivating lentivirus vector for safe and efficient in vivo gene delivery. *J. Virol.* **72**(12), 9873–80.

10. Dull, T., Zufferey, R., Kelly, M., et al. (1998) A third-generation lentivirus vector with a conditional packaging system. *J. Virol.* **72**(11), 8463–71.

11. Kogan, S. C., Ward, J. M., Anver, M. R., et al. (2002) Bethesda proposals for classification of nonlymphoid hematopoietic neoplasms in mice. *Blood* **100**(1), 238–45.

12. Morse, H. C. III, Anver, M. R., Fredrickson, T. N., et al. (2002) Bethesda proposals for classification of lymphoid neoplasms in mice. *Blood* **100**(1):246–58.

Chapter 11

Gene Expression Profiling of Leukemia Stem Cells

Andrei V. Krivtsov, Yingzi Wang, Zhaohui Feng, and Scott A. Armstrong

Summary

Characterization of gene expression programs and pathways important for normal and cancer stem cells has become an active area of investigation. Microarray analysis of various cell populations provides an opportunity to assess genomewide expression programs to define cellular identity and to potentially identify pathways activated in various stem cells. Here we describe methods to isolate a leukemia stem cell population, amplify RNA, and perform microarray analyses.

Key words: Stem cells, Leukemia stem cells, Gene expression profiling, Microarray, MLL-AF9, Leukemia, Gene expression, RNA amplification

1. Introduction

Gene expression is one of the major determinants of the biology of both normal and malignant cells. Gene expression profiling, which has enabled the measurement of expression of thousands of genes in an RNA sample, provides insight into the response of a cell to environmental stimuli, thereby facilitating our understanding of the molecular mechanisms underlying normal and dysfunctional biological processes. Gene expression profiling has also been shown to be very useful in identifying molecular features that distinguish leukemia stem cells (LSCs) from normal stem cells (1). Understanding the gene program of LSCs will be significant for the targeted therapy of leukemia. In this chapter, acute myeloid leukemia (AML) originating from MLL-AF9 transduced granulocyte-macrophage progenitors (GMPs) will be used to illustrate the methods utilized for identification, characterization, and microarray analysis of LSCs.

C.W.E. So (ed.), Leukemia, *Methods in Molecular Biology, vol. 538*
© Humana Press, a part of Springer Science + Business Media, LLC 2009
DOI: 10.1007/978-1-59745-418-6_11

2. Materials

1. pMSCV expression system (Clontech).

2. MLL-AF9 cDNA.

3. HEK 293T cells (ATCC CRL-1573).

4. Packaging plasmid: Ψ-Eco (Or any ecotropic retrovirus packaging system).

5. FuGENE 6 (Roche Molecular Biochemicals).

6. OptiMEM (Gibco/Invitrogen).

7. Fetal bovine serum (FBS, heat inactivated, Cellgro).

8. Penicillin/streptomycin (P/S) (Gibco/Invitrogen).

9. L-Gluamine (L-Glut) (Gibco/Invitrogen).

10. 2-Mercaptoethanol (Gibco/Invitrogen).

11. Iscove's Modified Dulbecco's Medium (IMDM) (Gibco/Invitrogen).

12. Dulbecco's Modified Eagle Medium (DMEM) (Gibco/Invitrogen).

13. 293T medium: DMEM supplemented with 10% FBS, 1% P/S, 1% L-Glut, 0.02% plasmocin.

14. Virus collection medium: IMDM supplemented with 15% FBS and 2-mercaptoethanol.

15. Polybrene (Sigma-Aldrich).

16. murine recombinant interleukin-3 (IL-3), IL-6, stem cell factor (SCF) (Peprotech).

17. Phosphate buffer saline (PBS) (Gibco/Invitrogen).

18. Antibodies for flow sorting and fluorescence-activated cell sorting (FACS): Nonlabeled CD3 (17A2); CD4 (GK1.5); CD8a (53-6.7); CD19 (6D5); B220 (RA3-6B2); Gr1 (RB-8C5); and TER-119 (TER-119); CD127 (A7R34); CD16/32-PE (Fc-RγII/III, clone 93); Sca1-PE/Cy7 (E13-161.7); Gr1-PE (RB-8C5); B220-PE (RA3-6B2); CD117-APC (c-Kit, 2B8); CD34-Pacific Blue (RAM34); CD3-Alexa647 (17A2); Mac1-APC (M1/70) from eBioscience. Dynal beads coated with goat-anti-rat IgG antibody (cat# 110.35) and goat-anti-rat IgG F(ab)$_2$ – Qdot605 (cat# Q11601MP) from Invitrogen.

19. Magnetic stand for beads separation (Cat# 120.01; Dynal/Invitrogen).

20. Viability stain, 7AAD (Molecular Probes/Invitrogen).

21. U-bottom 96-well plate (BD).

22. Cell strainer 70 μm (BD/Falcon).

23. Five milliliters FACS tubes (BD/Falcon REF352054).

24. C57BL/6 mice (Charles River Laboratories), 6–8 weeks old.

25. RBC lysis buffer (Puregene).

26. In vitro transcription (IVT) reagent (Ambion T7 Megascript Kit, Ambion).

27. Nanoprep RNA Isolation Kit (Stratagene).

28. RNeasy Mini Kit (Qiagen).

29. Tryzol (Invitrogen).

30. Chloroform (Sigma-Aldrich).

31. Glycogen (Invitrogen).

32. Ethanol (Sigma-Aldrich).

33. Phenol:chloroform:isoamyl alcohol (25:24:1, v/v) (Invitrogen).

34. RETRO*script* kit (Ambion).

35. RNase H (Sigma-Aldrich).

36. RNAse-Free DNAseI (Sigma-Aldrich).

37. T4 DNA polymerase (NEB).

38. *E. coli* DNA polymerase I (NEB).

39. NH_4OAc (Sigma-Aldrich).

40. Gamma Cell, ^{137}Cs γ-irradiator.

41. Cell sorter, FACSAria equipped with 407-, 488-, 640-nm layers.

3. Methods

The methods described below outline (1) identification of leukemia stem cells, (2) characterization of leukemia stem cells, (3) RNA isolation and amplification, and (4) microarray analysis.

3.1. Identification of Leukemia Stem Cells

Identification of LSCs is described in **Subheadings 3.1.1–3.1.4**. This includes (a) isolation of GMPs from 6- to 8-week-old C57BL/6 mice using FACS (*see* **Notes 1** and **2**) (we chose to initiate leukemia from GMPs since this population of committed myeloid progenitors cannot self-renew *(2)*, and introduction of MLL-ENL into committed myeloid progenitors (CMPs and GMPs) has been shown to induce leukemia *(3)*), (b) retroviral transduction of MLL-AF9 into GMPs (*see* **Note 3**), (c) transplantation of MLL-AF9 transduced GMPs into sublethally irradiated C57BL/6 mice, and (d) flow-sorting leukemia stem cells.

3.1.1. Flow-Sorting GMPs (4)

1. Harvest bone marrow (BM) cells from the tibia, femur, and humerus of 3–5 mice and filter through the cell strainer to prepare a single cell suspension *(5)*.

2. Pelletize the cells at 500g for 5 min at 4°C.

3. Lyse red blood cells (RBCs) in 3–5 mL of Puregene RBC lysis buffer on ice for 10 min.

4. Wash BM mononuclear cells with PBS to remove debris, and filter through a cell strainer.

5. Resuspend 5×10^6 cells in 300 μL of PBS supplemented with 0.1% of FBS (PBS–FBS) in a conical 15-mL tube.

6. Set aside approximately 1×10^6 cells to prepare "single color" controls for FACS.

7. Incubate BM cells for 30 min on ice with unlabeled lineage antibodies 2 μg/mL each: CD3, CD4, CD8, CD19, CD127, CD45R, Ter119, and Gr1.

8. Wash the cells with PBS, pelletize at 500g for 5 min at 4°C, and resuspend the cells in 300 μL of PBS–FBS.

9. While washing cells, wash Dynal magnetic beads with PBS-FBS twice.

10. Add the cell suspension to the magnetic beads and incubate with slow rotations at 4C for 40 min.

11. Collect the cell in suspension not bound to magnetic beads using a magnetic stand.

12. Pelletize the cells form the suspension at 500g for 5 min at 4°C, and resuspend in 300 μL of PBS–FBS.

13. Add 2 μL of Qdot605-labeled Goat F(ab')$_2$ anti-rat IgG (H + L) secondary antibody, and incubate on ice for 30 min.

14. Wash the cells with PBS, resuspend in 250 μL of PBS with 10 μL of rat IgG (20 mg/mL), and incubate on ice for 10 min.

15. Add 2 μL each of CD34-Pacific Blue, Sca1-PE/Cy7, Fc-RγII/III-PE, and c-Kit-APC, and incubate on ice for 30 min.

16. Wash cells with PBS, spin down cells, and resuspend in 300 μL of PBS.

17. Filter the cell suspension through a 70-μm cell strainer cap attached to a 5-mL FACS tube to remove cell clumps, and add 20 μL of 7-AAD (10 μg/mL) solution.

18. Adjust forward scatter and side scatter to bring the BM cells to the center of the axes; gate on the lymphocyte population.

19. Set up compensation using unstained and single-color stained cells (Qdot605, Pacific Blue, PE, 7AAD, PE/Cy7, and APC alone) *(see* **Note 2**).

20. Collect GMPs as 7AAD$^-$ Lin$^-$, Sca-1$^-$, c-Kit^{high}, CD34$^+$, Fc-RγII/III^{high} cells by flow-sorting *(see* **Fig. 1**) in PBS supple-

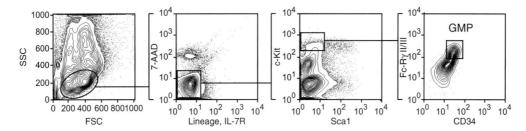

Fig. 1. Gating strategy for isolation of GMPs from murine bone marrow. GMPs are isolated as Lin⁻ Sca1⁻ c-Kit⁺ Fc-RγII/III⁺ CD34⁺ cells.

mented with 20% horse serum or FBS. If the cell sorted is properly aligned and controls are properly compensated, the double sorting does not increase purity.

3.1.2. Retroviral Transduction

The steps described in the following two subheadings outline the procedure for the production of retroviral supernatants and retroviral transduction of GMP (*see* **Note 3**).

Transfection of 293T Cells to Produce Retroviral Supernatants

1. Prepare "Fugene mix" by mixing 1.9 mL of OptiMEM and 95 μL of FuGENE.

2. Mix 10 μg of Ψ-Eco (or other packaging plasmid) and 10 μg of pMSCV-MLLAF9-MIG plasmids in a 15-mL conical tube.

3. Add 1.8 mL of FuGENE mix to the DNA mix and incubate at room temperature for 15 min.

4. Replace media in 30–50% confluent 293T plates with 4.2 mL of fresh 293T media and then gently apply 1.8 mL of the DNA/FuGENE mix to the plate to ensure uniform mixing.

5. Sixteen hours later (approximately next morning) remove the media from the plates and add 5 mL of the virus collection media to the cells.

6. After 8 h, harvest the first retroviral supernatant and add 6 mL of the virus collection media.

7. Filter the retroviral supernatant through a 0.45-μm filter, aliquot, and store at −70°C.

8. Repeat **steps 6** and **7** two more times at 8-h intervals.

Retroviral Infection of GMP

1. Pelletize 1–5×10^4 freshly sorted GMPs from **step 18** of **Subheading 3.1.1** by centrifugation (500*g*; 5 min), resuspend in 250 μL of retroviral supernatant, and transfer into a well in a 96-well plate.

2. Add 25 μL of 10× cytokine media (IMDM supplemented with 50% FBS, 200 ng/mL of SCF, 100 ng/mL of each IL-3, and IL-6) and 7 μg/mL of polybrene.

3. Centrifuge the plate for 1 h at 37°C and 600*g* and transfer the plate to a 37°C incubator for 16 h.

4. Next morning, remove 200 μL of the supernatant and add 200 μL of fresh IMDM media supplemented with 15% FBS, 20 ng/mL of SCF, 10 ng/mL of IL-3, and 10 ng/mL of IL-6. (Optional: repeat **steps 2–3** twice.)

5. Forty-two to 48 hours after the initiation of retroviral transduction, re-sort GFP$^+$ 7AAD$^-$ cells.

3.1.3. Transplantation of MLL-AF9 Transduced GMP

1. Irradiate syngeneic recipients (C57BL/6) with a single dose of 600 rad using a γ ^{137}Cs irradiator.

2. Transplant $1–10 \times 10^3$ GFP$^+$ 7AAD$^-$ cells resuspended in 250 μL PBS via the tail vein or retro-orbitally into the sublethally irradiated mice.

3. Monitor the mice daily for development of sickness; tail-bleed the mice weekly for peripheral white blood cell counts.

3.1.4. Isolation of Leukemia Stem Cells Using Flow Cytometry

This consists of the same steps as described in **Subheading 3.1.1** except that (1) normal bone marrow cells (BMCs) from C57BL/6 mice are used to set up the gates for flow-sorting LSCs (*see* **Figs. 1 and 2**), and (2) seven-color rather than six-color compensation is performed since leukemia cells are GFP$^+$.

3.2. Characterization of Leukemia Stem Cells – Transplantations into Secondary Recipient Mice

Using FACS we isolate several cell populations from bone marrow of mice with AML: GFP$^+$ Lin$^+$; GFP$^+$ Lin$^-$ Kit$^-$; GFP$^+$ Lin$^-$ Kit$^+$ Fc-Rγ$^+$ CD34$^+$. These cell populations are assayed for colony forming units (CFUs) in vitro and for the frequency of leukemia initiating cells in vivo by limiting dilution transplantation assay. The cell population with the most primitive immunophenotype, GFP$^+$ Lin$^-$ Kit$^+$ Fc-Rγ$^+$ CD34$^+$, similar to normal GMP, was found to contain the greatest percentage of CFUs and leukemia initiating cells (frequency of 1 in 6 ± 2 cells). This cell population is designated as leukemic GMPs (LGMPs). The immunophenotype of primary AML should be compared with that of secondary AML to determine whether the leukemia stem cell population recapitulates the primary AML.

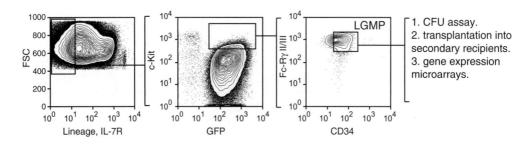

Fig. 2. LGMPs are expanded in bone marrow of mice with MLL-AF9 AML. Normal bone marrow cells are used to set up gates, and l-GMPs are identified in bone marrow cells from leukemic mice.

3.2.1. Transplantation of Leukemia Stem Cells

1. Irradiate syngeneic recipients (C57BL/6) with a single dose of 600 rad using a γ ^{137}Cs irradiator.

2. Transplant the purified LGMPs via tail vein or retro-orbitally into sublethally irradiated mice.

3. Monitor the mice daily for development of sickness; tail-bleed the mice weekly for peripheral white blood cell counts.

3.2.2. FACS Analysis

This step is performed to immunophenotypically compare AML from primary recipient mice with AML from secondary recipients.

1. Collect the BMCs from tibia, femur, and humerus of sick mice.

2. Lyse RBCs by incubating BMCs in Puregene RBC lysis on ice for 5–10 min.

3. Filter the cell suspension through a 70-μm cell strainer.

4. Count the viable cells and add 2×10^5 cells to each FACS tube.

5. Incubate the cells in each tube with one or two antibodies (e.g., Gr1-PE/Mac1-APC, CD3-APC/B220-PE).

6. Set appropriate compensations using single color controls.

7. FACS-analyze the stained cells using normal BMCs as a negative control (*see* **Fig. 3**).

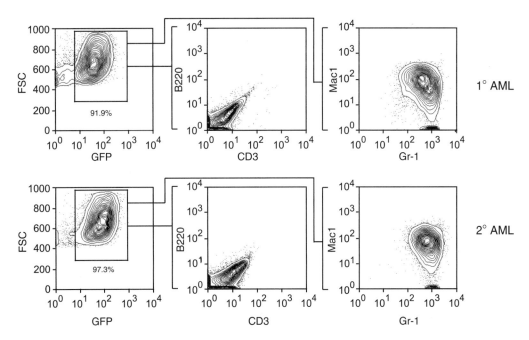

Fig. 3. The leukemias from the secondary (2°) recipient mice are immunophenotypically indistinguishable from the primary (1°) disease, demonstrating that LGMPs are enriched for leukemia stem cells.

3.3. RNA Amplification

Because of experimental limitation, number of cells is frequently limited for gene expression analysis. In our case, the sorted populations often contains $1-10 \times 10^4$ cells, which yield $1-10 \times 10^{-9}$ g of total RNA (**Subheading 3.3.1**). Generally, for hybridization with microarrays it is optimal to have 5 µg of biotinylated antisense RNA (aRNA). Therefore, to obtain enough labeled aRNA for hybridization it is necessary to perform RNA amplification. To increase the yield, two consecutive rounds of amplification are performed. The output RNA from round 1 is used as input RNA for round 2. Following is the description of RNA amplification by in vitro transcription (IVT) (*see* **Note 4**). We note that there are a number of recently developed commercial methods for RNA amplification that may work as well as what is described here.

3.3.1. Trizol-Based Isolation of RNA

1. Pelletize the cells of interest in a 1.5-mL Eppendorf-type tube at 500g, and aspirate the supernatant.
2. Add 1 mL of Tryzol reagent.
3. Mix by vortexing.
4. Incubate for 5 min at room temperature.
5. Add 200 µL of chloroform.
6. Vortex for 1 min.
7. Centrifuge at 13,000 g for 10 min at room temperature.
8. Gently aspirate the upper (clear) phase, transfer to a new 1.5-mL tube, and add 1 µL of glycogen (20 mg/mL).
9. Add 500 µL of isopropanol.
10. Precipitate RNA overnight at −20°C.
11. Pelletize RNA at 13,000g for 15 min at +4°C.
12. Wash the RNA pellet with 70% ethanol twice; air-dry the pellet.
13. Resuspend in 50 µL of diethylpyrocarbonate (DEPC) treated deionized water.
14. Spectrophotometrically measure the RNA concentration.

3.3.2. First Round of RNA Amplification

Round 1 of RNA amplification is described in the following subheadings (*see* **Fig. 4**), including (a) first-strand cDNA synthesis, (b) second-strand cDNA synthesis, (c) double-stranded cDNA (dscDNA) purification, (d) in vitro transcription (IVT) to synthesize antisense RNA (aRNA or cRNA), and (e) aRNA purification.

Reverse Transcription to Synthesize First-Strand cDNA Using Retroscript Kit

1. Add 1 µL of 100 µM T7 oligo (dT) primer in 9 µL of total RNA in DEPC-treated water.
2. Denature RNA by heating at 70°C for 10 min and anneal T-primer for 5 min at 42°C; then chill on ice.

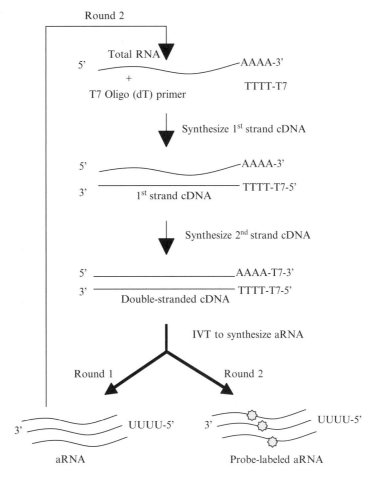

Fig. 4. Graphical representation of RNA amplification for microarray hybridization. dsDNA from the first round is used as input material for the second round of amplification. After the second round of amplification, the aRNA is used for labeling.

3. Add on ice to RNA/primer mixture (9 µL per tube): 4 µL of 5× first strand buffer, 2 µL of 0.1 M DTT (dithiothreitol), 1 µL of 10 mM dNTPs, 1 µL (200 U) of SuperScript III Reverse Transcriptase (RT enzyme), and 1 µL (40 U) of RNaseOUT.

4. Gently mix and incubate at 51°C for 1 h.

5. Heat-inactivate the RT enzyme at 70°C for 15 min, chill on ice, and proceed to dscDNA synthesis.

Second-Strand cDNA
Synthesis (Optional Stopping Point Used in These Experiments)

1. Add the following reagents to a tube containing freshly synthesized first-strand DNA (20 µL): 30 µL of 5× second-strand buffer, 3 µL of 10 mM dNTPs, 4 µL (40 U) of DNA polymerase I, 1 µL (10 U) of *E. coli* DNA ligase, 1 µL (2 U) of RNaseH, and 91 µL of DEPC water (130 µL total).

2. Incubate at 16°C for 2 h.

3. Add 10 U of T4 DNA polymerase and incubate at 16°C for 15 min.

Purification of Double-Stranded cDNA

1. Add equal volume buffer saturated phenol:chloroform:isoamyl alcohol (25:24:1, v/v) to dscDNA (approximately 154 μL).

2. Vortex and spin at 16,000g for 5 min.

3. Transfer the upper phase to a new 1.5-mL tube.

4. Add 0.5 volume (approximately 75 μL) of 7.5 M NH$_4$OAc, 1 μL (20 μg) of glycogen, and 2.5 volumes (375 μL) of 100% pre-chilled ethanol.

5. Vortex and chill at –80°C for 20 min.

6. Precipitate DNA by centrifuging for 20 min 16,000g at 4°C.

7. Wash the pellet with 80% ethanol, and spin at 16,000g for 2 min (optional: repeat this step twice).

8. Quick-spin and aspirate the remaining ethanol to allow the pellet to dry completely, and then resuspend it in IVT reagent mix.

In Vitro Transcription to Synthesize Antisense RNA Using Ambion T7 Megascript Kit

1. Thaw all reagents and keep them at room temperature to avoid precipitate formation (*see* **Note 5**).

2. Make an IVT mix (18 μL per reaction): 2 μL of 75 mM ATP, 2 μL of 75 mM GTP, 2 μL of 75 mM CTP, 2 μL of 75 mM UTP, 2 μL of 10× buffer, and 8 μL of DEPC water (all reagents are from the kit).

3. Resuspend purified dscDNA pellet in 18 μL of IVT master mix.

4. Add 2 μL of enzyme mixture and incubate at 37°C for 6 h.

aRNA Purification Using Nanoprep RNA Isolation Kit

1. Add an equal volume (approximately 100 μL) of 70% ethanol to the aRNA solution and vortex.

2. Transfer this mixture to an RNA-binding nano-spin cup and spin for 1 min 16,000g.

3. Remove the spin cup, discard the filtrate, and re-seat the spin cup in the same 2-mL collection tube.

4. DNase Treatment: Add 300 μL of 1× Low-Salt Wash Buffer to the spin cup, spin the sample for 1 min at 13,000g, discard the filtrate, re-seat the spin cup in the collection tube, transfer the cup to a new collection tube, and spin for 2 min to dry the RNA-binding matrix.

5. Prepare the DNase solution by combining 2.5 μL of reconstituted RNase-Free DNaseI with 12.5 μL of DNase Digestion Buffer for each sample.

6. Add the 15 µL of DNaseI solution directly onto the fiber matrix inside the spin cup and incubate the sample at 37°C for 15 min.

7. Pre-warm elution Buffer at 37°C, and elute the RNA in 50 µL of the elution buffer from the spin cups. (Optional: use the collected eluate for second elution of the remaining RNA from the spin cups.)

3.3.3. Second Round of RNA Amplification

The second round of RNA amplification is described in the following subheadings (*see* **Fig. 4**), including: (a) first-strand cDNA synthesis, (b) second-strand cDNA synthesis, (c) double-stranded cDNA (dscDNA) purification, (d) in vitro transcription (IVT) incorporating RNA labeling, and (e) the purification of probe-labeled aRNA.

Reverse Transcription to Synthesize First-Strand cDNA Using Retroscript Kit

1. Add 1 µg of random hexamer primers to 600 ng of aRNA (from **step** 7 in **Subheading** "aRNA Purification Using Nanoprep RNA Isolation Kit") in DEPC water and bring the total volume to 10 µL.

2. Heat at 70°C for 5 min, chill on ice for 3 min, spin, and warm up to room temperature.

3. Add (9 µL per tube) 4 µL of 5× first strand buffer, 2 µL of 0.1 M DTT, 1 µL of 10 mM dNTPs, 1 µL (200 U) of SuperScript III RT, and 1 µL (40 U) of RNaseOUT.

4. Mix, spin, heat at 25°C for 10 min increasing the temperature by 1°C every 12 s to 51°C, and incubate at 51°C for 1 h.

5. Add 1 µL (2 U) of RNAse H and incubate at 37°C for 20 min.

6. Inactivate RNAse H at 95°C for 2 min, chill on ice for 2 min, spin, and proceed to second strand cDNA synthesis.

Second-Strand cDNA Synthesis

1. Add 1 µL of 100 µM T7 oligo (dT) primer on ice.

2. Incubate at 70°C for 5 min, then at 42°C for 10 min, and chill on ice.

3. Make the master mixture (128 µL per tube): 30 µL of 5× second-strand buffer, 3 µL of 10 mM dNTPs, 4 µL (40 U) of DNA polymerase I, 1 µL (2 U) of RNase H, and 90 µL of DEPC water. Incubate at 16°C for 2 h.

4. Add 10 U of T4 DNA polymerase, incubate at 16°C for 15 min, and chill on ice.

Purification of Double-Stranded cDNA

1. Place all dscDNA solution and an equal volume (approximately 155 µL) of buffer saturated phenol:chloroform:isoamyl alcohol (25:24:1, v/v) into a Phase-Lock tube, vortex, and spin for 5 min (16,000*g*).

2. Transfer the upper phase to a new 1.5-mL tube.

3. Add 0.5 volume (75 µL) of 7.5 M NH_4OAc, 1 µL (20 µg) of glycogen, and 2.5 volumes (375 µL) of 100% cold ethanol mix and place at –80°C for 20 min.

4. Spin at 16,000g for 20 min at 4°C and discard the supernatant without disturbing the pellet.

5. Wash the pellet with 1 mL of 80% ethanol, spin at 16,000g for 2 min, discard the supernatant, and repeat the wash again.

6. Remove all ethanol, spin for 1 min, aspirate the remaining ethanol, and allow the pellet to dry completely; then resuspend in IVT reagent mix.

In Vitro Transcription to Synthesize Antisense RNA Incorporating RNA Labeling

1. Thaw and warm the reagents to room temperature (*see* **Note 5**).

2. Make IVT master mixture (18 µL per tube): 2 µL of 75 mM ATP, 2 µL of 75 mM GTP, 1.5 µL of 75 mM CTP, 1.5 µL of 75 mM UTP, 3.75 µL of 10 mM Bio-11-CTP, 3.75 µL of 10 mM Bio-16-UTP, 2 µL of 10× buffer (Ambion), and 1.5 µL of DEPC water.

3. Dissolve the dscDNA pellet in 18 µL of IVT master mix.

4. Add 2 µL of enzyme mix (Ambion), shake, and quick-spin.

5. Incubate at 37°C for 6 h.

Purification of Probe-Labeled aRNA Using Rneasy Mini Kit

1. Add 80 µL of DEPC water and 350 µL of RLT buffer to a tube with IVT reaction (20 µL) from the previous step.

2. Add 250 µL of 100% EtOH, mix well, and transfer the sample to RNeasy spin column.

3. Spin at 16,000g for 1 min, empty the collection tube, and add 500 µL of RPE buffer.

4. Spin at 16,000g for 1 min and empty the collection tube.

5. Add 500 µL of RPE buffer and spin at 16,000g for 2 min.

6. Transfer the spin column to a new capped collection tube.

7. Add 50 µL of DEPC water to the membrane and let it soak for 4 min; spin at max speed for 1 min.

8. Repeat **steps 1–7** using the first eluate for the second elution (optional).

9. Measure the optical density (OD) using a 1:50 dilution, and biotin-labeled aRNA is now ready for microarray hybridization.

3.3.4. Hybridization of Labeled aRNA to Affymetrix Microarrays

Usually, specially trained personnel at institutional core facilities perform microarray hybridizations and scanning since the equipment is rather expensive to purchase for individual laboratories. For our studies we used mouse 430 A 2.0 microarrays which includes approximately 22,000 probe sets. Affymetrix has released a newer version of mouse microarrays 430 2.0, which includes all probe sets from mouse 430 A 2.0 microarrays in addition to approximately new 17,000 probe sets, making it possible to analyze the expression of a total of approximately 39,000 transcripts. We would encourage using the newer version of the microarrays since the data generated with the new arrays is compatible with the old arrays.

3.4. Microarray Analysis

3.4.1. Data Normalization

After hybridization, the raw expression data generally has to be normalized to account for differences in chip intensities. We use dChip, a freely available software for data normalization and analysis that can be found at http://biosun1.harvard.edu/complab/dchip/. While we routinely use the Li and Wong method for data normalization found in dChip, there are a number of other approaches that may be useful for specific applications. However, we have found this method to work well for our analyses.

3.4.2. Data Analysis

For gene expression analysis, we routinely use either GenePattern, available from MIT (http://www.broad.mit.edu/tools/software.html), or cluster obtained from http://rana.lbl.gov/EisenSoftware.htm. First, we filter the data to remove probe sets that do not vary across the dataset or that have very low or high expression values. The preprocessing values we use are to set a minimum and maximum expression value, a max/min filter, and max – min filter. This filtering is performed in GenePattern, and the filtered data exported for analysis by other software. The filtering for the analyses shown in **Fig. 5** is max/min >2 and max – min >80.

The specific type of analysis is dependent on the question being addressed, and details of the decision process for computational analysis are beyond the scope of this chapter. However, the analysis described here will allow a first-pass assessment of gene expression in various populations of cells. One approach to determine global gene expression relationships between various samples is hierarchical clustering. When the question is solely the relationship between samples, one-dimensional clustering of the samples is performed (**Fig. 5a**). A number of unsupervised methods are available for clustering genes. We generally use K-means clustering (**Fig. 5b**). In this case, the number of clusters (K) was set at 10. Determining the "ideal" number for K in any experiment is a topic of considerable debate. The K-means and hierarchical clustering are performed with http://rana.lbl.gov/EisenSoftware.htm. Finally, in order to identify marker genes that distinguish two groups, we use the GenePattern software. We first filter the data as described above, and then compare the means of gene in the two groups using a signal-to-noise statistic (**Fig. 5c**). A first-pass assessment of significance is easily performed in gene pattern using the permutation analysis available in the

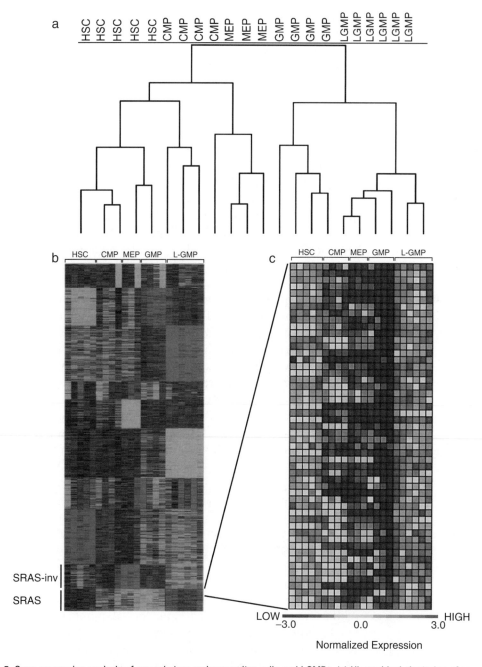

Fig. 5. Gene expression analysis of normal stem and progenitor cells and LGMPs. (**a**) Hierarchical clustering of samples identifies the gene expression profile of LGMPs as more similar to GMPs than any other population. (**b**) *K*-means analysis identifies a number of clusters of genes that have a similar gene expression pattern labeled 1–3. (**c**) Supervised marker gene analysis identifies the genes whose expression is most highly correlated with the distinction of interest, in this case cells with self-renewal potential. This is a black-and-white version of a figure taken from *(1)*.

software. For more details of these analyses the reader is referred to a number of sources *(6–9)*.

4. Notes

1. Dynabeads M-450 Sheep anti-rat IgG can be used for lineage depletion after the cells are labeled with the lineage-specific antibodies. The lineage-positive cells will bind to the magnetic beads, which can be removed in a magnetic field. The cells not expressing lineage markers will remain in the suspension. This procedure removes approximately 80–95% of the lineage-positive cells, which will dramatically reduce the time required for cell sorting.

2. Compensation is the process by which the fluorescence "spillover" originating from a fluorochrome other than the one specified for a particular channel detector is subtracted as a percentage of the signal from another channel detector. To set the fluorescence compensation, the percentage (%) compensation/subtraction is adjusted while observing a display of data being run on a two-color histogram for every channel. Compensation is correct when an imaginary line drawn across the top of the negatives and positives is level. Compensation may not be correctly set up with dimly stained cells. If the voltage is subsequently changed on any of the four detectors, or the detection filters are changed, the compensation procedure must be repeated.

3. Twenty-four hours prior to transfection, plate approximately 3–4 × 10⁶ 293 cells in 8 mL of 293T media in a 60-mm tissue culture dish. The culture should be approximately 40% confluent for transfection. Less or more confluence will reduce the transfection efficiency. It is necessary to wait for approximately 36 h post transfection to obtain high-titer retroviral supernatants. It may be possible to harvest and replenish the supernatant every 12 h up to 72 h post transfection without a significant drop in retroviral titer. Retroviral half-life is 3–6 h at 37°C *(10)*. To maintain high titers, supernatants should be aliquoted and frozen (–80°C) following harvest. Freezing does not appear to cause more than twofold drop in titer. To thaw frozen retroviral supernatants, warm for a few minutes in a 37°C water bath and immediately apply onto the cells.

4. aRNA quality is important to obtaining reproducible microarray data. The reverse transcription step of RNA amplification is the key for generating high yields of aRNA with minimal change to the initial representation of message abundance

in total RNA sample *(11)*. RNA with trace contaminants are poorly reverse-transcribed and yield less aRNA than pure samples. Therefore it is critical to use a purification method that yields RNA free of contaminants. The protocols used in this report have been optimized and the two rounds of reactions are carried through, facilitating potent amplification of total RNA from samples containing as few as 5×10^3 cells. Moreover, it is important to ensure that each reaction sample contains the same mass amount of total RNA. Differences in the amount of total RNA will affect aRNA yields and amplification efficiency. Furthermore, there are commercial kits such as Ribo-SPIA RNA amplification kit (Nugen) and MessageAmp II aRNA Amplification Kit (Ambion) that also work well for RNA amplification.

5. Heat 10× buffer (Ambion) at 55°C to dissolve precipitates, and then cool to room temperature.

Acknowledgments

We thank all the members of the Armstrong lab for their help in developing these protocols. Also, we would like to thank members of the Broad Institute cancer program and Todd R. Golub for help in developing these approaches and for ongoing collaborative efforts.

References

1. Krivtsov AV, Twomey D, Feng Z, et al. (2006) Transformation from committed progenitor to leukaemia stem cell initiated by MLL-AF9. *Nature* **442**(7104):818–22.

2. Na Nakorn T, Traver D, Weissman IL, Akashi K. (2002) Myeloerythroid-restricted progenitors are sufficient to confer radioprotection and provide the majority of day 8 CFU-S. *J Clin Invest* **109**(12):1579–85.

3. Cozzio A, Passegue E, Ayton PM, Karsunky H, Cleary ML, Weissman IL. (2003) Similar MLL-associated leukemias arising from self-renewing stem cells and short-lived myeloid progenitors. *Genes Dev* **17**(24):3029–35.

4. Akashi K, Traver D, Miyamoto T, Weissman IL. (2000) A clonogenic common myeloid progenitor that gives rise to all myeloid lineages. *Nature* **404**(6774):193–7.

5. Coligan JE, Kruisbeek AM, Margulies DH, Shevach EM, Strobber W. (1994) Current protocols in immunology, isolation of murine macrophages. New York: Wiley,

6. Eisen MB, Spellman PT, Brown PO, Botstein D. (1998) Cluster analysis and display of genome-wide expression patterns. *Proc Natl Acad Sci U S A* **95**(25):14863–8.

7. Golub TR, Slonim DK, Tamayo P, et al. 1999 Molecular classification of cancer: class discovery and class prediction by gene expression monitoring. *Science* **286**(5439):531–7.

8. Tamayo P, Scanfeld D, Ebert BL, Gillette MA, Roberts CW, Mesirov JP. Metagene projection for cross-platform, cross-species characterization of global transcriptional states. *Proc Natl Acad Sci U S A* 2007;**104**(14): 5959–64.

9. Reich M, Liefeld T, Gould J, Lerner J, Tamayo P, Mesirov JP. (2006) GenePattern 2.0. *Nat Genet* **38**(5):500–1.

10. Sanes JR, Rubenstein JL, Nicolas JF. (1986) Use of a recombinant retrovirus to study post-implantation cell lineage in mouse embryos. *EMBO J* **5**(12):3133–42.

11. Van Gelder RN, von Zastrow ME, Yool A, Dement WC, Barchas JD, Eberwine JH. (1990) Amplified RNA synthesized from limited quantities of heterogeneous cDNA. *Proc Natl Acad Sci U S A* **87**(5):1663–7.

Chapter 12

Humanized Model to Study Leukemic Stem Cells

Dominique Bonnet

Summary

The xenotransplantation model has been instrumental for the identification and characterization of human leukemic stem cells. In this chapter we will discuss the development of the immunodeficient model in the understanding of leukemogenesis, describe the different models of immunodeficiency now available and their values, as well as describe the methods used for the purification of LSCs. We will concentrate on the model of acute myeloid leukemia, as it was the first type of leukemia for which the xenotransplantation model was developed.

Key words: Hematopoietic stem cell (HSC), Xenotransplantation, Immunodeficient mice, Leukemic stem cell (LSC)

1. Introduction

The adaptation of xenotransplantation assays to examine the propagation of AML in vivo has been instrumental in the identification and characterization of the leukemic initiating cells. Transplantation of primary AML cells into NOD/SCID mice led to the finding that only rare cells, termed *AML-initiating cells* (AML-IC), are capable of initiating and sustaining growth of the leukemic clone in vivo, and serial transplantation experiments showed that AML-IC possess high self-renewal capacity, and thus can be considered to be the leukemic stem cells. By leukemic stem cell (LSC) we refer to a cell that has self-renewal and differentiation potential and is able to reinitiate the leukemia when transplanted into NOD/SCID mice. This definition does not preclude the nature of the cells that is being transformed. Indeed, it is still unclear about the nature of the cells responsible

C.W.E. So (ed.), Leukemia, *Methods in Molecular Biology, vol. 538*
© Humana Press, a part of Springer Science + Business Media, LLC 2009
DOI: 10.1007/978-1-59745-418-6_12

for the leukemic transformation (i.e. normal HSC, progenitors, or mature cells).

The confusion regarding the origin of the AML-IC may be due to the extreme heterogeneity of AML. Given the various possible routes to AML from a normal hematopoietic cell, it is not surprising that there is great heterogeneity in AML. Indeed, AML may be thought of as a large collection of different diseases that merely share a similar morphology. Indeed, the most effective risk stratification approach so far has been to examine the genetic abnormalities associated with a particular case of AML and compare with previous experience of AML cases with the same abnormality (1, 2). Although cytogenetic analysis allows the definition of the hierarchical groups with favorable, intermediate, and poor prognosis, the intermediate-risk group contains patients with variable outcomes. Assessing the prognosis of this large group of patients is currently difficult.

The ability of a particular AML to engraft in the NOD/SCID model is related to the prognosis of individual AML cases (3). Specifically, examination of the follow-up of younger patients with intermediate-risk AML revealed a significant difference in overall survival between NOD/SCID-engrafting and non-engrafting cases. No differences have been detected between engrafting and non-engrafting cases in various engraftment variables, including homing ability, AML-IC frequency, immune rejection by the host, or alternative tissue sources. Hence, the ability to engraft NOD/SCID recipients seems to be an inherent property of the cells that is directly related to prognosis.

Other mouse models have been developed to support the growth of human hematopoietic cells, but less is known about the ability of these new models to sustain AML engraftment. The NOD/SCID-β_2 microglobulin null ($\beta2m^{-/-}$) mouse has a further defect in NK cell activity and is more tolerant of human grafts than the NOD/SCID model (4–6). However, the percentage of AML samples that engraft in $\beta2m^{-/-}$ is similar to the level achieved using the NOD/SCID mice. Thus it does not appear that the $\beta2m^{-/-}$ is superior for the engraftment of AML samples (3). Furthermore, both NOD/SCID and $\beta2m^{-/-}$ are susceptible to developing lymphomas overtime, limiting their lifespan and preventing long-term reconstitutional assessment. These hurdles have recently been overcome in three new strains: NOD/Shi-Scid Il2Rg^{null} (7, 8), NOD/SCID IL2Rg^{null} (9, 10), and BALB/c-Rag2^{null} IL2Rg^{null} (11), which all lack the IL-2 family common cytokine receptor gamma chain gene. The absence of functional receptors for IL-2, IL-7, and other cytokines may prevent the expansion of NK cells and early lymphoma cells in NOD/SCID IL2Rg^{null} mice, resulting in better engraftment of transplanted human cells and longer lifespan of the mice. It was reported recently that human HSCs and progenitor cells engraft successfully in these mice and produce all human myeloid and lymphoid lineages. T and B cells migrate into lymphoid organs and mount HLA-dependent allogeneic responses, and generate antibodies against T-cell-dependent antigens, such as ovalbumin and tetanus toxin *(11, 12)*. Whether these mice will be superior for leukemic engraftment needs to be evaluated.

To exclude stem cell homing interference and focus on the intrinsic capacity of a cell to self-renew, a few groups recently developed a highly sensitive strategy based on direct intra-bone marrow (IBM) injection of the candidate human stem cell *(13–15)*. IBM injection was found to be a more sensitive and adequate means to measure human HSC capacity. Nevertheless, we recently demonstrated that non-engrafting AML samples still do not engraft even after intra-bone injection, demonstrating that the efficiency of homing to the bone marrow is not related to the capacity of leukemic samples to engraft *(3)*.

Importantly, AML-IC can be prospectively identified and purified as CD34$^+$/CD38$^-$ cells in AML patient samples, regardless of the phenotype of the bulk blast population, and represent the only AML cells capable of self-renewal *(16)*.

The phenotype of AML-IC has been extended via the use of immunodeficient mice to include an absence of CD71, HLA-DR, and CD117, but include expression of CD123 *(17–20)*. In a recent study this phenotype was further extended to include expression of CD33 and CD13 on AML-IC from the vast majority of patients *(21)*. Hence, the immunophenotype of the LSC as defined by in vivo propagation is CD34$^+$/CD38$^-$/CD71$^-$/HLA-DR$^-$/CD117$^-$/CD33$^+$/CD13$^+$/CD123$^+$. However, the exclusivity of some markers is debatable. For instance, CD123 is indeed expressed on AML-IC, but is also expressed on the vast majority of AML blasts (unpublished observations) from most patients and hence, could be excluded from the above phenotype of AML-IC.

In addition to the use of these surrogate markers, alternative methods to identify hematopoietic stem cells have been developed. Aldehyde dehydrogenase (ALDH) is a cytosolic enzyme that is responsible for the oxidation of intracellular aldehydes. This enzyme is thought to have an important role in oxidation of alcohol and vitamin A, and in cyclophosphamide chemoresistance *(22, 23)*. Elevated levels of ALDH have been demonstrated in murine and human progenitor cells when compared with other hematopoietic cells *(24)*. More recently, a method has been developed for the assessment of ALDH activity in viable cells. This non-cytotoxic method utilizes a cell-permeable fluorescent substrate to identify cells with high ALDH activity *(25)*. Substrate converted by ALDH is a charged molecule and is unable to leave the cell as freely as the unconverted substrate. In this way, converted ALDH substrate accumulates in cells with a high

ALDH activity. This approach has allowed the analysis of viable murine and human ALDH+ progenitors by flow cytometry.

Using aldehyde dehydrogenase-1 activity from various AML samples, AML-IC can also be enriched. It seems that in approximately one-third of patients, a subset of AML-IC possess a high ALDH activity that is detectable using the fluorescent ALDH substrate (26).

It is clear nevertheless that despite the different isolation strategies employed, considerable heterogeneity within the AML-IC compartment exists. Lentiviral gene marking to track the behavior of individual LSCs, following serial transplantation, has revealed heterogeneity in their ability to self-renew, similar to what is seen in the normal HSC compartment (27).

2. Materials

1. Immunodeficient mice NOD/SCID, $\beta2m^{-/-}$ or NOD/SCID IL2Rg^{null} can be purchased from Jackson Laboratory (Bar Harbor, ME).

2. 29 ½-gauge needle/syringe from Kendall Monoject Insulin syringe (Tyco Healthcare, Basingstoke, Hampshire, UK).

3. Phosphate buffered saline (PBS): Either commercially available or prepared as described. Prepare 10× stock with 1.37 M NaCl, 27 mM KCL, 100 mM Na_2HPO_2, 18 mM KH_2PO_4 (adjust to pH 7.4 if necessary) and autoclave before storage at room temperature. Prepare working solution by diluting one part with nine parts of water.

4. Acidified water: A solution of HCl at a final pH 2.8–3.2.

5. Ketaset solution (Fort Dodge Animal Health Ltd., Southampton, UK).

6. Rompun 2% solution (Bayer Plc, Newbury, UK).

7. Vetergesic (Alstoe Animal Health, Melton Mowbray, Leicestershire, UK).

8. Purified rat anti-mouse CD122 antibody (BD Pharmingen, Oxford, UK – clone TbM1).

9. Antibodies against human anti-CD45, CD34, CD38, CD33, and CD19 (BD Pharmingen, Oxford, UK clones: HI30, 8G12 or 581, HB7, HIM3-4 and HIB19 respectively).

10. Ficoll Hypaque (Stem Cell Technologies, Meylan, France).

11. Lineage cocktail antibodies (BD Pharmingen, cat 340546),

12. Aldefluor reagent (Becton, Dickinson [BD] Biosciences, Oxford, UK).

13. Ammonium chloride solution (Stem Cell Technologies, Vancouver, BC, Canada).

14. 4′,6-diamidino-2-phenylindole (DAPI, UV excited, Sigma-Aldrich, St Louis 100 ng/ml final concentration).

15. TOPRO-3 200 ng/ml final concentration (HeNe (633 nm) excitable, Molecular Probes Inc., Eugene, Or).

16. SSC/NP-40 (Sigma-Aldrich).

17. Karnoy's fixative (Sigma-Aldrich).

18. A FACS analyzer and a FACS sorter, e.g. LSRII and Aria (BD Biosciences, Oxford, UK).

3. Methods

3.1. Preparation of the Immunodeficient Mice

All the animals used have some impairment in their immune system and may succumb to infections not affecting normal mice. They thus should be kept in pathogen-free status within barrier systems to protect them from inter-current infections.

3.1.1. Sublethal Irradiation of the Mice

The mice are sublethally irradiated before the adoptive transfer of cells. The dose of irradiation depends on the mouse strains used and also on the source and irradiator used. It usually varies from 300 to 375 cGy (see **Notes 1** and **2**). Any mouse receiving irradiation should be maintained on acidified water at least 1 week before the irradiation and 2 weeks after the irradiation dose to prevent diarrhea or weight loss possibly arising through epithelial damage of the intestines. Any animal showing persistent weight loss exceeding 20% of body weight and/or other signs of illness (rough fur, inappetance, inability to groom, immobility, tympany) should be sacrificed. Experience shows that with these measures, the above side effects rarely arise (average 0.5%).

Full body irradiation may cause the mice to appear anaemic within the first 3 weeks after irradiation. Previous experience has shown that the anaemia is transient and last for approximately five consecutive days. During the first 3 weeks after irradiation the mice should be monitored closely (see **Note 3**).

3.1.2. General Anaesthesia of the Mice (Only for Intra-Bone Injection and Biopsy)

The mice are injected intra-peritoneally with a dose of 0.2–0.25 ml of anaesthetic solution (see **Note 4**). General anaesthesia suppresses the heat regulating mechanisms of the body. This is overcome by intra- and post-operative maintenance of body temperature in appropriate thermostatically-controlled incubators or by other heat sources. During recovery, animals should be kept under regular observation until full mobility is regained. At this stage, animals should receive at least one dose of post-operative analgesic following bone marrow injection (100 µl of analgesic solution (Vetergesic diluted 1/10) *see* **Note 5**).

3.2. Preparation of the Cells

Fresh peripheral blood or bone marrow samples are usually used to test for the engraftment ability of the samples. For this pre-screening, 5–10 millions of mononuclear cells are injected per mouse (4–5 mice are tested). After 8–10 weeks, the mice are sacrificed and the AML engraftment analysis is performed as indicated below. If the AML sample engrafts, purification of the AML-IC can be performed using Lin-CD34+CD38- or ALDH staining and cell sorting (see below).

3.2.1. Purification Strategy Using Surface Markers

1. Mononuclear cells from peripheral blood or bone marrow aspirated from newly diagnosed patients are extracted using Ficoll-Hypaque separation. Briefly, each sample is diluted in IMDM medium (2:1 – vol:vol) before layering the cells gently over 15 ml of Ficoll-Hypaque in 50-ml conical tubes. The cells are centrifuged for 30 min at $440 \times g$ at room temperature (RT) with brake off. Most of the upper layer is carefully removed and the cells at the interface with the ficoll are extracted gently using a Pasteur pipette. These cells are diluted in IMDM (5:1 – vol:vol) in order to remove the Ficoll and pelleted by centrifugation for 10 min at $440 \times g$ at RT. The mononuclear cells are now ready to be used or if necessary can be frozen at this stage for future use.

2. Mononuclear cells from AML samples can be stained using a combination of antibodies. The most commonly used are the lineage cocktail antibodies (5 µl/million – available only as FITC-conjugated), anti-CD34 (5µl/million, suggested fluorochrome: PerCp), and anti-CD38 (5 µl/million, suggested Fluorochrome: PE). The cells are stained at 4°C for 25–30 min in the presence of each of these antibodies. After the incubation period, the cells are washed twice in PBS-2%FCS. After washing, the cells (with addition of DAPI, 200 ng/ml, for staining dead cells) are ready to be sorted through a cell sorter (FACS Aria, BD, or others).

3. A typical diagram showing the resultant staining is showed in **Fig. 1**. The heterogeneity of AML samples becomes apparent from this staining.

3.2.2. Purification Strategy Using ALDH Staining

1. Cells are labeled with Aldefluor reagent as described by the manufacturer. Briefly, mix cells with 0.5 ml of Aldelfluor reagent and incubate 15–30 min at 2–8°C. Add 0.5 ml of Aldefluor assay buffer to all tubes and centrifuge cells at $250 \times g$ for 5 min.

2. Cells are washed and resuspended in PBS with 2% fetal calf serum and DAPI (200 ng/ml).

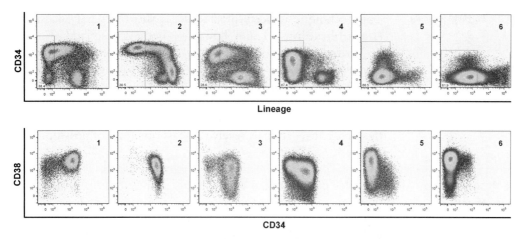

Fig. 1. Phenotypic heterogeneity in AML samples. FACS analysis of six different AML patient samples based on the expression of lineage, CD34 and CD38 antigen expression.

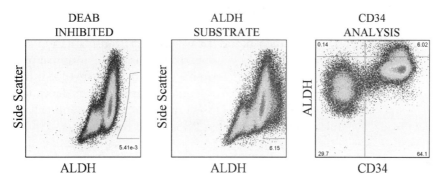

Fig. 2. Example of AML samples stained with ALDH. The *left panel* represents the ALDH staining of this specific AML patient. The *middle panel* shows the specificity of the staining based on the disappearance of the staining using DEAD inhibitor. The *right panel* represents the co-staining between CD34 and ALDH.

3. Cells are then analyzed on a BD LSR flow cytometer or sorted using a FACS Aria cell sorter. Aldefluor reagent was excited at 488 nm. Gates are set up to exclude non-viable cells and debris.

4. A typical diagram showing the resultant staining is shown in **Fig. 2**.

3.3. Adoptive Transfer of Cells

Mice that have been subjected to sublethal irradiation will receive cell preparations (unpurified or purified cell fraction, genetically modified or not). This may be performed on the same day as, or up to 72 h following, irradiation.

3.3.1. Intravenous Injection

Cells will be injected intravenously via the tail vein (maximum volume 1% body weight) using a syringe with a 29 ½-gauge needle.

3.3.2. Intra-Bone Injection

This technique is performed under a short general anaesthesia (*see* **Subheading 3.1.2**) following a method described originally by Verlinden et al. *(28)* (*for a diagram of this technique confer to this original paper*). A syringe with a 29 ½-gauge needle (maximum) is inserted into the joint surface of the right or left tibia/ femur, and cells to a maximum volume of 40 µl suspension are injected into the bone marrow cavity of the tibia or femur. After this procedure, animals receive at least one dose of post-operative analgesic (*see* **Note 5**).

3.4. Analysis of the Engraftment

3.4.1. Bone Marrow Aspiration

Samples can be taken under general anaesthesia, as described previously, on up to four occasions per mouse at least 14 days apart, alternatively from the left and right femur. Bone marrow will be aspirated by puncture through the knee joint using a 29 ½-gauge needle. The maximum amount taken per sample should not exceed 30 µl. The first sample should be taken at least 16 h after adoptive transfer of cells. After this procedure, animals receive at least one dose of post-operative analgesic (*see* **Note 5**).

3.4.2. Sacrificing the Mice

Mice between 6 and 14 weeks after transplantation will be sacrificed either using cervical dislocation or terminal anaesthesia. When work under terminal anaesthesia is involved, the level of anaesthesia should be maintained at sufficient depth for the animal to feel no pain. Dissect the femurs, tibias, and pelvis from the mice and store at RT in PBS before flushing.

3.4.3. Preparation of the Mouse Bone Marrow

Place 1 ml of RT PBS in a 5 ml snap-top polystyrene tube. Cut both ends of each bone to provide an opening. To flush, insert a PBS-containing insulin syringe into one end of each bone and wash the lumen of the bone with a medium pressure. Repeat twice for both ends of the bone or until the bone appears relatively white.

3.4.4. Preparation of the Cells for FACS Analysis

To lyse red blood cells, first cool the cell suspension for 5 min on ice, then add 3 ml of cold ammonium chloride solution to the 1 ml PBS/cell suspension, mix, and leave for 5 min at 4°C. Add 0.5 ml of FCS, spin down cells at 1,200 rpm 250 g for 5 min, remove the supernatant, and resuspend the cells in 1 ml of cold PBS-containing 2% FCS. Count the cells using a hematocytometer. Store on ice and it is ready for antibody labeling.

3.4.5. Staining Procedure

1. Prepare a mix of human-specific FITC-conjugated anti-CD19, PE-conjugated anti-CD33, and PerCP-conjugated anti-CD45 antibodies (5 µl/sample/antibody for all stains and compensation/isotype controls).

2. Also prepare FITC, PE, and PerCP single color compensation control tubes (5 ml snap-top polystyrene as before) and a combined FITC/PE/PerCP matched isotype control tube.

3. Distribute 15 µl of the antibody mix into each fresh tube for antibody labeling.

4. Dispense 40 µl of each cell suspension into the appropriate antibody labeling tube and leave to label for 30 min at 4°C.

5. Wash cells in 2 ml of PBS–2%FCS and resuspend in 500 µl of PBS–2%FCS supplemented with a cell impermeant DNA dye for live/dead discrimination, either 100 ng/ml DAPI, (UV excited), or TOPRO-3 (HeNe (633 nm) excitable).

3.4.6. FACS Analysis

1. To analyze this combination of fluorochromes you will require a 488-nm excitation source and either a UV or HeNe (633 nm) source depending on your choice of live/dead discriminator. For emission collection you will need a 440/40 bandpass (bp) filter for analysis of DAPI, a 530/30 bp filter for FITC, a 575/26 bp for PE, a 695/40 bp for PerCP and a 660/20 bp for TOPRO-3.

2. Set the photomultiplier gains so that the background signal from the combined isotype control gives 1–5% positive cells in each collection channel. Set the compensation amount according to the detected spectral overlap.

3. To analyze the engraftment, draw four dotplots A, B, C, and D as in **Fig. 1** (440/40 nm vs. side-scatter (SSC), forward scatter (FSC) vs. SSC, 695/40 nm vs. SSC and 530/30 nm vs. 575/26 nm).

4. First, exclude dead cells from the analysis via a region (R1) around the live, unstained cells as in **Fig. 3a** (left panel: bone marrow of a mice injected with 10^7 AML MNC. As control, right panel represents a FACS analysis of a mouse transplanted with 5×10^6 MNC from umbilical cord blood).

5. Next, display these cells on a FSC vs. SSC plot and select the lymphoid and myeloid cells for further analysis, but exclude debris via a region (R2) as in **Fig. 3b**.

6. Display cells that fall into the first two regions on a 695/40 nm vs. SSC plot and draw a generous region around the CD45-PerCP positive cells as in **Fig. 3c** (R3).

7. Display these CD45$^+$ cells on a CD19-FITC vs. CD33-PE (530/30 nm vs. 575/26 nm) dotplot and draw a quadrant to define FITC$^+$/PE$^-$ cells and FITC$^-$/PE$^+$ cell subsets as in **Fig. 3d**.

8. The number of events that fall within these regions may be used to calculate the percentage of live, debris-free cells (R2) that are human cells.

9. In addition, the scatter characteristics of cells may be confirmed as consistent with myeloid (high FSC and SSC, example in **Fig. 3e**) and lymphoid (low FSC and SSC, example in **Fig. 3f** (in this example there are no CD19$^+$ cells).

10. Engraftment is classed as myeloid leukemia if a population of CD45$^+$/CD33$^+$ cells is present without an accompanying CD45$^+$CD19$^+$/CD33$^-$ cell population.

3.4.7. Fluorescent In Situ Hybridization Analysis (FISH)

To confirm the leukemic origin of the myeloid cells present in the bone marrow of engrafted mice and if the AML sample originally has a known translocation, it is possible to sort human CD45$^+$ cells and perform a fluorescent in situ hybridization analysis of the cells as stipulated below.

1. If starting with sorted cells, wash around 10^5 cells in PBS, resuspend in 1 ml of PBS and 5%FCS.

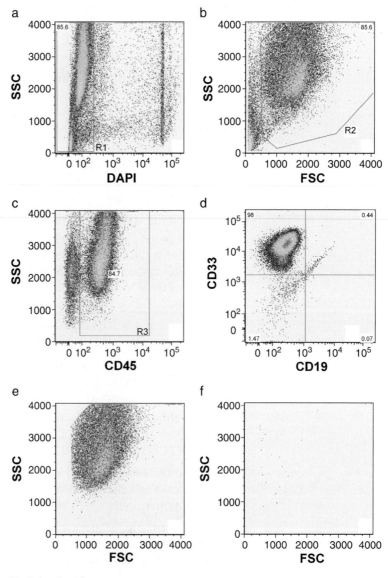

Fig. 3. (continued)

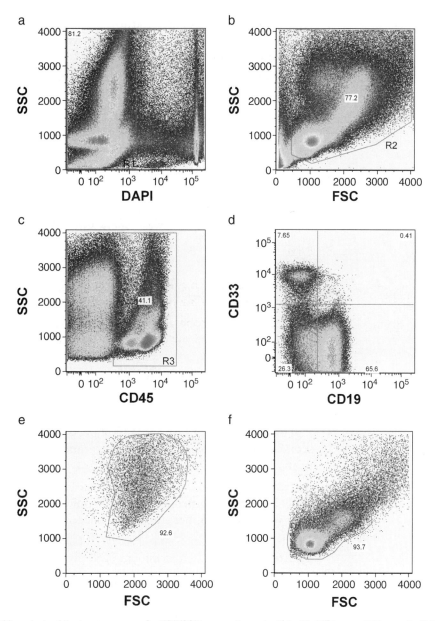

Fig. 3. FACS analysis of the bone marrow of a NOD/SCID mouse transplanted with 10^7 human AML sample (*left panel*) or 5 × 10^6 umbilical cord blood mononuclear cells (*right panel*). Dead cells are excluded using the DAPI staining (region (R1) in (**a**)). The lymphoid and myeloid cells are selected using the FSC vs. SSC plot for further analysis, excluding debris via a region (R2) as in (**b**). The human CD45-PerCP positive cells are selected in region (R3) in (**c**). (**d**) displays these CD45$^+$ cells on a CD19-FITC vs. CD33-PE dotplot. In addition, the scatter characteristics of these cells may be confirmed as consistent with myeloid (high FSC and SSC, example in (**e**)) and lymphoid (low FSC and SSC, example in (**f**)).

2. Pre-warm cells to 37°C and add 10 ml of 37°C KCl (excess). Incubate at 37°C for 10 min.

3. Spin off KCl at RT on a reasonably slow spin (≈250 × *g*, pellet will be diffused).

4. Resuspend in 1 ml of RT Karnoy's fixative (in fume cupboard, break up pellet first, add drop-wise while agitating firmly but not too vigorously).

5. Spin at $\simeq 350 \times g$ (RT, no longer class 2). Resuspend in 1 ml of Karnoy's fixative as before.

6. Repeat this procedure twice more, finally resuspend in fixative (suspension may be stored in a small sealed tube at 4°C for 2 years).

7. Apply a drop ($\simeq$100 µl) of distilled water (DW) onto prewashed slides (see below).

8. Apply 20 µl of cell suspension in the DW drop and place slide on a preheated slide warmer/heating block at 45°C.

9. Keep slide flat throughout and allow to dry on the block for 10 min.

10. Keep the slide for 16 h at RT in dust free environment (slides can be stored at 4°C for 6 months) before the hybridization step.

11. Thaw the FISH probe and buffer at RT, vortex, and pulse spin. Mark cell area on underneath of slide with diamond cutter.

12. Dehydrate slide at RT: 2 min in each of 70, 85, and 100% ethanol (leave in 100% until ready to use).

13. Prepare the probe mix in the dark. For Vysis LSI probes add 7 µl of buffer, 2 µl of DW and 1 µl of probe. For other probe sets follow the manufacturer's recommendation. Protect probe from light from this point onwards.

14. Air dry the slide on 45°C block, once dried immediately apply 5 µl of probe mix per slide and apply coverslip and seal with vulcanizing rubber – allow rubber to dry on the block.

15. Incubate at 73°C for 5 min exactly and switch to 37°C for 12–16 h in a humid environment (LSI probes).

16. Peel off rubber cement, remove the coverslip and place in preheated (73°C) 0.4%-SSC/0.3%NP-40 for 2 min exactly.

17. Wash slides in RT 2× SSC, 0.1% NP-40 for 1 min.

18. Dehydrate slides at RT for 2 min in each of 70, 85, and 100% ethanol (leave in 100% until ready to use) and finally air dry at RT.

19. Apply $\simeq$ 10 µl of DAPI supplemented anti-fade mountant (125 ng/ml in vectorshield or Vysis anti-fade).

20. Apply coverslip and seal with rubber or acrylic varnish and allow DAPI to diffuse into nuclei from 1 h to overnight (best results if left overnight).

21. The label will last for 2 years if sealed at 4°C in the dark. Analyse the slides as described below.

An example of a FISH analysis is presented in **Fig. 4**. The sample analyzed is an AML sample from a patient with the trans-location t[8,21]. The Vysis LSI t[8,21] (AML1/ETO) probe (cat no. 32-191006) labels the AML-1 (21q22) with Spectrum-Green™ and the ETO (8q22) with SpectrumOrange™. Images were acquired on a Carl-Zeiss Axioplan-2 fluorescence micro-scope equipped with an Axiocam Mrc digital camera and 10× ocular lens. **Figure 4a, b** were generated with a Plan-Apochro-mat 100×/1.4na DIC oil objective lens. **Figure 4c** was generated via a Plan-Neofluar 40×/0.75na air objective lens. In **Fig. 4a**, the cell on the left is positive for the rearrangement and exhibits

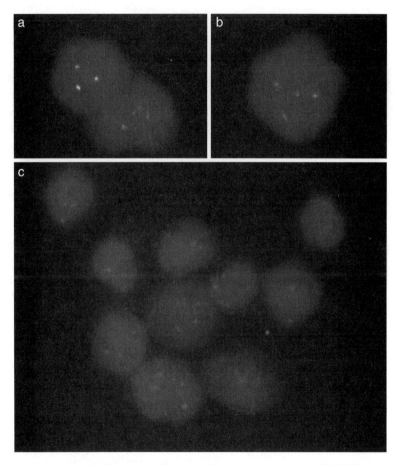

Fig. 4. Example of FISH analysis of human AML blasts recovered from NOD/SCID mice 12 weeks post-transplant. Dual fusion, dual fluorescent in situ hybridization of a t(8, 21) (AML/ETO) AML-M2 sample. In (**a**), the cell on the left is positive for the rearrangement and exhibits 1 *green*, 1 *red*, and 2 *orange spots* whereas the cell on the right is an exam-ple of an inconclusive result and as such is excluded from counts. An example of a cell that is positive for the rearrangement but the resolution of the microscope is sufficient to resolve the co-localised dots as separate *red* and *green dots* rather than a composite *yellow dot* (**b**). A lower power image showing a complete field of view, in which the majority of cells are positive for the t[8,21] rearrangement (**c**). (*see* Color Plates)

1 green, 1 red and 2 orange spots whereas the cell on the right is an example of an inconclusive result and as such is excluded from counts. An example of a cell that is positive for the rearrangement but the resolution of the microscope is sufficient to resolve the co-localised dots as separate red and green dots rather than a composite yellow dot (**Fig. 4b**). A lower power image showing a complete field of view, in which the majority of cells are positive for the t[8,21] rearrangement (**Fig. 4c**).

4. Notes

1. The mice should be treated for at least 8 days with acidified water before the irradiation.

2. The sublethal irradiation dose (between 320 and 375 cGy) should be adapted to the irradiator used. It indeed depends on the dose rate/minute of irradiation. If the dose rate is initially too high, the time should be increased (by using appropriate shielding), to reduce the impact on internal organs. Gamma radiation primarily damages cells dividing at a high rate, such as gut epithelium or cells of the hemopoietic system. Damage to gut epithelium may result in mal-absorption, resulting in weight loss, and it allows the overgrowth of microorganisms, resulting in enteritis. These may enter the circulation resulting in bacteraemia or even septicaemia. Damage to the hemopoietic system may cause bone marrow depression in low doses and its destruction in high doses resulting in increased susceptibility of infections, leucopoenia, platelet deficiency resulting in haemorrhages (immediately) and anaemia. It may also cause skin haemorrhages (petechiae) and hyperaemia (erythema), especially in SCID animals, possibly resulting in dermatitis. Adverse effects of whole body irradiation are noticed in ~1% of animals undergoing the procedure. To minimise the presence of potentially pathogenic agents, mice of the cleanest available health status are used and held within barrier protection (such as isolator, filter cages, barrier rooms or at least maximal hygienic measures) at all times.

3. General health monitoring: Mice should be monitored daily and might be culled if they show signs of ill health, such as piloerection and hunched posture, inactivity or inappetance for a period of 48 h. In addition, any animal that loses 20% body weight or that develops more serious clinical signs, such as diarrhoea or dyspnoea should also be sacrificed.

4. Anaesthetic solution: Mix 1 ml of Ketaset with 0.5 ml of Rompun 2% and dilute with 8.5 ml of PBS. This solution can be kept at least 1 month at 4°C.

5. Analgesic: Vetergesic should be diluted 1/10 in PBS and injected at 100 µl subcutaneously per mouse.

Acknowledgments

The author thanks Mr. Christopher Ridler and Dr. Daniel Pearce for their assistance in the preparation of this manuscript.

References

1. Grimwade, D., Walker, H., Harrison, G., Oliver, F., Chatters, S., Harrison, C. J., et al. (2001). The predictive value of hierarchical cytogenetic classification in older adults with acute myeloid leukemia (AML): analysis of 1065 patients entered into the United Kingdom Medical Research Council AML11 trial. *Blood* **98**, 1312–1320.

2. Grimwade, D., Walker, H., Oliver, F., Wheatley, K., Harrison, C., Harrison, G., et al. (1998). The importance of diagnostic cytogenetics on outcome in AML: analysis of 1,612 patients entered into the MRC AML 10 trial. *The Medical Research Council Adult and Children's Leukaemia Working Parties. Blood* **92**, 2322–2333.

3. Pearce, D. J., Taussig, D., Zibara, K., Smith, L. L., Ridler, C. M., Preudhomme, C., et al. (2006). AML engraftment in the NOD/SCID assay reflects the outcome of AML: implications for our understanding of the heterogeneity of AML. *Blood* **107**, 1166–1173.

4. Christianson, S. W., Greiner, D. L., Hesselton, R. A., Leif, J. H., Wagar, E. J., Schweitzer, I. B., et al. (1997). Enhanced human CD4+ T cell engraftment in beta2-microglobulin-deficient NOD-scid mice. *J Immunol* **158**, 3578–3586.

5. Glimm, H., Eisterer, W., Lee, K., Cashman, J., Holyoake, T. L., Nicolini, F., et al. (2001). Previously undetected human hematopoietic cell populations with short-term repopulating activity selectively engraft NOD/SCID-beta2 microglobulin-null mice. *J Clin Invest* **107**, 199–206.

6. Kollet, O., Peled, A., Byk, T., Ben-Hur, H., Greiner, D., Shultz, L., et al. (2000). beta2 microglobulin-deficient (B2m(null)) NOD/SCID mice are excellent recipients for studying human stem cell function. *Blood* **95**, 3102–3105.

7. Hiramatsu, H., Nishikomori, R., Heike, T., Ito, M., Kobayashi, K., Katamura, K., et al. (2003). Complete reconstitution of human lymphocytes from cord blood CD34+ cells using the NOD/SCID/gammacnull mice model. *Blood* **102**, 873–880.

8. Yahata, T., Ando, K., Nakamura, Y., Ueyama, Y., Shimamura, K., Tamaoki, N., et al. (2002). Functional human T lymphocyte development from cord blood CD34+ cells in nonobese diabetic/Shi-scid, IL-2 receptor gamma null mice. *J Immunol* **169**, 204–209.

9. Ishikawa, F., Yasukawa, M., Lyons, B., Yoshida, S., Miyamoto, T., Yoshimoto, G., et al. (2005). Development of functional human blood and immune systems in NOD/SCID/IL2 receptor {gamma} chain(null) mice. *Blood* **106**, 1565–1573.

10. Shultz, L. D., Lyons, B. L., Burzenski, L. M., Gott, B., Chen, X., Chaleff, S., et al. (2005). Human lymphoid and myeloid cell development in NOD/LtSz-scid IL2R gamma null mice engrafted with mobilized human hemopoietic stem cells. *J Immunol* **174**, 6477–6489.

11. Traggiai, E., Chicha, L., Mazzucchelli, L., Bronz, L., Piffaretti, J. C., Lanzavecchia, A., et al. (2004). Development of a human adaptive immune system in cord blood cell-transplanted mice. *Science* **304**, 104–107.

13. Mazurier, F., Doedens, M., Gan, O. I., and Dick, J. E. (2003). Rapid myeloerythroid repopulation after intrafemoral transplantation of NOD-SCID mice reveals a new class of human stem cells. *Nat Med* **9**, 959–963.

14. Wang, J., Kimura, T., Asada, R., Harada, S., Yokota, S., Kawamoto, Y., et al. (2003).

SCID-repopulating cell activity of human cord blood-derived CD34- cells assured by intra-bone marrow injection. *Blood* **101**, 2924–2931.

15. Yahata, T., Ando, K., Sato, T., Miyatake, H., Nakamura, Y., Muguruma, Y., et al. (2003). A highly sensitive strategy for SCID-repopulating cell assay by direct injection of primitive human hematopoietic cells into NOD/SCID mice bone marrow. *Blood* **101**, 2905–2913.

16. Bonnet, D., and Dick, J. E. (1997). Human acute myeloid leukemia is organized as a hierarchy that originates from a primitive hematopoietic cell. *Nat Med* **3**, 730–737.

17. Blair, A., Hogge, D. E., Ailles, L. E., Lansdorp, P. M., and Sutherland, H. J. (1997). Lack of expression of Thy-1 (CD90) on acute myeloid leukemia cells with long-term proliferative ability in vitro and in vivo. *Blood* **89**, 3104–3112.

18. Blair, A., Hogge, D. E., and Sutherland, H. J. (1998). Most acute myeloid leukemia progenitor cells with long-term proliferative ability in vitro and in vivo have the phenotype CD34(+)/CD71(-)/HLA-DR. *Blood* **92**, 4325–4335.

19. Blair, A., and Sutherland, H. J. (2000). Primitive acute myeloid leukemia cells with long-term proliferative ability in vitro and in vivo lack surface expression of c-kit (CD117). *Exp Hematol* **28**, 660–671.

20. Jordan, C. T., Upchurch, D., Szilvassy, S. J., Guzman, M. L., Howard, D. S., Pettigrew, A. L., et al. (2000). The interleukin-3 receptor alpha chain is a unique marker for human acute myelogenous leukemia stem cells. *Leukemia* **14**, 1777–1784.

21. Taussig, D. C., Pearce, D. J., Simpson, C., Rohatiner, A. Z., Lister, T. A., Kelly, G., et al. (2005). Hematopoietic stem cells express multiple myeloid markers: implications for the origin and targeted therapy of acute myeloid leukemia. *Blood* **106**, 4086–4092.

22. Wang, J. S., Fang, Q., Sun, D. J., Chen, J., Zhou, X. L., Lin, G. W., et al. (2001). Genetic modification of hematopoietic progenitor cells for combined resistance to 4-hydroperoxycyclophosphamide, vincristine, and daunorubicin. *Acta Pharmacol Sin* **22**, 949–955.

23. Duester, G. (2000). Families of retinoid dehydrogenases regulating vitamin A function: production of visual pigment and retinoic acid. *Eur J Biochem* **267**, 4315–4324.

24. Kastan, M. B., Schlaffer, E., Russo, J. E., Colvin, O. M., Civin, C. I., and Hilton, J. (1990). Direct demonstration of elevated aldehyde dehydrogenase in human hematopoietic progenitor cells. *Blood* **75**, 1947–1950.

25. Jones, R. J., Barber, J. P., Vala, M. S., Collector, M. I., Kaufmann, S. H., Ludeman, S. M., et al. (1995). Assessment of aldehyde dehydrogenase in viable cells. *Blood* **85**, 2742–2746.

26. Pearce, D. J., Taussig, D., Simpson, C., Allen, K., Rohatiner, A. Z., Lister, T. A., et al. (2005). Characterization of cells with a high aldehyde dehydrogenase activity from cord blood and acute myeloid leukemia samples. *Stem Cells* **23**, 752–760.

27. Hope, K. J., Jin, L., and Dick, J. E. (2004). Acute myeloid leukemia originates from a hierarchy of leukemic stem cell classes that differ in self-renewal capacity. *Nat Immunol* **5**, 738–743.

28. Verlinden, S. F., van Es, H. H., and van Bekkum, D. W. (1998). Serial bone marrow sampling for long-term follow up of human hematopoiesis in NOD/SCID mice. *Exp Hematol* **26**, 627–630.

Chapter 13

Model Systems for Examining Effects of Leukemia-Associated Oncogenes in Primary Human CD34+ Cells via Retroviral Transduction

Mark Wunderlich and James C. Mulloy

Summary

The use of primary human cells to model cancer initiation and progression is now within the grasp of investigators. It has been nearly a decade since the first defined genetic elements were introduced into primary human epithelial and fibroblast cells to model oncogenesis. This approach has now been extended to the hematopoietic system, with the first described experimental transformation of primary human hematopoietic cells. Human cell model systems will lead to a better understanding of the species and cell type specific signals necessary for oncogenic initiation and progression, and will allow investigators to interrogate the cancer stem cell hypothesis using a well-defined hierarchical system that has been studied for decades. The molecular and biochemical link between self-renewal and differentiation can now be experimentally approached using primary human cells. In addition, the models that result from these experiments are likely to generate highly relevant systems for use in identification and validation of potential therapeutic targets as well as testing of small molecule therapeutics. We describe here the methodologies and reagents that are used to examine the effects of leukemia fusion protein expression on primary human hematopoietic cells, both in vitro and in vivo.

Key words: Human HSPC, CD34, Retroviral transduction, Leukemia fusion genes, Differentiation, NOD/SCID, Xenograft

1. Introduction

Many different systems are now available for modeling leukemia, but by far the most popular model is the mouse, using either genetically engineered mice or a bone marrow transduction and transplantation system (1) (refer to Chapter "Retroviral/Lentiviral Transduction and Transformation Assay"). However, it

C.W.E. So (ed.), Leukemia, *Methods in Molecular Biology, vol. 538*
© Humana Press, a part of Springer Science + Business Media, LLC 2009
DOI: 10.1007/978-1-59745-418-6_13

is becoming increasingly clear that there are important differences between murine and human cells with respect to cellular transformation *(2–4)*. Species-specific differences in ras signaling as well as in telomerase and telomere length regulation limit the conclusions that can be reached when using murine cells to model human cancer *(5–7)*. The inbred nature of the mouse strains used for these studies further complicates the extrapolation of results to humans. For these reasons, some labs are now using human cells to study oncogenesis, and the controlled transformation of primary human fibroblasts and epithelial cells has been previously reported *(8, 9)*. Similar studies have been pursued using hematopoietic stem and progenitor cells (HSPCs) to model preleukemia *(10–14)*, and recently the experimental transformation of a primary human HSPC has been accomplished in the laboratory *(15, 31)*.

The strategy that is used in these studies with primary human HSPC necessarily involves the introduction of oncogenes using retroviral or lentiviral delivery systems. The specific HSPC that is used, whether the cord blood, bone marrow or mobilized CD34+ (or lineage negative) cell, may alter the results that are obtained, since it is now recognized that these cells differ significantly in their properties *(16)*. In addition, many delivery options are available using different viral promoters, marker genes, and viral envelopes. These options give great flexibility to the investigator for pursuing different experimental approaches as well as in using combinations of genes together in the same experiment. The in vitro and in vivo systems in which to examine the phenotype upon oncogene expression are also expanding. As we learn more about the specific signals that are important in self-renewal divisions of the human HSPC, we strive to mimic these signals in vitro, to expand normal or preleukemic cells for analysis and therapeutic purposes. The strains of immunodeficient mice are continually improving, allowing greater sensitivity for xenograft analysis and ultimately for in vivo drug treatment studies. With the defined transformation of primary human cells of hematopoietic origin now in hand, we can use these systems to study the cell type specific signals involved in oncogenesis and identify the critical pathways that can be therapeutically targeted in these cancers.

2. Materials

2.1. Isolation of Human CD34+ Cells

1. Human umbilical cord blood (UCB) derived CD34+ cells. Selected, cryopreserved cells are available commercially from multiple vendors. Acquiring umbilical cord blood from donors is a cost effective alternative (*see* **Note 1**).

2. Dulbecco's Phosphate Buffered Saline (DPBS), without calcium and magnesium (Mediatech). Ca^{2+} and Mg^{2+} aid in cell-to-cell adhesion and clumping and thus should be avoided.

3. Ficoll-Paque PLUS (GE Healthcare).

4. Selection buffer: DPBS, 0.5% BSA, 2 mM ethylenediamine tetraacetic acid (EDTA), 50 U/mL each penicillin and streptomycin (antibiotics). Filter-sterilize and store at 4°C.

5. CD34+ selection kit. Either EasySep human CD34 Positive Selection kit (StemCell Technologies) or human CD34 MicroBead Kit (Miltenyi Biotech) works well. Both kits utilize antibodies to CD34 that are directly or indirectly linked to magnetic particles. Use of either kit requires a specialized magnet, available separately from the manufacturers.

6. Counting solution: Trypan blue dye solution, 3% acetic acid.

7. Hetastarch freezing media solutions (Store at 4°C). Hetastarch solution 1: 50% Hetastarch solution (6% stock solution in 0.9% NaCl) (Baxter Healthcare Corp, Deerfield IL), 30% Iscove's Modified Dulbecco's Eagle's Medium (IMDM), and 20% BSA fraction V solution (25% stock solution). Hetastarch solution 2: 10% DMSO, 50% hetastarch solution (6% stock solution in 0.9% NaCl), 20% IMDM, and 20% BSA fraction V solution (25% solution) (*see* **Note 2**).

2.2. Virus Preparation

1. Producer cells. These are generally 293T cells (ATCC) or derivatives.

2. 293T Media: Dulbecco's Modified Eagle's Medium (DMEM), 10% fetal bovine serum (FBS), and antibiotics.

3. Trypsin-EDTA: Hank's balanced salt solution (without calcium and magnesium), 0.05% trypsin, 0.5 mM EDTA. Store at 4°C, or at –20°C for long-term storage.

4. Poly-L-lysine: 0.1 mg/mL solution of poly-L-lysine is prepared in water and stored at 4°C.

5. Calcium phosphate precipitation reagents: Kits are commercially available; however the components are easily made. Three solutions are required: (1) Sterile, nuclease-free water. (2) 2 M $CaCl_2$. (3) 2× HEPES buffered saline (2× HBS): 50 mM HEPES, 280 mM NaCl, 1.5 mM Na_2HPO_4, pH 7.10. A large batch can be prepared and aliquots can be stored long-term at –20°C. The pH of the 2× HBS solution is critical. Each batch of reagent should be tested prior to use.

6. Virus collection media: IMDM, 10% FBS, antibiotics. Alternatively, FBS can be replaced with BIT (BSA, Insulin, Transferrin) serum substitute (StemCell Technologies) at a final concentration of 20% (*see* **Note 3**).

7. Large syringes (10–60 mL).

8. Syringe filters, 0.45 μm.

9. Tubes for concentration of virus. These are protein purification columns with a 100-kD molecular weight cutoff (Centricon Plus concentrators, Millipore). Viral particles are retained when the supernatant is spun at 2,000 × g in these columns.

10. HT1080 cells (ATCC).

2.3. Transduction of Human CD34+ Cells

1. Prestimulation media: IMDM, 10% FBS (*see* **Note 4**), 10^{-4} M β-mercaptoethanol (BME) (*see* **Note 5**), antibiotics, and 100 ng/mL each of the human cytokines stem cell factor (SCF), megakaryocyte growth and differentiation factor (MGDF), and FMS-like tyrosine kinase-3 ligand (Flt3L). All cytokines used in these procedures are available for purchase (Peprotech, Rocky Hill, NJ).

2. RetroNectin (TaKaRa): Prepare a 24 μg/mL solution by dissolving RetroNectin into water. Aliquot and store at –20°C. Six-milliliter aliquots will be sufficient for coating an entire six-well nontissue culture treated plate.

3. DPBS containing 2% BSA. Sterilize by vacuum filtration with a low protein binding filter such as SFCA. Store the solution at 4°C.

4. Hank's balanced salt solution (HBSS) containing 2.5% (v/v) 1 M HEPES. Ensure sterility by vacuum filtration. Store at room temperature.

5. Polybrene (hexadimethrine bromide). Prepare an 8-mg/mL solution in water. Store at 4°C or –20°C for long-term storage.

6. Six-well nontissue culture treated plate.

7. Non-enzymatic cell dissociation buffer (Gibco Invitrogen).

2.4. In Vitro Culture of Transduced Cells

1. Myeloid culture media. This is the same media as that used for prestimulation prior to transduction with the exception that cytokines (10 ng/mL) are SCF, MGDF, Flt3L, interleukin-3 (IL-3), and interleukin-6 (IL-6).

2. B-cell culture media: Minimum essential medium α (MEMα), 10% FBS, antibiotics, and 10 ng/mL of each of the human cytokines SCF, Flt3L, Interleukin-7 (IL-7).

3. MS-5 mouse stroma cell line.

4. MS-5 media: MEMα, 10% FBS, antibiotics.

5. Methylcellulose media: 40 mL Base Methylcult H4100 (StemCell Technologies), 20% FBS (20 mL), 2 mM l-glutamine, 10^{-4} M BME, antibiotics. IMDM (~20 mL) is added to bring the volume to 80 mL. All calculations should be based on a final volume of 100 mL, which includes the cell suspension (20% of the final volume) when performing the assay.

6. Methylcellulose cytokine cocktail. Make a 20× concentrated cytokine cocktail by adding each human cytokine into IMDM. Our typical cytokines and final concentrations are granulocyte colony stimulating factor (G-CSF), SCF, IL-3, and IL-6 (all at 10 ng/mL), and erythropoietin (EPO, 6 U/mL).

7. 16-gauge needles.

8. 3-mL syringes.

9. 35-mm tissue culture plate with grid lines.

2.5. Injection of Transduced Cells into Immunodeficient Mice

1. A strain of immunodeficient NOD/SCID mice (Jackson Laboratories, Bar Harbor, ME).

2. Doxycycline-treated chow (Purina prolab RMH 1500 with 0.0625% doxycycline, which provides approximately 2–3 mg of doxycycline per adult mouse per day; Harlan Teklad, Indianapolis, IN).

3. Bactrim-treated chow (Teklab 2018 with 0.373% Bactrim; Harlan Teklad).

4. Isoflurane.

5. Anesthesia machine.

6. Buprenex.

7. Betadine (povidone–iodine, 10%; Purdue Pharma).

8. Alcohol wipes.

9. 25-gauge needles, 5/8 in.

10. Insulin syringe (28 gauge, ½ in.).

11. Ammonium chloride solution: 150 mM NH_4Cl, 100 nM $KHCO_3$, 10 nM Na_4EDTA, pH 7.3 +/– 0.1. Generally, a 10× concentrated solution is prepared that is diluted with water before use. Store at 4°C.

12. Murine anti-F_c receptor γ antibody clone 2.4G2 (BD F_c Block™, Pharmingen).

3. Methods

We typically use cord blood CD34+ cells in our protocols, as these cells have been shown to give the most robust engraftment in immunodeficient mice (17). However, whether these fetal/infant cells are representative of the bulk of human leukemia, which occurs in the adult, remains an open question, and it will be necessary to perform comparative experiments to answer these questions. Our system is focused on retroviral constructs rather than lentiviral, and it remains to be determined whether the strong viral promoters that are present in these constructs are contributing to the phenotypes obtained, presumably through retroviral insertional activation of endogenous oncogenes. It will also be interesting to examine whether lentiviral transduction of quiescent, noncycled human HSPC will increase the transduction frequency of the most primitive cells. The optimal viral envelope for use in human CD34+ experiments is also a variable that has been analyzed in some studies, with varying and sometimes contradictory results (18–20). As more labs become proficient in the growth, transduction, and transplantation of human CD34+ cells, it is likely that these questions will be answered.

The specific conditions that are used for the transduction of the human CD34+ cells depend upon the ultimate use of the cells upon transduction. If the cells are to be propagated in vitro, and will not be injected into immunodeficient mice, it is less critical that the cytokines IL-3 and IL-6 are excluded from the prestimulation mix. Including these cytokines will increase cell yield and transduction efficiency, and typically does not negatively impact on the overall expansion and proliferation of the cells in vitro. The choice of immunodeficient mouse, and the route of delivery as well as the age at which to transplant, depends upon the availability of the strains and the expertise of the lab. Intravenous injection of 6- to 8-week-old NOD/SCID or NOG mice (both commercially available strains) is the most popular approach, but the use of newborn pups, cranial facial vein injection, intrafemoral injection, and the newer strains of immunodeficient mice (e.g., NOD/SCID-SGM3 mice for myeloid biased grafts) are gaining popularity, and only time will tell which approach will be superior for studying normal human hematopoiesis as well as leukemogenesis in the mouse.

3.1. Isolation of Human CD34+ Cells

1. Mix the whole blood in an equal volume of sterile PBS in a 50-mL tube, layer slowly onto 0.5 volumes of Ficoll-Paque PLUS solution, spin at $250 \times g$ for 30 min to 1 h at 18–20°C. The majority of red blood cells and granulocytes will be pelleted while mononuclear cells including CD34+ cells will form a white interface just above the ficoll. Serum is left above the interface.

2. Harvest the mononuclear cells (MNC) from the interface, transfer to a 50-mL tube, wash cells in at least 3 volumes of selection buffer, centrifuge at $500 \times g$ for 15 min at 18–20°C.

3. Resuspend the pellet in 5 mL of selection buffer and transfer to a 15-mL tube. Rinse the 50-mL MNC wash tube with an additional 5 ml of selection buffer and transfer to the 15-mL tube to make 10 mL of total volume.

4. Take 10 μL of MNC and mix with 90 μL of counting solution (*see* **Note 6**).

5. Spin at $700 \times g$ for 8 min, aspirate the supernatant, resuspend the MNC in selection buffer at the density recommended by the manufacturer of the selection kit.

6. CD34+ cells are positively selected from this population using either the Miltenyi Macs CD34 Microbead Kit or the Stem Cell Technologies CD34 EasySep procedure. Both protocols are successful and give comparable yields and purity of CD34+ cells (**Fig. 1a**). Each protocol is followed according to the manufacturer's recommendations (*see* **Note 7**).

7. After selection of CD34+ cells, count the cells and centrifuge at $700 \times g$ for 10 min to pellet them. Aspirate the supernatant. Cells can either be used immediately as described in **Subheading 3.3** below, or viably frozen by resuspending the pellet in 300–500 μL of hetastarch solution 1 and transferring to a cryovial. An equal volume of hetastarch solution 2 is then added dropwise (10^5 to 2×10^6 cells per vial).

3.2. Virus Preparation and Titer

1. Either the 293T or Phoenix cell line is used for transient virus production using a plasmid transfection procedure. The "strain" of Phoenix cell line used depends on the species of

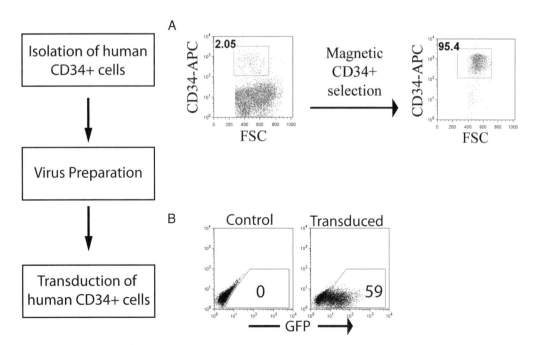

Fig. 1. Overview of the model system for retroviral transduction of human CD34+ cells. (**a**) Human CD34+ cells are purified by magnetic selection, and purity is confirmed by flow cytometric analysis. (**b**) A transduction of human CD34+ cells is shown, with a non-transduced control. GFP expression is visualized by flow cytometry.

the cells that will be targeted (*see* **Note 8**). Virus production is best done in batches that are titered and aliquoted for future use. 10-cm tissue culture dishes are coated with poly-L-lysine by adding 3 mL of solution to the dish, swirling to cover the whole bottom, and transferring to subsequent dishes. 5 million cells are then plated to each dish (day 1). To ensure even distribution, do not swirl the media, but rock the dishes twice side-to-side and twice to-and-fro. The dishes are placed in the incubator overnight (37°C, 5% CO_2).

2. Virus production is initiated by transfecting the cells in the 10-cm dish with three plasmids:

   (a) Retroviral vector 12 µg

   (b) Gag/Pol vector 10 µg

   (c) Envelope vector 3 µg

   All three plasmids are used in the transfection, even if a Phoenix cell line already contains the gag/pol or envelope plasmids as stable integrants. The quality of the plasmid used in the transfection is critical for maximal uptake by the cells. Only DNA from a maxiprep should be used for virus production. Different transfection protocols can be used, but one of the most reliable and cost-efficient is the calcium phosphate method (*see* **Note 9**).

3. Transfect the cells the afternoon of day 2. The cells should be approximately 75% confluent. All solutions should be at room temperature. For calcium phosphate transfection, a final volume of 1-mL transfection mix is needed per 10-cm dish. The volumes can be scaled up if multiple dishes are transfected with the same retroviral vector. Add plasmids to ddH_2O to a final volume of 438 µL and mix by brief pipeting. Next, add 62 µL of 2 M $CaCl_2$ and mix. Then add this solution dropwise to a Falcon 2054 polystyrene tube containing 500 µL of 2× HBS (pH 7.10). The solution should appear somewhat cloudy after this step. Some investigators prefer to vortex while adding the DNA mixture, others prefer to bubble air through the 2× HBS during the addition. Results seem to be comparable using the two techniques in our experience.

4. Remove dishes from the incubator and slowly add 1 mL of the DNA–CaPO$_4$ mixture solution directly on top of the cells. Use a 1-mL pipetman with the tip beneath the media to discharge the mixture while moving the tip around, blanketing the entire cell layer. Return the dishes to the incubator. Some investigators prefer to incubate the mixture for 15–45 min before adding to the cells, but we find that this increases the size of the precipitate which decreases the transduction efficiency. Very fine black particles (visible at 20× power under a microscope) are the best precipitate for transfection.

5. On the morning of Day 3 (12–16 h after initiating transfection), remove dishes from the incubator and aspirate the media by gently tipping the dish at a 45° angle and touching the tip of the aspirating device to the side of the dish. Slowly add 6–7 mL of warmed collection media to the side of the angled dish, so as not to disturb the cell monolayer. The media that is used depends on the target cells that will be transduced and should be the optimal media for these cells. Ideally, virus-containing supernatant is now collected at 12-h intervals, for a total of 4–5 collections. Fresh warm collection media is replaced each time, gently, to prevent disruption of the cell monolayer. Virus supernatant can be kept overnight on ice at 4°C to allow concentration of the supernatant in one step. Producer cells should be visualized under the fluorescent microscope, if a fluorescent marker protein is used (i.e., EGFP). At least 50% of cells should be transfected to justify proceeding with the collections (*see* **Note 10**).

6. Combine virus collections, filter through a 0.45-μm filter (0.2 μm can also be used with no loss of virus and less risk of producer cell contamination), and concentrate using a protein purification column with a molecular weight cutoff of 100-kD. The specific fold concentration depends on the needs of the investigator and the transgene used, but can range between 5 and 100× or more. These filters can be re-used for the same virus supernatant. Aliquot and freeze concentrated virus at –80°C. Keep a very small aliquot for determining viral titer. Depending on the envelope used, viral titer will drop by one-half for each freeze-thaw cycle. (*see* **Note 11**).

7. To titer the virus, we use the HT1080 adherent cell line (for a human-tropic virus). These cells are available from ATCC.

8. Remove sub-confluent HT1080 cells from the plate with trypsin–EDTA and plate in six-well plates at 2.5×10^5 cells per well, in DMEM 10% FBS (Day 1).

9. The following day, dilute viral supernatant by taking 30 μL of virus and mixing with 3 mL of DMEM 10% FBS. This is a 10^{-2} dilution. Make tenfold serial dilutions by taking 300 μL of the 10^{-2} dilution and adding to 2.7 mL of DMEM 10% FBS (10^{-3}), repeating this three more times until a 10^{-6} dilution is reached. Aspirate the media from the six-well plate of HT1080 cells, add 2 mL of the 10^{-6} dilution to a single well, and continue for each of the remaining dilutions. Use a new pipet and add 2 mL of DMEM 10% FBS to the final well of the six-well plate (no-virus control well). Add 2 μL of an 8 mg/mL polybrene solution to each well (final concentration is 8 μg/mL). Incubate overnight at 37°C in a 5% CO_2 incubator.

10. On day 3, aspirate the medium from each well. Add 2 mL of complete media. If the retrovirus contains a drug-selectable cassette, add the working solution of drug in complete media at this time (*see* **Note 12**).

11. After 10–14 days, fix the colonies of cells that have formed by adding ice-cold methanol for 5–10 min and then rinse once with distilled deionized water. Stain the colonies with an aqueous solution of 0.4% methylene blue for one minute, wash twice with water and dry the plate upside down. Calculate the titer. The best dilution for calculations will be one that gives between 10 and 100 colonies.

12. For viral vectors that contain a fluorescent marker, collect cells two days after the end of transduction (day 5) and analyze by flow cytometry.

13. Viral particle number is calculated by multiplying the percentage marked cells by the total number of target cells present at the time of incubation with virus (day 2; a replicate well is included, and this is counted at the time of incubation with virus) (It is important that the dilution that is used for the calculation of titer has given a transduction efficiency of less than 37%, to ensure single hit kinetics). Multiplying this number by the dilution factor for that well (e.g., 100 for a 10^{-2} dilution) will give the titer of the virus per mL. We have found that the viral titer should not be less than 10^5/mL for successful transduction of human CD34+ cells.

3.3. Transduction of Human CD34+ Cells

1. To thaw frozen human CD34+ cells, agitate the vial rapidly in a 37°C water bath until only a small piece of ice remains. Add 2 mL of room temperature HBSS + 2% BSA to the vial, mix, and transfer to a 15-mL tube. Rinse the vial and cap with HBSS + 2% BSA and increase the volume in the 15-mL tube to 10 mL. Centrifuge at 4°C, $500 \times g$ for 10 min, flick the tube with index finger to disperse the cell pellet, and resuspend in prestimulation media to give a final concentration of 10^6 cells per mL (*see* **Note 13**).

2. Culture the cells for 1.5–2 days to ensure that a population of cells are replicating (essential for transduction with retrovirus).

3. Prepare a RetroNectin-coated plate the day before transduction. Incubate a six-well nontissue culture treated plate with RetroNectin solution (2 h, room temperature), then PBS containing 2% BSA (30 min, room temperature), and finally with HBSS containing 2.5% HEPES (quick wash). Although plates can be stored for months at 4°C, we have found that a fresh treatment is superior to stored plates. The primary solution of RetroNectin can be used in a secondary (and tertiary) treatment, and these plates can be used for transduction of less critical cell lines if desired.

4. Count the cells. The cell number should be approximately equal to the number when cells were thawed (*see* **Note 14**).

5. Precoat the RetroNectin well with 2–4 mL of unconcentrated viral supernatant or 1 mL of concentrated supernatant. Centrifuge the plate for 45 min at 2,000 × g at room temperature. Aspirate the solution and repeat the spin with additional virus supernatant. After the second treatment, add approximately 1 million prestimulated cells in an equal volume of fresh prestimulation media to the viral supernatant in the well, and incubate at 37°C for 4–8 h (during the day), with 8 μg/mL polybrene (*see* **Note 15**).

6. At the end of the day, carefully aspirate the majority of the media (cells should be predominantly attached to the Retro-Nectin-coated plastic) and add 2 mL of fresh prestimulation media. Allow the cells to recover in the incubator overnight.

7. The next morning, add 2–4 mL (unconcentrated) or 1 mL (concentrated) of virus and polybrene. Do not centrifuge. At the end of the day, remove the cells from the plate by collecting the media and detaching the cells from the plate using a non-enzymatic cell dissociation buffer. Centrifuge at 500 × g for 7 min and resuspend in the appropriate media at a density of 10^6 cells per mL.

8. Two days later, cells can be analyzed by flow cytometry (if a fluorescent co-marker was present in the retroviral construct; **Fig. 1b**) to determine the transduction frequency, or drug selection can begin if a drug-selectable construct was used (*see* **Note 16**).

3.4. In Vitro Culture of Transduced Cells

1. The choice of culture medium will depend on the specific lineage that is desired and the oncogene that is used in the transduction. For culture under *myeloid* conditions, a complex mixture of cytokines is most likely to allow the greatest diversity in terms of myeloid potential for the cells. After transduction, cells can be cultured in a five-cytokine cocktail of SCF, MGDF, Flt3L, IL-6, and IL-3. The specific concentrations to use can be determined empirically and may differ depending on the transgene. We have found that 10 ng/mL of each is sufficient for the AML1-ETO, CBFB-SMMHC, and MLL-AF9 fusion protein-expressing long-term cultures (*12, 21, 22, 31, 32*). Typically the control-transduced CD34+ cells will proliferate for 8–12 weeks under these conditions, while the oncogene-transduced cultures grow for varying lengths of time, depending on the specific oncogene.

2. Count cells weekly and seed at $4 × 10^5$ cells/mL, in a volume that will give the desired number of cells after the 1-week expansion period (*see* **Note 17**). During the first 3–4 weeks, cells will expand approximately tenfold each week, and

supplementation of the medium may be needed on day 4 or 5 to prevent depletion of the medium. Under these conditions, the control cultures will maintain a population of CD34+ cells of approximately 2–10%, depending on the specific cord blood. The remainders of the cells are at various stages of myelopoiesis. A layer of adherent cells will slowly form over time, and the suspension cells can be moved to a new well each week if desired. Toward the end of the proliferative period (weeks 7–12 depending on the cord blood), cells will double only once or twice per week, and the majority of the cells will be monocyte/macrophage. Expression of the fluorescent marker, if present in the retroviral construct, can be monitored during this time, to determine effects of the transgene on proliferation and/or differentiation. An example of a myeloid culture of cells expressing AML1-ETO in shown in **Fig. 2a**.

3. For expansion of *B-lymphoid* cells in vitro, the use of a stroma coculture will give the best growth and the most reliable and reproducible results. We use the MS-5 murine stroma cell line *(23)* (*see* **Note 18**). Immediately after transduction, seed 1 × 10^5 cells onto a monolayer of MS-5 stroma cells formed in a T25 culture flask with 5 mL of B-cell media. Some cells will invade the stroma layer and grow beneath the stroma as "phase-dark" cells, meaning that they will appear as dark, nontranslucent cells through the phase-contrast microscope. Under B-cell growth conditions, these cells will typically form organized areas known as cobblestone areas, and will also appear dispersed throughout the monolayer in addition to growing in loosely organized areas. An example of a typical cobblestone area forming cells is shown in **Fig. 2b**. The majority of cells will grow as suspension cells or weakly attached to the topside of the stroma. The dilution to make during weekly passage of cells will depend upon the individual capacity of each cord blood preparation, which demonstrates large proliferative variations under B-cell growth conditions (*see* **Note 19**). For the first 2–3 weeks of growth, only myeloid cells (CD33+) will be present in the suspension. At weeks 3–4, a small population of CD19+ cells will form, which can become the majority population by 5–6 weeks of culture. Most of the CD19+ B-cells will co-express CD10, and a percentage (10–50%) will co-express CD20, but in our hands the B-cells that develop under these conditions do not express surface Ig (**Fig. 2c**).

4. The methylcellulose assay is a convenient and powerful way to determine the effects of a particular transgene on hematopoietic differentiation and proliferation. For the most quantitative assay, transduced cells should be sorted or drug selected prior to use in a methylcellulose assay. Typically, after transduction, cells are washed with IMDM without cytokines or FBS and counted. Then, 8,000 cells are deposited into a 15-mL tube in

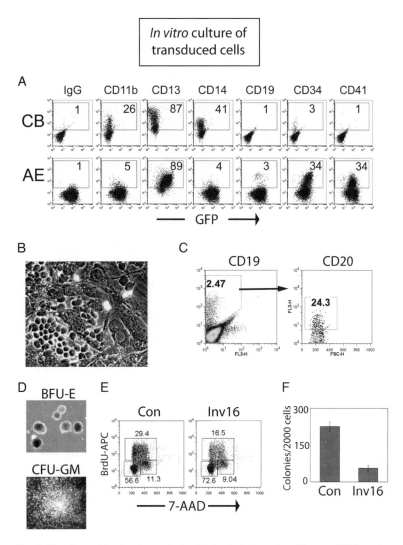

Fig. 2. Overview of the in vitro analysis of retrovirally transduced human CD34+ cells. (**A**) Representative long-term myeloid cultures (6 weeks) of control CB cells and cells expressing the AML1-ETO oncogene (AE). This phenotype is preserved throughout the 6–8 months of growth. (**B**) Example of a cobblestone area that forms upon coculture of human CD34+ cells with the MS-5 stroma cell line. (**C**) B cells can be expanded from the transduced CD34+ cultures upon coculture with MS-5 and the cytokines Flt3L, SCF and IL-7. Shown is a CBFB-SMMHC-transduced culture that was 12 weeks posttransduction. Cells were cultured on MS-5 for an additional 4 weeks. A fraction of the CD19+ cells also express the CD20 B-cell marker. (**D**) A clonogenic methylcellulose assay is shown, with representative BFU-E (red cell colony) and CFU-GM (myeloid colony) that result from the growth of a single cell. (**E**, **F**) Expression of a fusion oncogene frequently leads to loss of clonogenic potential immediately upon transduction, and this effect is due to a G0/G1 cell cycle block for cells expressing the inv16 fusion protein CBFB-SMMHC.

a final volume of 800 µL IMDM (enough cells to give triplicate methylcellulose plates with 2,000 cells each, and allowing for pipetting error by calculating for four plates). The cells are mixed with 3.2 mL of methylcellulose media while vortexing at high speed. The methylcellulose is easiest to measure and manipulate using a 3-mL syringe with a 16 gauge needle (fill the syringe with methylcellulose solution from the bottle, discharge to clear the air void, and completely fill the syringe by slowly withdrawing the plunger fully. This will give a volume of approximately 3.2 mL). After mixing, rest the syringe and needle in the falcon tube for approximately 5 min to allow the air bubbles to rise.

5. Draw up 3 mL of methylcellulose/cell suspension, and add 1 mL to each of triplicate 35-mm dishes that contain 50 μL of 20× cytokine cocktail (*see* **Note 20**). Tilt and rotate the dish to distribute the solution over the entire bottom. Incubate the dishes for 2 weeks in a humidified chamber to prevent drying of the methylcellulose media (*see* **Note 21**). Minimize disturbance or movement of the dishes during this time.

6. After two weeks, count the colonies and score the colony type. We typically will score three types of colonies, including granulocyte/macrophage (GM), burst forming unit-erythroid (BFU-E), and granulocyte/erythroid/macrophage/megakaryocyte (GEMM) colonies (**Fig. 2d**). Transgene expression in human CD34+ cells could affect the size, the number as well as the specific type of colonies present. For example, expression of the CBFB-SMMHC oncogene causes a G0/G1 arrest, and the number of colonies that are present after 2 weeks are severely decreased (**Fig. 2e and 2f**). The expected number of colonies from 2,000 input cells varies greatly depending on the particular cord blood as well as the timing of the experiments. Numbers could range from 50–400 colonies per dish. The best growth/differentiation will typically occur when colony number is around 100–200 per dish.

3.5 Injection of Transduced Cells into Immunodeficient Mice

1. If cells are going to be used for injection into immunodeficient mice, the culture medium for prestimulation should have only minimal cytokines to preserve the primitive nature of the cells as much as possible. The cytokines SCF, TPO, and Flt3L should be sufficient to promote cell cycle entry and survival; IL-3 should be avoided, since this cytokine has been found to promote differentiation and loss of SCID repopulating potential.

2. Cells should be injected into animals as soon after thaw as possible. Our usual approach would be to prestimulate for 1.5 days, transduce cells for 0.5–1.0 days (1–2 incubations with virus, 4–6 h each) and then immediately inject into animals, so that only two or three days pass from initial thaw. A small aliquot can be retained in vitro to verify transduction and calculate efficiency.

3. The best characterized animal model for xenograft of human hematopoietic cells is the NOD/SCID mouse. A number of variants are now available, including the NOD/SCID-β_2M$^{-/-}$, NOD/SCID-IL2R$\gamma_c^{-/-}$ (NOG), and NOD/SCID-SGM3 mice. The latter two strains are just becoming widely used, and limited information is available in the literature for these mice. The NOG mouse should be highly immunocompromised and possess no residual NK activity and may be defective for dendritic cell and macrophage function as well *(24)*. The SGM3 mouse is transgenic for the myeloid-promoting cytokines SCF, GM-CSF, and IL-3 and skews the human graft towards myeloid differentiation, but has also been documented to promote loss of the normal human graft, possibly due to mobilization and differentiation of the primitive human cells in the mouse bone marrow *(25, 26)*.

4. The number of human cells that must be injected to ensure a reliable hematopoietic graft will vary depending on the mouse strain and sub-strain that is used. A good rule of thumb for regular NOD/SCID mice, with injection of prestimulated, cycling cells, is to use 300,000 cells per mouse, calculated based on the starting number of the CD34+ population. For example, if 9×10^5 CD34+ cells are prestimulated, and after 4 days have doubled in number to 1.8×10^6, this would be enough cell number for three mice (900,000 starting cells/300,000 = 3). If the cells tripled in this time to 2.7×10^6, this would still be enough cell number for only three mice. (*see* **Note 22**).

5. Mice (6–8 weeks old on the day of injection) should be prepared for injection by feeding with doxycycline-treated chow for 1 week before irradiation, and continued on this chow for 1 week after irradiation (we have recently found that we achieve better results using Bactrim-treated chow for 2 weeks post-irradiation, with doxycycline-treated chow for 1 week before irradiation. It is possible that this treatment needs optimization for individual animal facilities, and procedures may need to be altered if mouse loss becomes unacceptable after irradiation). This minimizes the loss of mice due to radiation illness. The dose of radiation needs to be determined empirically for each colony, and the dose may need to be recalculated as the colony ages. We have found that our colony gave very good results using 375 Gy initially, but we now use 280 Gy (2 years after establishing the colony) with similar survival numbers (approximately 10–20% of mice will be lost in each experiment due to radiation illness).

6. Mice are irradiated up to 24 h in advance of injection. For intravenous injection, a volume of 300 µL works well (cells in a PBS solution). For intrafemoral injection, a volume of 25 µL or less should be used. (*see* **Note 23**).

7. To inject cells intravenously, place mice under a heat lamp for several minutes. This will allow easier visualization of the tail vein. Injection is easiest with immobilized mice, either by containment in a mouse restraint device or by anesthetization with isoflurane. After cleaning the tail with an alcohol wipe, inject the cells into the tail vein with an insulin syringe taking special care to avoid injection of any air bubble (this will kill the mouse). You will be able to see the clear PBS-cell mixture travel through the vein. If the needle is not in the vein, the plunger will not easily be depressed and a bump will form in the tail of the mouse. Attempt the initial injection midway down the tail so that if this occurs, another attempt can be made closer to the body of the mouse.

8. To inject intrafemorally, anesthetize the mouse with isoflurane. Give the mouse painkiller such as Buprenex (buprenorphine) by injecting under the skin of the back. Place the mouse on its back, and insert the snout of the mouse into a tube for constant delivery of isoflurane during the procedure. Clean the leg with an alcohol wipe and Betadine. Insert a 25 gauge needle (5/8 in.) attached to a 1-mL syringe into the femur (*see* **Note 24**). Remove the needle slowly, while keeping the leg steady and remaining fully focused on the location of the hole. Insert the insulin syringe containing the cells and slowly inject the mixture into the hole. Move the mouse back to its cage where it will regain consciousness within 5 min.

For measurement of a graft due to the most primitive human cells, it is recommended that the mice be monitored at 9–12 weeks post injection. It is often difficult to measure human cells in the peripheral blood in these mice, but depending on the size of the graft it is possible. We use the CD45, CD33 and CD19 antibodies to determine total cell graft, myeloid and B-lymphoid populations respectively. To block non-specific staining of murine hematopoietic cells that express F_cR, the use of 1 µL of F_c block is recommended per 1×10^6 cells. For surface staining of PB, red cells should be lysed in an ammonium chloride solution, and the residual red blood cells should be excluded from the viable cell gate during flow to determine an accurate percentage of human white blood cells in the mouse.

9. When the experiment is to be ended, the bone marrow, spleen and peripheral blood of the animal should be processed and analyzed for human cells. The four long bones of the hind legs are removed, and either crushed using mortar and pestle or flushed using an insulin syringe and IMDM media after cutting the ends of the bones with scissors. Either way, cells are then filtered through a 40 µm filter, and red blood cells are lysed. The spleen or other organs can be crushed through a 40 µm filter, using the flat end of a 3 mL syringe, and red cells are then lysed. Cells are stained for surface markers to determine the lineage composition

of the human graft (**Fig. 3a** and **3b**). Expression of a leukemia fusion gene can specifically affect the composition of the graft, as shown by expression of the inv16 oncogene CBFB-SMMHC, which leads to a myeloid-dominated graft with very few CD19+ cells and a decreased number of CD34+ cells

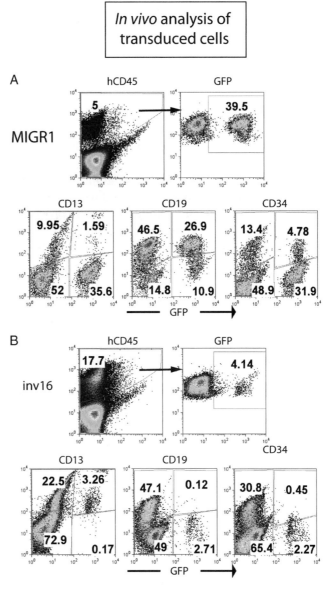

Fig. 3. Overview of the in vivo analysis of retrovirally transduced human CD34+ cells. (**A, B**) Analysis of the bone marrow of a NOD/SCID-β2M−/− mouse that was injected with control transduced (MIGR1) and CBFB-SMMHC-transduced (inv16) cells. 8.5 weeks after injection, the human graft in the bone marrow of the mouse was readily detectable, and GFP+ cells were present in both mice. Most of the human cells in the control mouse were CD19+ B-cells, as is typical, but for the CBFB-SMMHC-expressing cells, there is a loss of the B-cell fraction, and essentially all of the cells express the myeloid marker CD13.

(**Fig. 3a** and **3b**). Methylcellulose assays using human-specific cytokines can be performed to determine the progenitor activity, using the protocol described earlier. Cells can be viably frozen for later use. To show self-renewal of the human cells using the most stringent criteria, a secondary transplant is performed, following the same procedures as for the primary transplant. Secondary mice are analyzed at 6–12 weeks for the presence of human cells..

4. Notes

1. The quality of the whole blood sample should be considered prior to proceeding with the selection protocol. We have found that a significant drop in yield occurs at volumes smaller than 80 mL and we generally do not proceed with these samples. Additionally, the procedure should begin within 48 h of collection. The samples can be stored at room temperature in the presence of anticoagulants. Samples with obvious clumps or a very dark color should be avoided.

2. Solutions should be prepared without including the BSA. Solutions can then be stored at 4°C for months. Withdraw an aliquot of each solution and add BSA to each immediately before use.

3. The choice of virus collection media will depend on which culture condition is preferred (serum or serum-free) for culture of the CD34+ cells after transduction. Phoenix-GP producer cells produce adequate viral particles in either virus collection media.

4. The response of CD34+ cells to FBS culture conditions can vary significantly depending on the lot of serum. For this reason, it is important to carefully test several lots before purchase. We generally perform methylcellulose colony assays of UCB CD34+ cells with several lots of serum before purchasing a bulk quantity of a satisfactory lot (most colonies, with good growth and multilineage differentiation, with performance at least as good as the current or past lots).

5. A typical stock BME solution is 14.4 M. To prepare aliquots of 500× concentrated BME, dilute 35 μL of stock BME into 10 mL water and sterilize with a 0.2-μm syringe filter. This yields a 10^{-2} M solution (500×, add 1 mL to a 500-mL bottle IMDM) that can be aliquoted and stored at –20°C. Solutions are generally stable for 1 month at 4°C, wrapped in foil.

6. The acetic acid/trypan blue solution will allow easy counting of nucleated cells. The red blood cells will be lysed in this solution. Depending on the number of cells in the preparation, a larger or smaller dilution of the suspension may be needed.

7. The yield and quality of cells from these procedures can vary significantly, due to sample differences. From an average UCB of 100 mL, the expected yield of CD34+ cells should be between 0.5 and 1.5 million cells. Occasionally far more CD34+ cells can be recovered, but typical recovery is approximately 50% of the CD34+ cells present in the MNC fraction. The purity of the selected cells should be confirmed by flow cytometry and the cell counts adjusted to represent the actual number of CD34+ cells. We routinely achieve purities of greater than 90% using these methods (**Fig. 1a**). A small aliquot of the selected cells can be tested for growth and viability by culturing in myeloid media and monitoring cell counts or by performing methylcellulose assays.

8. The Phoenix cells, based on the 293T cell line, are available through ATCC in an agreement with Dr. Garry Nolan. The cells can be obtained with only the gag and pol genes (Phoenix-GP), or additionally with the ecotropic or amphotropic envelopes (Phoenix-E or Phoenix-A). We typically use Phoenix-GP and transfect additional gag/pol helper plasmid, as this has been shown to be the limiting construct in viral preparations. Full details on these cell lines are available upon purchase from ATCC.

9. Many methods of transfection exist. The amounts of DNA required by these methods vary. The DNA amounts presented here are optimized for the calcium phosphate precipitation method. In using different methods of transfection we have found that the ratio of the different plasmids is an important factor and should be preserved if the total amount of DNA is altered.

10. The fluorescent intensity of EGFP may not be impressive on the first day after transfection, but by day 2 it should be readily visible, especially from the control cells transfected with empty vector. It is possible that the transgene in the viral construct will severely diminish the intensity of the EGFP. We have found that this is transgene-specific but often occurs when large genes or oncogenes are used. In this case, the intensity of the EGFP will not correlate with the viral titer.

11. The rule of thumb is that approximately 50% of viral titer is lost for each freeze/thaw cycle when using amphotropic or ecotropic envelopes. We have not formally tested this. When using the feline endogenous virus (RD118) or the vesicular stomatitus virus envelope (VSV-G), there is little to no loss of virus titer. These two envelopes are also reported to allow concentration of virus particles by ultracentrifugation without loss of viral titer.

12. For HT1080, use the following concentrations for commonly used drugs. G418 for neomycin resistance, 800 µg/mL,

(10–14 days, with a media change at day 5); hygromycin B, 500 µg/mL, (7–10 days); puromycin, 1 µg/mL (4–7 days).

13. Media is IMDM with 10% heat-inactivated FBS, 50 U/mL penicillin, 50 U/mL streptomycin, 2 mM l-glutamine, 10^{-4} M β-mercaptoethanol. Alternatively, if serum-free conditions are preferred, the FBS is substituted with the BIT supplement from Stem Cell Technologies, supplied as a 5× concentrate. If the transduced cells will be used in vivo (in immunodeficient mice), the human cytokines SCF, TPO (MGDF), and FLT3L are included at 100 ng/mL. For in vitro applications only, the addition of human IL-3 at 20 ng/mL and IL-6 at 100 ng/mL will increase growth and transduction efficiency but will also promote differentiation.

14. Some cells will die during the prestimulation period, and some cells will begin to divide. This typically results in approximately an equal viable population relative to the starting number on Day 0. If the number is lower than 50% of the viable cell number on Day 0 it is often not worth proceeding with the transduction, since the cells that do recover are usually less hardy and long-lived and may not represent the expected population of human CD34+ cells.

15. Ensure that cells have adhered to the RetroNectin-coated plastic after approximately 15 min of incubation. This is essential for good transduction by all pseudotypes of virus with the exception of VSV-G; if the virus is pseudotyped with VSV-G, no RetroNectin is used for transduction (27, 28).

16. Working concentrations for human CD34+ cells for some common drugs are: G418 (for neomycin), 800 µg/mL (will take approximately 1.5 weeks; fresh drug should be added at day 4 or 5); hygromycin B, 300 µg/mL (will take approximately 1 week); puromycin, 0.5 µg/mL (will take 3–5 days for selection). Nontransduced cells should be incubated with drug, and selection is complete when all of these cells are dead. As a note of caution, it is possible that some transgenes will have deleterious effects on human CD34+ cells, and selection with drug resistance may be impossible. A fluorescent marker is more useful in this case; cells can be sorted after transduction and analyzed for these effects.

17. We find the cells grow best when we use six-well plates, for reasons we have not determined. Cultures can reach a density of 2 million cells/mL without significant loss of viability, and a volume of up to 8 mL can be used for each well of the plate.

18. The MS-5 cell line is grown in α-MEM medium with 10–20% FBS. Cells are never allowed to become confluent. A large number of viably frozen vials should be made to ensure a

reliable stock of cells that are at an early passage. Over time in vitro, the phenotype/morphology of the cells can become more fibroblastoid, and these cultures are less able to support hematopoiesis and also tend to lose contact inhibition. The MS-5 cells do not need to be irradiated for use as a feeder layer. If cells will not be used for experiments within 2–3 weeks, it is better to discontinue the culture and thaw a new vial rather than to continue passage of cells during this time.

19. A typical cell split would include a gentle agitation of the flask to loosen the hematopoietic cells that are weakly attached to stroma cells, followed by removal of 50% of the volume with replacement by fresh media. This procedure is frequently referred to as demi-depopulation. Care must be taken to ensure that the stroma does not loosen, which becomes more likely with each passing week.

20. The cytokines to use in a methylcellulose assay that will permit the broadest range of colony types includes 10 ng/mL G-CSF, 20 ng/mL each of SCF, IL-3 and IL-6, and 6 U/mL of Epo.

21. Large 500 cm² square tissue culture dishes can be used to create a humidified chamber. Fill both halves of two 60-mm culture plates with sterile water and place one piece into each corner of the dish (use each lid and the bottom separately). This chamber can hold approximately twenty 35-mm methylcellulose cultures. The chambers are sterilized and reused.

22. There is great variability in the engraftment of different cord blood preparations and also large variability mouse to mouse from the same cord blood. This biological variability is impossible to control at this time, and means that a large number of mice must be used for experiments.

23. We have found that the intrafemoral route, although significantly more time-consuming and requiring more practice, results in a significantly superior graft. It has also been shown that the cell number can be markedly reduced given the superiority of this route of injection (29, 30). It is likely that with the newly available NOG mice, and the intrafemoral route of injection, the number of CD34+ cells that are needed for each mouse will be less than tenfold what is currently recommended.

24. While looking at the mouse knee, locate the highest point (just above the white connective tissue of the joint; it is easier for some investigators if the hair at the knee joint is removed, by simply plucking it off with gloved index finger and thumb). Insert the needle just above that point and slightly to the outside of the leg. The inside of the bone will have a gritty texture that can be sensed by moving the needle

up and down slightly. Before attempting this procedure on live mice, it is best to obtain the skill by practicing with sacrificed mice. Try inserting a colored dye into the femur; e.g., trypan blue. Dissection will confirm injection and allow a certain amount of trial and error that is required to successfully and consistently perform the procedure.

References

1. Sharpless NE, Depinho RA. (2006). The mighty mouse: Genetically engineered mouse models in cancer drug development. *Nat Rev Drug Discov*;5(9):741–54.
2. Rangarajan A, Weinberg RA. (2003). Opinion: Comparative biology of mouse versus human cells: Modelling human cancer in mice. *Nat Rev Cancer*;3(12):952–9.
3. Rangarajan A, Hong SJ, Gifford A, Weinberg RA. (2004). Species- and cell type-specific requirements for cellular transformation. *Cancer Cell*;6(2):171–83.
4. Drayton S, Peters G. (2002). Immortalisation and transformation revisited. *Curr Opin Genet Dev*;12(1):98–104.
5. Smogorzewska A, de Lange T. (2002). Different telomere damage signaling pathways in human and mouse cells. *Embo J*;21(16):4338–48.
6. Hamad NM, Elconin JH, Karnoub AE, et al. (2002). Distinct requirements for Ras oncogenesis in human versus mouse cells. *Genes Dev*;16(16):2045–57.
7. Lim KH, Baines AT, Fiordalisi JJ, et al. (2005). Activation of RalA is critical for Ras-induced tumorigenesis of human cells. *Cancer Cell*;7(6):533–45.
8. Hahn WC, Counter CM, Lundberg AS, Beijersbergen RL, Brooks MW, Weinberg RA. (1999). Creation of human tumour cells with defined genetic elements. *Nature*;400(6743):464–8.
9. Hahn WC, Weinberg RA. (2002). Rules for making human tumor cells. *N Engl J Med*;347(20):1593–603.
10. Pereira DS, Dorrell C, Ito CY, et al. (1998). Retroviral transduction of TLS-ERG initiates a leukemogenic program in normal human hematopoietic cells. *Proc Natl Acad Sci U S A*;95(14):8239–44.
11. Grignani F, Valtieri M, Gabbianelli M, et al. (2000). PML/RAR alpha fusion protein expression in normal human hematopoietic progenitors dictates myeloid commitment and the promyelocytic phenotype. *Blood*;96(4):1531–7.
12. Mulloy JC, Cammenga J, MacKenzie KL, Berguido FJ, Moore MA, Nimer SD. (2002). The AML1-ETO fusion protein promotes the expansion of human hematopoietic stem cells. *Blood*;99(1):15–23.
13. Buske C, Feuring-Buske M, Antonchuk J, et al. (2001). Overexpression of HOXA10 perturbs human lymphomyelopoiesis in vitro and in vivo. *Blood*;97(8):2286–92.
14. Daga A, Podesta M, Capra MC, Piaggio G, Frassoni F, Corte G. (2000). The retroviral transduction of HOXC4 into human CD34(+) cells induces an in vitro expansion of clonogenic and early progenitors. *Exp Hematol*;28(5):569–74.
15. Barabe F, Kennedy JA, Hope KJ, Dick JE. (2007). Modeling the initiation and progression of human acute leukemia in mice. *Science*;316(5824):600–4.
16. Bowie MB, Kent DG, Dykstra B, et al. (2007). Identification of a new intrinsically timed developmental checkpoint that reprograms key hematopoietic stem cell properties. *Proc Natl Acad Sci U S A*;104(14):5878–82.
17. Holyoake TL, Nicolini FE, Eaves CJ. (1999). Functional differences between transplantable human hematopoietic stem cells from fetal liver, cord blood, and adult marrow. *Exp Hematol*;27(9):1418–27.
18. Kelly PF, Carrington J, Nathwani A, Vanin EF. (2001). RD114-pseudotyped oncoretroviral vectors. Biological and physical properties. *Ann N Y Acad Sci*;938:262–76; discussion 76–7.
19. Kelly PF, Vandergriff J, Nathwani A, Nienhuis AW, Vanin EF. (2000). Highly efficient gene transfer into cord blood nonobese diabetic/severe combined immunodeficiency repopulating cells by oncoretroviral vector particles pseudotyped with the feline endogenous retrovirus (RD114) envelope protein. *Blood*;96(4):1206–14.
20. Hanawa H, Kelly PF, Nathwani AC, et al. (2002). Comparison of various envelope proteins for their ability to pseudotype lentiviral vectors and transduce primitive hematopoietic cells from human blood. *Mol Ther*;5(3):242–51.

21. Wunderlich M, Krejci O, Wei J, Mulloy JC. (2006). Human CD34+ cells expressing the inv(16) fusion protein exhibit a myelomonocytic phenotype with greatly enhanced proliferative ability. *Blood*;**108**(5):1690–7.

22. Mulloy JC, Cammenga J, Berguido FJ, et al. (2003). Maintaining the self-renewal and differentiation potential of human CD34+ hematopoietic cells using a single genetic element. *Blood*;**102**(13):4369–76.

23. Itoh K, Tezuka H, Sakoda H, et al. (1989). Reproducible establishment of hemopoietic supportive stromal cell lines from murine bone marrow. *Exp Hematol*;**17**(2):145–53.

24. Ito M, Hiramatsu H, Kobayashi K, et al. (2002). NOD/SCID/gamma(c)(null) mouse: an excellent recipient mouse model for engraftment of human cells. *Blood*;**100**(9):3175–82.

25. Nicolini FE, Cashman JD, Hogge DE, Humphries RK, Eaves CJ. (2004). NOD/SCID mice engineered to express human IL-3, GM-CSF and Steel factor constitutively mobilize engrafted human progenitors and compromise human stem cell regeneration. *Leukemia*;**18**(2):341–7.

26. Feuring-Buske M, Gerhard B, Cashman J, Humphries RK, Eaves CJ, Hogge DE. (2003). Improved engraftment of human acute myeloid leukemia progenitor cells in beta 2-microglobulin-deficient NOD/SCID mice and in NOD/SCID mice transgenic for human growth factors. *Leukemia*;**17**(4):760–3.

27. Haas DL, Case SS, Crooks GM, Kohn DB. (2000). Critical factors influencing stable transduction of human CD34(+) cells with HIV-1-derived lentiviral vectors. *Mol Ther*;**2**(1):71–80.

28. Sandrin V, Boson B, Salmon P, et al. (2002). Lentiviral vectors pseudotyped with a modified RD114 envelope glycoprotein show increased stability in sera and augmented transduction of primary lymphocytes and CD34+ cells derived from human and nonhuman primates. *Blood*;**100**(3):823–32.

29. Wang J, Kimura T, Asada R, et al. (2003). SCID-repopulating cell activity of human cord blood-derived CD34- cells assured by intra-bone marrow injection. *Blood*;**101**(8): 2924–31.

30. Yahata T, Ando K, Sato T, et al. (2003). A highly sensitive strategy for SCID-repopulating cell assay by direct injection of primitive human hematopoietic cells into NOD/SCID mice bone marrow. *Blood*;**101**(8):2905–13.

31. Wei J, Wunderlich M, Fox C, Alvarez S, Cigudosa JC, Wilhelm JE, Zheng Y, Cancelas JA, Gu Y, Jansen M, DiMartino JF and Mulloy, JC (2008) Microenvironment Determines Lineage Fate in a Human Model of MLL-AF9 Leukemia. *Cancer Cell;* **13**(6): 483–495.

32. Mulloy JC, Wunderlich M, Zheng Y, Wei J. (2008) Transforming Human Blood Stem and Progenitor Cells: A New Way Forward in Leukemia Modeling. *Cell Cycle;* **7**(21): 57–52.

Chapter 14

Ex Vivo Assays to Study Self-Renewal and Long-Term Expansion of Genetically Modified Primary Human Acute Myeloid Leukemia Stem Cells

Jan Jacob Schuringa and Hein Schepers

Summary

With the emergence of the concept of the leukemia stem cell, assays to study them remain pivotal in understanding (leukemic) stem cell biology. Although the in vivo NOD-SCID xenotransplantation model is still the favored model of choice in most cases, this system has some limitations as well, such as its cost-effectiveness, duration, and the lack of engraftability of cells from subsets of acute myeloid leukemia (AML) patients. Here, we have described an ex vivo bone marrow stromal coculture system in which CD34+ cells, but not CD34− cells, from the bone marrow or peripheral blood of AML patients can give rise to long-term cultures (LTC) that can be maintained for over 20 weeks. Long-term expansion is associated with the formation of leukemic cobblestone area (L-CA) formation underneath the stroma. Self-renewal within these L-CAs can be determined by sequential passaging of these L-CAs onto new MS5 stromal layers, which results in the generation of second, third, and fourth L-CAs that are able to sustain long-term expansion and generate high numbers of immature undifferentiated suspension cells. Furthermore, we have optimized lentiviral transduction procedures in order to stably express genes of interest or stably downmodulate genes using RNAi in AML CD34+ cells, and this method has also been described here. Together, these tools should allow a further molecular elucidation of derailed signal transduction in AML stem cells.

Key words: Acute myeloid leukemia, Leukemic stem cell self-renewal, Ex vivo assay, MS5 bone marrow stromal coculture, Lentiviral transduction

1. Introduction

With the development of NOD-SCID-leukemia and later the NOD-SCID-β2-microglobulin−/−-leukemia xenotransplantation models, it has been possible to firmly establish the concept of the leukemic stem cell (1–3). As in the normal hematopoietic system,

C.W.E. So (ed.), Leukemia, *Methods in Molecular Biology, vol. 538*
© Humana Press, a part of Springer Science + Business Media, LLC 2009
DOI: 10.1007/978-1-59745-418-6_14

it has been recognized that in AML the developing malignant clone is comprised of a heterogeneous group of cells that differ in their differentiation status *(2, 4, 5)*. Only a rare subset of the most immature cells, termed the AML SCID-Leukemia Initiating Cells (AML SL-ICs) that are present in 0.2–100 per 10^6 mononuclear cells, are capable of initiating and sustaining growth in vivo in SCID or NOD-SCID mice *(1, 2)*. These SL-ICs have high self-renewal capacity as demonstrated in serial transplantation experiments *(2, 6)*. Besides leukemic stem cells, AML colony forming units (AML-CFU) have been identified in acute leukemias, which form small clusters or colonies in semisolid methylcellulose medium with frequencies of 1 in 10^2–10^4 primary AML mononuclear cells *(7–9)*. However, the majority of these leukemic progenitors do not contain significant self-renewal capacity, as the AML-CFUs are incapable of giving rise to secondary colonies upon serial replating *(10)*. Furthermore, it has been attempted to grow AML cells on bone marrow stromal layers, and indeed a subset was capable of initiating long-term growth (leukemic long-term culture initiating cells (AML LTC-ICs)) *(11, 12)*. In these assays, AML cells were plated onto stromal cell layers for a period of 5 weeks, after which methylcellulose was added to the wells for an additional 2 weeks to determine the AML LTC-IC frequencies. The AML LTC-IC represents a rare subpopulation within the AML clone, ranging from 1.6 to 37 in 10^5 mononuclear cells *(11, 12)*, but this frequency is higher than the reported SL-IC frequencies, suggesting that slightly different cell populations are being monitored in these assays.

The NOD-SCID model has been used so far as the favored model of choice in most cases, although this system has some limitations as well, such as its cost-effectiveness, duration, and the lack of engraftability of cells from large subsets of AML patients *(13)*. Thus, it would be of great value to obtain information of a larger number of AMLs with regard to the stem cell characteristics. Also, in order to further understand the differences in molecular mechanisms that are involved in the leukemic transformation of hematopoietic stem cells, accessible assays are required in which gene-function analyses in the leukemic stem cell can be performed and in which phenotypes such as long-term expansion, self-renewal, and apoptosis can be monitored. Moreover, it has been postulated that self-renewal of normal stem cells heavily depends on interactions with stromal cells in the bone marrow microenvironment, but very little is known about how leukemic stem cells interact with stromal cells and depend on a bone marrow microenvironment for self-renewal. We have developed an AML LTC-IC assay using MS5 bone marrow stromal cells in which long-term leukemic expansion for 7–24 weeks could be established in 75% of the studied cases (n = 50 until date of publication) *(14)*. Self-renewal was addressed by serial replating of cultures onto new stroma. Also, we were able to introduce or downmodulate genes in the AML LTC-ICs by lentiviral (RNAi) approaches *(14–18)* and detailed information on our lentiviral transduction protocols are described in the second part of the chapter.

2. Materials

2.1. Isolation of AML CD34+ Cells

1. Lymphocyte separation medium (LSM1077; PAA Laboratories GmbH, Cölbe, Germany).

2. Minimum essential medium (MEM) alpha media (αMEM; Cambrex, Verviers, Belgium), phosphate buffered saline (PBS).

3. Fetal calf serum (FCS) and fetal horse serum are obtained from Sigma (Zwijndrecht, The Netherlands).

4. AML CD34+ and CD34− cells are sorted on a MoFlo cell sorter (DakoCytomation, Carpinteria, CA). Anti-CD34-PE antibodies (clone 581) are obtained from Becton Dickinson (BD, Alphen a/d Rijn, The Netherlands). In some cases, we have utilized the MiniMACS system from Miltenyi to isolate CD34+ AML cells (130-056-701, Miltenyi Biotec, Amsterdam, The Netherlands).

2.2. Long-Term Coculture of AML Cells on Bone Marrow Stroma

1. MS5 murine bone marrow stromal cells (ACC 441) can be obtained from the Deutsche Sammlung von Mikroorganismen und Zellkulturen (DSMZ GmbH, Braunschweig, Germany).

2. MS5 growth medium for propagation: αMEM supplemented with heat-inactivated 10% FCS, penicillin and streptomycin (Sigma), and 2 mM Glutamine (Sigma).

3. LTC medium: αMEM supplemented with heat-inactivated 12.5% FCS, heat-inactivated 12.5% Horse serum, penicillin and streptomycin, 2 mM glutamine, 57.2 μM β-mercaptoethanol (Sigma), and 1 μM hydrocortisone (Sigma). Furthermore, IL-3, G-CSF and TPO (20 ng/ml each) are added to the LTC medium.

4. Gelatin (Sigma) was prepared as 0.1% stock solutions in PBS which is used to coat flasks or plates prior to plating MS5 stromal cells. AML LTCs are typically performed in 12-well plates or T25 flasks. Prior to plating of MS5, plates or flasks are precoated with 0.1% gelatin in PBS for 2 h at room temperature (in order to firmly attach the MS5 to the plates or flasks). Then, gelatin is removed and MS5 cells are plated in αMEM (10% FCS) such that confluency is reached within 24 h.

We do not routinely irradiate the MS5 stroma, although this is optional to further prevent overgrowth of stromal cells.

2.3. Replating of MS5 Cocultures

To isolate human cells from trypsinized MS5 bone marrow stroma, we used anti-human CD45 antibodies from Becton Dickinson.

2.4. Lentiviral Transductions: Preparation of Particles

1. HEK 293T cells (ATCC number CRL-11268).
2. Dulbecco's Modified Eagle Medium (DMEM + Glutamax and 4.5 g/l D-Glucose, Gibco, Breda, The Netherlands).
3. Hematopoietic progenitor growth medium (HPGM) (Cambrex).
4. Fugene 6 (Roche, Almere, The Netherlands).
5. We used a third-generation lentiviral packaging system with the following vectors: Packaging construct (pCMVΔ 8.91), a vector encoding the VSV-G glycoprotein envelop (pMD2.G), and various lentiviral vectors with the gene of interest (GOI) or an shRNA-expressing cassette, and a marker gene such as GFP, YFP, or the truncated NGF receptor *(14–16)*.
6. Millex HV low protein binding filters (Millipore).
7. Leica DM-IL fluorescence microscope (Leica Microsystems, Rijswijk, The Netherlands) with a 20×/0.30 or 40×/0.60 objective.

2.5. Lentiviral Transductions: Transduction of AML CD34+ Cells

1. Retronectin (Takara, Tokyo, Japan) is dissolved in H_2O at a stock concentration of 1 mg/ml, which was stored at –20°C. Prior to use, the retronectin stock is diluted in PBS to a final concentration of 25–50 µg/ml. Plates are coated with retronectin for 2 h at room temperature, and the diluted stock was stored at 4°C and reused for about four times within a period of 2 weeks.
2. Polybrene (Hexadimethrin Bromid, Sigma) is prepared as a stock concentration of 4 mg/ml in PBS which was used 1:1,000.

3. Methods

3.1. Isolation of AML CD34+ Cells

1. Peripheral blood or bone marrow cells from AML patients are studied after informed consent. Mononuclear cells (MNC) are harvested by density-gradient centrifugation over lymphocyte separation medium according to the manufacturer's instructions. MNCs are routinely cryopreserved in aliquots of 50–100 × 10^6 cells in 80% αMEM, 10% dimethylsulfoxide (DMSO), and 10% FCS in liquid nitrogen. The recovery rate is typically in the range of 50–80%.

2. Upon thawing, DMSO is removed by resuspending cells in 6 ml serum in the presence of 200 µl of 1 mg/ml DNAse and 200 µl of 25 mM $MgCl_2$, followed by centrifugation for 5 min at $800 \times g$.

3. To sort AML $CD34^+$ and $CD34^-$ cells, $50-100 \times 10^6$ AML cells are incubated with 10 µl anti-CD34-PE antibodies in 200 µl PBS for 30 min at room temperature. Cells are washed once with PBS, and followed by cell sorting on a MoFlo. In some cases, we have utilized the MiniMACS system from Miltenyi to isolate $CD34^+$ AML cells. Then, $50-100 \times 10^6$ AML cells were incubated with 100 µl MultiSort CD34 MicroBeads and isolation was performed according to the manufacturer's instructions (*see* **Note 1**).

3.2. Long-Term Coculture of AML Cells on Bone Marrow Stroma

1. MS5 murine bone marrow stromal cells are routinely propagated in αMEM (10% FCS and pen/strep). Cells are subcultured three times a week and should never be grown to full confluency during passaging, as MS5 overgrowth or detachment might occur later during LTCs.

2. Typically, 4×10^4 AML $CD34^+$ cells are plated per well in gelatin-coated 12-well plates, while 2×10^5 AML $CD34^+$ cells are plated in gelatin-coated T25 flasks. AML cells are plated in LTC medium supplemented with cytokines (*see* **Note 2** and **3**).

3. Cultures are kept at 37°C and 5% CO_2 and are weekly demidepopulated. Plates or flasks are swirled gently, and half of the medium is collected and is set aside for analysis. Fresh LTC medium including cytokines are added back to the cultures. The harvested cells are spun down, counted, and can be analyzed by e.g., FACS, Western blotting, or q-PCR. Examples of expansion profiles are shown in **Fig. 1a**. Our experience so far indicates that in about 75% of the investigated cases ($n = 50$) the AML $CD34^+$ fraction contains cells that can give rise to expanding LTCs on MS5. Furthermore, AML cells that are capable of initiating LTCs reside predominantly in the $CD34^+$ fraction, while the $CD34^-$ fraction only gives rise to transiently expanding cultures (**Fig. 1b**).

4. While normal $CD34^+$ cells derived from cord blood or bone marrow give rise to phase-dark cobblestone area forming cells (CAFCs) only after 5 weeks of plating onto MS5, we typically observed leukemic cobblestone areas (L-CAs) earlier in the cultures, ranging from 1 to 5 weeks when the first L-CAs arise. An example of those L-CAs is shown in **Figs. 1c** and **2b**.

3.3. Addressing Self-Renewal: Replating of Long-Term AML Cocultures onto New Bone Marrow Stroma

1. Self-renewal is addressed by serial replating of cultures. Typically, cultures are replated at week 5, but in case high numbers of L-CAs arise early on in the cultures or when a lot of suspension cells are produced and the MS5 stroma no longer seems capable of sustaining the cultures, we have replated cultures earlier than week 5, at week 3 or 4.

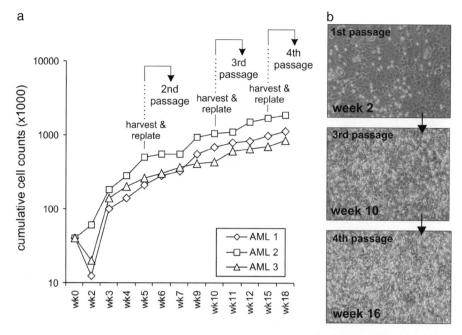

Fig. 1. Establishing of long-term AML cocultures on bone marrow stroma. (**a**) Three representative examples of AML LTCs. CD34+ cells were isolated from the peripheral blood of AML patients and cultured on MS5 stroma. Cultures were weekly demidepopulated, suspension cells were analyzed and the cumulative expansion of suspension cells is shown. At weeks 5, 10, and 15 the suspension and human CD45+ adherent cells were collected and replated onto new MS5 stroma to give rise to second, third, and fourth passage cultures. (**b**) AML cells (n = 9) were sorted into CD34+ and CD34− populations and LTCs were initiated as in (**a**). (**c**) Representative examples of third and fourth passages on MS5 stroma. Phase-dark L-cobblestone area – forming cells (L-CAs) underneath the MS5 stroma as well as nonadherent suspension cells are clearly visible.

2. Harvest suspension cells, wash adherent layer twice with PBS and collect all fractions.

3. Trypsinize adherent cells for 5 min at 37°C.

4. Collect adherent fraction in PBS.

5. Stain human cells with an antibody recognizing human CD45, and sort cells on a MoFlo (*see* **Note 4**).

6. Combine the sorted CD45+ human AML cells with the suspension cells, and replate 1/20–1/3 of the total cells onto a new 12-well plate or T25 flask that was precoated with new MS5 the day before. We have also replated adherent and suspension cells separately onto new stroma. We found that the majority of replating activity resides in the adherent L-CA population, but some replating activity is also present in the suspension cells in some cases.

7. At weeks 10 and 15 (or at earlier timepoints when MS5 stromal cells deteriorate due to high numbers of leukemic cells) **steps 2–6** can be repeated to initiate third and fourth cultures. Expansion in replating experiments for three AMLs is shown

in **Fig.1a** and a typical example of the morphology of replated cocultures is shown in **Fig.1b** (*see* **Note 5** and **6**).

3.4. Lentiviral Transductions: Preparation of Particles

Detailed molecular analysis of signal transduction pathways in human leukemic stem cells depend upon efficient delivery of gene targeting vectors, by which loss-of-function and gain-of-function analyses can be performed. The efficient delivery involves optimal preparation of lentiviral particles, which takes about 4 days. Each day is described below in detail.

3.4.1. Day 1

1. Coat 10-cm dishes for 2 h with 0.1% gelatin at room temperature.
2. Remove gelatin, plate 2.5×10^6 293T cells in 10 ml DMEM plus 10% FCS per group, incubate overnight at 37°C, 5% CO_2. Multiple plates can be seeded at the same time and later harvested into one large batch of virus, but the detailed protocol below describes the procedure for one plate. Obtaining a larger batch of virus can be useful from the point of experiment to experiment consistency as well as reducing the overall amount of work, since fewer preparations need to be done.

3.4.2. Day 2

1. Transient transfection of 293T cells using fugene. Prepare two tubes according to the following table according to the manufacturers recommendations

Tube 1	
DMEM without FCS and penicillin/streptomycin	100 µl
Packaging construct (pCMV Δ8.91)	3 µg
Glycoprotein envelop plasmid (pMD2.G)	0.7 µg
Vector construct containing gene of interest (GOI) and e.g. GFP	3 µg
Tube 2	
DMEM without FCS and Penicillin/Streptomycin	400 µl
Fugene6	21 µl

2. Add tube 1 to tube 2, flick gently and allow complex formation for 20 min at room temperature.
3. After 20 min add mixture dropwise to 293T cells, swirl gently and incubate cells overnight at 37°C, 5% CO_2.

3.4.3. Day 3

Check the transfection efficiency of the 293T cells. If the 293T cells are still solidly attached and a bright GFP signal is observed through the fluorescent microscope, the medium on the 293T cells can be changed to 4.5 ml HPGM and cells can be incubated overnight at 37°C, 5% CO_2. If 293T cells are detaching or a weak

GFP signal is observed, an optimization of the growth and transfection procedure is necessary to obtain higher viral titers, mandatory for efficient AML transduction (*see* **Note** 7 and **8**).

3.4.4. Day 4

After an ~12 h of virus production into HPGM medium, virus can be harvested by removing 4.5 ml medium from 293T cells and filtering over low protein binding filters Millex HV filters to remove residual 293T cells. As we have observed that some 293T cells might be detaching during the harvest period, this step is necessary. After filtering, use virus directly for infection of AML cells or freeze virus containing supernatant in aliquots of 500 µl in cryotubes in −80°C and thaw upon use.

3.5. Lentiviral Transductions: Transduction of AML CD34+ Cells

The procedure for AML CD34+ transduction takes 3 days to complete and can be started on day 4 of the lentiviral preparation. A typical AML transduction involves three rounds of infection of ~8–12 h and we have reached transduction efficiencies ranging from 25 to –80%, depending upon AML sample, viral preparations and the vector of interest.

3.5.1. Day 1

1. Typically, 1.5×10^6 AML CD34+ cells are isolated with MACS columns or sorted by MoFlo and incubated at a cell density of 0.5×10^6 cell/ml in LTC medium supplemented with IL-3, G-CSF and TPO (each 20 ng/ml) for 4 h at 37°C, 5% CO_2.

2. During this incubation period, wells from a 12-well plate are coated with 0.5 ml of retronectin (50 µg/ml in PBS) at room temperature (one well per group). After 2 h retronectin is removed and the wells are blocked immediately with 2% BSA/PBS for 30 min. Wash the plate twice with PBS and keep at 4°C until use. In case, if high mortality of AML cells is observed during the transduction period we have also used retronectin-coated 96-well plates for transduction as well to plate cells at higher densities.

3. After 4 h, the preincubated AML CD34+ cells are split in various groups that will be transduced with lentiviral batches of interest. Use at least 1.5×10^5 cells per group, but not more than 5×10^5 in 500 µl per well in 12-well plates. In 96-well plates, we used 0.5 to 1.5×10^5 cells per group in 100–200 µl per well. Make sure to include both an empty vector control group that only expresses your marker gene, as well as a no virus control group which will not be transduced but will be used for setting FACS gates and also allow a comparison of the growth of nontransduced AMLs with empty vector-transduced AMLs.

4. Per transduction group, plate 500 µl AML cell suspension per well in the retronectin-coated 12-well plates. Add 500 µl lentivirus supernatant to each well. In the no virus control

group, add 500 µl HPGM. Furthermore, add the following to each group: 110 µl FCS (final concentration 10%), 20 ng/ml hIL-3, 20 ng/ml TPO, 20 ng/ml G-CSF, and 4 µg/ml polybrene. Incubate overnight at 37°C, 5% CO_2. This will be the first round of transduction.

5. Meanwhile, MS5 stromal cells need to be cultured as described earlier in α-MEM supplemented with 10% FCS, so that e.g.,

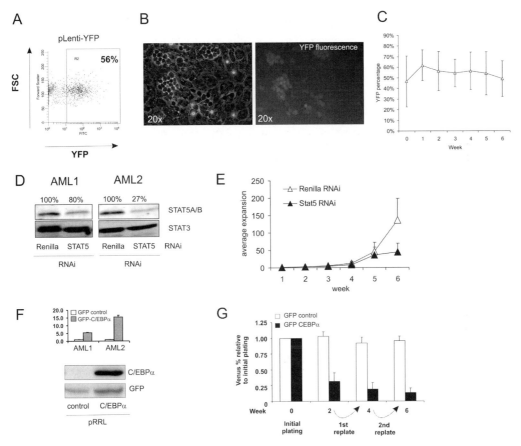

Fig. 2. Lentiviral transduction of AML CD34+ cells. (**A**) Typical transduction efficiency plot from AML CD34+ cells transduced with YFP-expressing vectors after 1 week of culture on MS5 stromal cells. (**B**) Phase-dark and YFP fluorescent images of transduced AML cultures, demonstrating the ability to transduce cells capable of initiating Leukemic Cobblestone Areas. (**C**) YFP expression remains stable over a 6 weeks period. The average YFP percentage of seven control transduced AML cultures is shown. (**D**) AML CD34+ cells were transduced with lenti shRNA vectors targeting Renilla luciferase (control) or STAT5. The STAT5 expression levels could be reduced from 80% up to 27% of the original expression levels as determined by Western blotting, whereas the related STAT3 protein levels were unaffected. (**E**) Transduced cells were plated on MS5, cultures were weekly demidepopulated, and harvested cells were analyzed by FACS for relative expansion of transduced and nontransduced cells. The average expansion of STAT5 RNAi cells vs. Renilla luciferase cells is shown in the panel. (**F**) Lentiviral vectors were used to over express C/EBPα in AML CD34+ cells. Overexpression levels were determined by quantitative PCR (*upper panel*) as well as by Western blotting (*lower panel*). (**G**) Example of serial replating experiments of 6 AML cultures indicate that control transduced cells contribute equally in generating new AML cultures, whereas cells transduced with a C/EBPα rapidly loose the competition from nontransduced cells as measured by a loss of YFP fluorescence of subsequent cultures. Part of this data was originally published in Experimental Hematology and Blood *(14–16)* (© by the American Society of Hematology).

a T75 reaches 80% confluency at day 2, which should be sufficient for three T25 flasks (in case you want to plate a no virus control group, an empty vector control group and an experimental group).

3.5.2. Day 2

1. Repeat transduction procedure in the morning (round 2). Add 500 μl new viral supernatants (or HPGM) to the wells as well as FCS, growth factors, and polybrene at concentrations indicated above. Washing of cells or removal of the first 500 μl of viral supernatant that was added in round 1 is not necessary and will only lead to loss of cells. Incubate for 8 h at 37°C, 5% CO_2.

2. Transduction round 3 should be started in the evening by adding another 500 μl of viral supernatant, as well as FCS, growth factors, and polybrene at concentrations indicated earlier.

3. Furthermore, coat three T25 flasks with 0.1% gelatin for 2 h at room temperature. After that, trypsinize an 80% confluent T75 flask with MS5, resuspend in 15 ml α-MEM with 10% FCS and plate 5 ml per gelatin-coated per T25 (these MS5 cultures will reach confluency on day 3, optimal for seeding with AML cells). When more than three T25 are required, make sure to prepare multiple T75 flasks with MS5 that reach 80% confluency at day 2.

3.5.3. Day 3

1. The transduced AML CD34+ cells from each group are washed 3–5 times with PBS and are resuspended in 1.5 ml of LTC medium supplemented with IL-3, G-CSF and TPO (each 20 ng/ml).

2. Take a 50 μl aliquot for FACS to assess transduction efficiency (use cells from the no virus group to set the gates).

3. Plate equal amounts of AML CD34+ cells on MS5 in LTC medium (at least 1.5×10^5 cells per T25, not more than 5×10^5). MoFlo sorting of transduced cells can be performed, but is not strictly necessary as the untranduced cells within each culture can serve as an internal control. However, note that, e.g., GFP/YFP expression usually does not reach steady state levels until 2 days after the infection procedure; hence, analyzing a small sample after 2 days of expansion on MS5 stromal layers will give a more reliable transduction efficiency. **Figure 2a** demonstrates a typical FACS profile from transduced AML cultures after 1 week on MS5 stromal cells and **Fig. 2b** displays the ability of this protocol to transduce cells capable of forming leukemic cobblestone areas (L-CAs) (*see* **Note 9**).

3.6. Loss- and Gain-Of-Function Studies with Long-Term Coculture of Transduced AMLs on MS5

LTCs of transduced AML cells are essentially the same as long-term cocultures of nontransduced AML cells as described in **Subheading 3.2**. Remove half of the suspension (2.5 ml) from the cultures weekly and add 2.5 ml fresh LTC medium supplemented with IL-3, G-CSF, and TPO (each 20 ng/ml). The removed half can be used for FACS analysis, cell count, cytospins etc. Determining the percentage of marker genes such as GFP or YFP as well as the use of differentiation makers in FACS analyses on these weekly demipopulations give a rapid insight in growth and differentiation characteristics of transduced cells. We typically compared GFP/YFP-expressing cells with the nontransduced cells within each group as negative controls, as well as with the control group that contains AML cells that were not transduced at all. Stable marker gene expression was obtained for over 10 weeks, and an example of some empty vector control experiments are shown in **Fig. 2c** using YFP as a marker gene *(14)*. Also note the rise in the percentage of YFP-positive cells from week 0 to week 1, indicating the delayed expression of YFP, as mentioned above. **Figure 2d** demonstrates that lentiviral short hairpin vectors against STAT5 can specifically knockdown the target gene STAT5 in various primary AML CD34$^+$ cells, which results in a reduced expansion as compared to controls (**Fig. 2e**) *(15)*. Gain-of-function studies can also be efficiently performed, as demonstrated in **Fig. 2f**, where C/EBPα was overexpressed. **Figure 2g** depicts serial replatings from control-transduced AML CD34$^+$ cells and AML CD34$^+$ cells transduced with C/EBPα *(16)*. In such a setting it could rapidly be determined that the cells with restored C/EBPα loose the competition from GFP-transduced or nontransduced cells, indicating our ability to modify the self-renewal potential of AML CD34$^+$ cells, by attenuating genes that have been suggested to play a mayor role in the process of leukemogenesis.

4. Notes

1. Instead of sorting CD34$^+$ AML cells on the MoFlo, we have been utilizing the MiniMACS columns using anti-CD34 magnetic beads as well (Miltenyi Biotec). It must be taken into account that the maximum binding capacity of the columns is (in our experience) around 20–30×10^6 cells, so when the CD34 percentage of an AML is high, the flow through cannot be considered as CD34$^-$.

2. The culture system obviously also allows for sorting on the basis of different markers, and we have been able to use CD34, CD38, CD123, D117, and HLA-DR as potential markers to identify leukemic stem cells. While the AML cells that give rise to LTCs almost always reside in the CD34$^+$, and are absent from the CD34$^-$ fraction *(14)*, we have observed in our analyses of various AML samples a much more heterogeneous expression pattern of the other markers on cells that can initiate LTCs on MS5 stroma.

3. Instead of using 12-well plates, we have been able to initiate long-term AML cocultures on 96-well plates coated with MS5 using as little as 20 AML cells per well, allowing more high-throughput analyses.

4. Upon replating of cocultures, we have been able to use human CD45 MicroBeads (130-045-801) from Milteny as well instead of sorting by MoFlo in order to isolate human AML cells from the adherent fraction. However, it must be taken into account that some MS5 cells will contaminate your CD45 isolation as it is difficult to deplete all MS5 cells from the column during the wash steps. Alternatively, we have been able to remove the majority of MS5 stromal cells from AML cells by preplating of trypsinized adherent fractions on T75 flasks in 15 ml αMEM (10% FCS) for 5 min. The majority of MS5 cells will attach to the plastic within this period while the AML cells do not and can be harvested from the nonadherent suspension fraction.

5. An important issue is how to deal with leukemic vs. normal stem cells that might obviously be present in the CD34 isolation steps as well. We established the leukemic origin of the expanding cultures by performing PCR analysis for the presence of genetic markers, such as the Flt3-ITD and by the fact that cultures generate second, third and fourth L-CAs, a feature of self-renewing cells that we do not observe with normal cord blood (CB) stem cells. Also, L-CAs derived from PB should represent leukemic cells as the PB of healthy donors typically do not contain significant numbers of stem/progenitor cells that give rise to cobblestone areas on stroma.

6. We have observed that around 75% of all investigated AMLs (~50 until date of publication) can give rise to long-term expanding cultures on MS5 stroma. The growth characteristics were categorized into the risk groups according to the new World Health Organization classification, but no significant differences were observed. It was intriguing, however, that out of the AMLs under investigation that belonged to the good risk group (containing either AML1-ETO or INV (16) translocations), no AML LTC-ICs could be established, suggesting that good risk AMLs do not perform well in our ex vivo assay.

7. When transducing AML CD34+ cells, efficient transduction can be achieved when using viral supernatants that contain a titer of ~10^7 viral particles per ml (TU/ml). By infecting 293T cells using a standard viral titration protocol this number can be easily calculated. If titers are low, this might have been due to low transient transfection efficiencies of 293T cells. Ensure that the producing 293T cells are proliferating optimally, and that cells are attached and correct Fugene6/DNA complexes are used. Use clean DNA to transfect the 293T cells with an OD 260/280 of >1.8. Furthermore, the ratio of the various

plasmids in the DNA/Fugene6 complex as described above may vary when slightly different plasmids are used. The protocol described earlier has been optimized for various plasmids, but we have observed (unpublished results) that different promoters, different plasmid sizes, and different sizes of the gene of interest can also influence transfection and transduction efficiencies. In such cases, transfections need to be optimized with different ratios of plasmid vs. Fugene6.

8. Another possibility when low viral titers are obtained is to concentrate the virus particles. Standard concentration of virus involves ultracentrifugation for several hours but an easier and faster method can be employed when using Centriprep columns (YM-50, Amicon, Millipore). Following the manufacturer's instructions, 15 ml of virus supernatant can be concentrated 15–20× in two rounds of 20 min of centrifugation using any normal centrifuge. This method is therefore ideally suited when an expensive ultracentrifuge is not at hand and ensures that virus can be frozen or used as fast as possible without risk of losing virus due to a possible short half life.

9. Since the transductions are performed in the absence of stromal cells and the efficient culture of AML cells is dependent upon interactions with stroma, an important point of interest is how many AML cells die during the transduction procedure. During most of our transductions we have observed that the number of AML cells after transductions is ~20–50% lower than what was plated upon the start of the transduction procedure, while only in some exceptional cases we have observed a slight expansion during the transduction procedures. We have therefore always counted viable cells after the transduction procedure, before subjecting them to long-term stromal cultures, ensuring that we had equal numbers of AML cells at the start of the culture. To ensure that LTCs are not dying during the first week of culture, a minimum of 1.5×10^5 cells was plated per T25. In the first 1 or 2 weeks, an initial drop in cell number is usually observed, but in all LTCs with transduced AML CD34[+] cells we have performed till date ($n = 21$) rapidly expanding cultures could be established within a few weeks after plating.

Acknowledgements

We acknowledge Prof. Dr. Edo Vellenga and all members of the hematology lab for helpful discussions. This work was supported by a NWO-VENI (Nederlandse organisatie voor Wetenschappelijk Onderzoek-VENI) grant (J.J.S.).

References

1. Lapidot, T., Sirard, C., Vormoor, J., Murdoch, B., Hoang, T., Caceres-Cortes, J., Minden, M., Paterson, B., Caligiuri, M. A., and Dick, J. E. (1994) A cell initiating human acute myeloid leukaemia after transplantation into SCID mice. *Nature* **367**, 645–648.

2. Bonnet, D. and Dick, J. E. (1997) Human acute myeloid leukemia is organized as a hierarchy that originates from a primitive hematopoietic cell. *Nat. Med.* **3**, 730–737.

3. Kollet, O., Peled, A., Byk, T., Ben Hur, H., Greiner, D., Shultz, L., and Lapidot, T. (2000) beta2 microglobulin-deficient (B2m(null)) NOD/SCID mice are excellent recipients for studying human stem cell function. *Blood* **95**, 3102–3105.

4. Warner, J. K., Wang, J. C., Hope, K. J., Jin, L., and Dick, J. E. (2004) Concepts of human leukemic development. *Oncogene* **23**, 7164–7177.

5. Wang, J. C. and Dick, J. E. (2005) Cancer stem cells: lessons from leukemia. *Trends Cell Biol.* **15**, 494–501.

6. Hope, K. J., Jin, L., and Dick, J. E. (2004) Acute myeloid leukemia originates from a hierarchy of leukemic stem cell classes that differ in self-renewal capacity. *Nat. Immunol.* **5**, 738–743.

7. Moore, M. A., Williams, N., and Metcalf, D. (1973) In vitro colony formation by normal and leukemic human hematopoietic cells: characterization of the colony-forming cells. *J. Natl. Cancer Inst.* **50**, 603–623.

8. Minden, M. D., Buick, R. N., and McCulloch, E. A. (1979) Separation of blast cell and T-lymphocyte progenitors in the blood of patients with acute myeloblastic leukemia. *Blood* **54**, 186–195.

9. Vellenga, E., Young, D. C., Wagner, K., Wiper, D., Ostapovicz, D., and Griffin, J. D. (1987) The effects of GM-CSF and G-CSF in promoting growth of clonogenic cells in acute myeloblastic leukemia. *Blood* **69**, 1771–1776.

10. McCulloch, E. A. (1983) Stem cells in normal and leukemic hemopoiesis (Henry Stratton Lecture, 1982). *Blood* **62**, 1–13.

11. Ailles, L. E., Gerhard, B., and Hogge, D. E. (1997) Detection and characterization of primitive malignant and normal progenitors in patients with acute myelogenous leukemia using long-term coculture with supportive feeder layers and cytokines. *Blood* **90**, 2555–2564.

12. Sutherland, H. J., Blair, A., and Zapf, R. W. (1996) Characterization of a hierarchy in human acute myeloid leukemia progenitor cells. *Blood* **87**, 4754–4761.

13. Pearce, D. J., Taussig, D., Zibara, K., Smith, L. L., Ridler, C. M., Preudhomme, C., Young, B. D., Rohatiner, A. Z., Lister, T. A., and Bonnet, D. (2006) AML engraftment in the NOD/SCID assay reflects the outcome of AML: implications for our understanding of the heterogeneity of AML. *Blood* **107**, 1166–1173.

14. Gosliga van, D., Schepers, H., Rizo, A., Kolk van der, D., Vellenga, E., and Schuringa, J. J. (2007) Establishing long-term cultures with self-renewing acute myeloid leukemia stem/progenitor cells. *Exp. Hematol.* **35**, 1538–1549.

15. Schepers, H., Gosliga van, D., Wierenga, A. T., Eggen, B. J., Schuringa, J. J., and Vellenga, E. (2007) STAT5 is required for long-term maintenance of normal and leukemic human stem/progenitor cells. *Blood* **110**, 2880–2888.

16. Schepers, H., Wierenga, A. T., Gosliga van, D., Eggen, B. J., Vellenga, E., and Schuringa, J. J. (2007) Reintroduction of C/EBPalpha in leukemic CD34+ stem/progenitor cells impairs self-renewal and partially restores myelopoiesis. *Blood* **110**, 1317–1325.

17. Fuhler, G. M., Drayer, A. L., Olthof, S. G., Schuringa, J. J., Coffer, P. J., and Vellenga, E. (2008) Reduced activation of protein kinase B, Rac and F-actin polymerisation contribute to an impairment of SDF-1-induced migration of CD34$^+$ cells from patients with Myelodysplasia. *Blood* **111**, 359–368.

18. Rozenveld-Geugien, M., Baas, I. O., Gosliga van, D., Vellenga, E., and Schuringa, J. J. (2007) Expansion of normal and leukemic human hematopoietic stem/progenitor cells requires rac-mediated interaction with stromal cells. *Exp. Hematol.* **35**, 782–792.

Chapter 15

Identification and Characterization of Hematopoietic Stem and Progenitor Cell Populations in Mouse Bone Marrow by Flow Cytometry

Jenny Yeung and Chi Wai Eric So

Summary

The study of key mechanisms and molecules involved in the regulation of hematopoiesis in mouse models has been greatly facilitated by multi-parameter flow cytometry. Subpopulations of hematopoietic stem and progenitor cells can be identified and characterized using this technique. Furthermore, fluorescence-activated cell sorting (FACS) can prospectively isolate functionally-defined subpopulations of hematopoietic cells for use in further in vitro or in vivo analysis. The chapter describes methodology for preparing samples from mouse bone marrow, staining cells with fluorochrome conjugated antibodies, enrichment of HSC and progenitors, and finally data analysis.

Key words: Hematopoietic stem cells (HSCs), Progenitors, CMP, GMP, CLP, Flow cytometry, FACS

1. Introduction

Hematopoietic stem cells (HSCs) are rare cells within the mouse bone marrow that are able to give rise to progeny and generate all the mature cells within the hematopoietic system. A hierarchy exists within the hematopoietic system whereby HSCs give rise to progeny that progressively lose self-renewal capacity and become restricted to one lineage (**Fig. 1**). The HSCs at the top of this hierarchy are defined by their abilities to self-renew and differentiate into committed progenitors. The lineage-restricted progenitors in turn gain proliferative potential and eventually give rise to terminally-differentiated mature cells. Long-term

C.W.E. So (ed.), Leukemia, *Methods in Molecular Biology, vol. 538*
© Humana Press, a part of Springer Science + Business Media, LLC 2009
DOI: 10.1007/978-1-59745-418-6_15

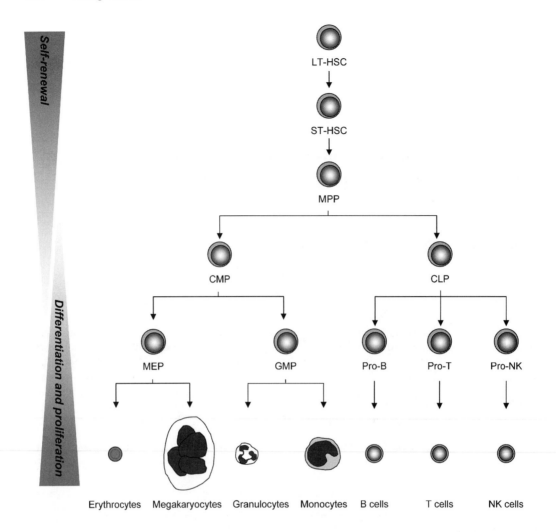

Fig. 1. Hematopoiesis in the mouse bone marrow. HSCs can generate all the cells of different lineage of the hematopoietic system in a hierarchical manner. HSCs can produce progeny that can undergo self-renewal or differentiate to produce more lineage-committed cells with greater proliferative potential. *LT-HSC* long-term HSC; *ST-HSC* short-term HSC; *MPP* multipotent progenitor; *CMP* common myeloid progenitor; *CLP* common lymphoid progenitor; *MEP* megakaryocyte/erythrocyte progenitor; *GMP* or granulocyte/macrophage progenitors; *NK* natural killer.

HSCs (LT-HSCs) are defined by their ability to confer long-term reconstitution of all the lineages of the hematopoietic system to a lethally irradiated mouse, and subsequently to a secondary recipient. Short-term HSCs (ST-HSCs) have more limited self-renewal capacity and are capable of giving rise to short-term reconstitution for up to several months after transplantation into lethally irradiated recipients, but cannot reconstitute a secondary recipient. Downstream of HSCs are non-self-renewing multipotent progenitors (MPPs), and further downstream of these are lineage-restricted progenitors, which include common lymphoid progenitors (CLPs) and common myeloid progenitors (CMPs). CLPs generate T cells, B cells, and natural killer (NK) cells *(1)*, while CMPs give rise to either megakaryocyte/erythrocyte or granulocyte/macrophage progenitors *(2)*. Characterization and isolation of these distinctive populations of hematopoietic cells by flow cytometry have been instrumental towards our understanding of the hematopoietic system. In addition, many mouse models have been generated in order to study the regulation of hematopoiesis, in which flow cytometry has been an extremely valuable tool to interrogate and analyze any perturbation within the hematopoietic systems. Different populations of stem cells or progenitors can be identified and isolated, from both wild type and genetically modified mice, based on their unique expression of a combination of surface markers *(3–5)* are discussed in this chapter.

2. Materials

2.1. Isolating Bone Marrow Cells

1. Phosphate-buffered saline (PBS): 1.54 mM KH_2PO_4, 155 mM NaCl, 2.71 mM Na_2HPO_4. Adjust to pH 7.2 and autoclave to sterilize.

2. Suspension medium (SM): 0.2% Fetal calf serum in PBS. Filter fetal calf serum with a 0.22-μm syringe filter prior to addition to sterile PBS. Store at 4°C.

3. Erythrocyte lysis buffer: 10 mM $KHCO_3$, 150 mM NH_4Cl, 0.1 mM EDTA (pH 8.0). Autoclave to sterilize and store at 4°C.

4. 0.4% Trypan blue solution.

2.2. Antibody Staining of Mouse Bone Marrow Cells

1. Rat immunoglobulin G (IgG) from serum (Technical grade) (Sigma).

2. 96-well V-bottom plates.

3. Anti-rat Ig, k CompBead set (BD).

4. 5-mL round-bottom polystyrene tubes (12 × 75 mm).

5. 1 mg/mL propidium iodide (PI): Dissolve powder in double distilled water (ddH_2O) and store in the dark at 4°C.

6. For analysis, a thirteen parameter BD LSRII flow cytometer equipped with a 488 nm laser (6 color octagon), a 405 nm laser (2 color trigon), and a 633 nm laser (3 color trigon) was used. For sorting, either a ten parameter BD FACSVantage DiVa sorter equipped with a 488 nm laser (4 colors), a 333.6–363.8 nm multi-line UV laser (2 colors), and a 633

nm laser (2 colors) or a nineteen parameter BD FACSAria sorter equipped with a 355 nm laser (2 color trigon), a 405 nm laser (5 color octagon), 488 nm laser (2 color octagon), a 638 nm laser (3 color trigon), and a 532 nm laser (5 color octagon) was used. BD FACSDiva™ flow cytometry software was used with all machines.

7. Unconjugated, purified rat antibodies (clone number in parentheses): Anti-CD11b (M1/70), anti-Gr-1 (RB6-8C5), anti-CD3ε (145-2C11), anti-Ter119 (Ter-119), anti-CD4 (RM4-5), anti-B220 (RA3-6B2), and anti-CD8a (53-6.7) (*see* **Note 1**).

8. Conjugated rat antibodies (clone number in parentheses): Anti-Sca1-Pacific Blue (D7), anti-c-Kit-PE-Cy7 (2B8), anti-CD34-FITC (RAM34), anti-CD16/32 ($F_c\gamma R$)-APC (2.4G2), anti-IL7-Rα-Biotin (A7R34), and anti-Flt3-PE (A2F10) (*see* **Note 1**).

9. Goat F(ab')$_2$ anti-Rat IgG (H + L)-Tri-Color® (also called PE-Cy5) (Invitrogen).

10. Streptavidin-Alexa Fluor 700® conjugate (Invitrogen).

2.3. Deletion of Lineage-Positive Cells from Mouse Bone Marrow

1. Dynabeads® sheep anti-rat IgG (Invitrogen).

2. Dynal MPC-L magnet (Invitrogen).

3. Methods

Hematopoietic stem and progenitor cells express a unique combination of antigens on their cell surface that can be recognized by specific antibodies. Antibodies conjugated with different fluorochromes can be excited to emit specific signals for detection using a flow cytometer. Depending on the availability of antibody-fluorochrome combinations and the configuration of the flow cytometer (lasers and detectors), multiple subpopulations can be determined by multiplex antibody-staining in a single reaction tube given accurate color compensation. This is particularly useful when analyzing mice carrying severe defects in the hematopoietic system and, as a consequence, may have a greatly reduced total number of bone marrow cells.

This section describes (i) the procedures required to analyze mouse bone marrow cells using a multi-parameter flow cytometer from the preparation of the sample to the analysis of the data and (ii) a protocol for enriching the HSC and progenitor fraction of the bone marrow to facilitate the sorting of these populations using a FACS sorter.

3.1. Preparation of a Single-cell Suspension of Mouse Bone Marrow Mononuclear (BMN) Cells

1. Sacrifice the animal according to procedures recommended by local institution (e.g., CO_2 inhalation).

2. Dissect out the tibia and femur from both legs and remove the muscle from the bones.

3. Trim the ends of the bones to make small openings for subsequent bone marrow flushing. Keep bones in a container containing cold PBS on ice.

4. Place a 40-μm nylon cell strainer into a 50-mL tube.

5. Flush out bone marrow from the four bones using 10 mL of cold SM with a 10-mL syringe and a 21-gauge (G) needle on to the cell strainer. Insert the needle into the shaft of the bone and flush with SM until all the bone marrow is expelled and appears white (*see* **Note 2**).

6. Gently push any bone marrow aggregates through the cell strainer using the plunger from a syringe and flush the cells through with 1–2 mL of SM. Recover any medium and residual cells from underneath the cell strainer.

7. Pellet the cells by centrifugation at $300 \times g$ for 5 min at 4°C.

8. Aspirate or carefully decant the supernatant.

9. Resuspend the cell pellet in 1 mL of erythrocyte lysis buffer and incubate at room temperature for 10 min or 4°C for 15 min (*see* **Note 3**).

10. Add 10 mL of cold SM to dilute the erythrocyte lysis buffer.

11. Pellet the cells by centrifugation at $300 \times g$ for 5 min at 4°C.

12. Resuspend cells in 1 mL of cold SM and determine the viable cell count using a hemocytometer and trypan blue.

13. Keep cells on ice until use.

3.2. Antibody Staining and Flow Cytometry for Subpopulation Analysis

1. Resuspend 3×10^6 to 5×10^6 BMN cells in 200 μL of cold SM containing 1:40 dilution of each of the purified unconjugated rat antibodies anti-Gr-1, -CD11b, -B220, -Ter119, -CD3ε, -CD4, and -CD8a (*see* **Note 4**), and transfer to a well of a 96-well V-bottom plate (*see* **Note 5**). Keep some unstained bone marrow for setting up compensations (see below).

2. Incubate on ice for 30 min.

3. Pellet the cells by centrifugation at $300 \times g$ for 5 min at 4°C.

4. To remove the supernatant, quickly invert the plate and flick the plate once over a sink.

5. Add 200 μL of cold SM to the cells and pellet the cells by centrifugation at $300 \times g$ for 5 min at 4°C.

6. Repeat wash **steps 4–5** and remove supernatant.

7. Resuspend the cells in 200 µL of cold SM containing 1:50 dilution of goat anti-rat IgG-Tri-Color conjugate and incubate on ice for 30 min in the dark.

8. Pellet the cells by centrifugation at $300 \times g$ for 5 min at 4°C, and wash as described in **steps 4–6**.

9. Resuspend cells in 100 µL of neat rat IgG for 30 min on ice in the dark (*see* **Note 6**).

10. Wash cells as described in **steps 3–6**.

11. Resuspend cells in 200 µL of cold SM containing the following antibodies (their final dilution given in parentheses): anti-CD34-FITC (1:25), anti-Flt3-PE (1:50), anti-CD16/32-APC (1:75), anti-c-Kit-PE-Cy7 (1:100) anti-Sca1-Pacific Blue (1:50), and anti-IL-7Rα-Biotin (1:100) (*see* **Note 7**).

12. Incubate on ice for 30 min in the dark.

13. Compensation samples can be prepared concurrently using the BD anti-rat Ig, k CompBead set (*see* **Note 8**). Resuspend the CompBeads in 200 µL of SM for each of the fluorochrome-conjugated antibodies (and use second step reagents where necessary).

14. Pellet the cells by centrifugation at $300 \times g$ for 5 min at 4°C, and wash as described in **steps 4–6**.

15. Resuspend the cells in 200 µL of cold SM containing 1:200 dilution of streptavidin-Alexa Fluor 700 in order to visualize the anti-IL-7Rα-Biotin.

16. Incubate on ice for 30 min in the dark.

17. Pellet the cells by centrifugation at $300 \times g$ for 5 min at 4°C, and wash as described in **steps 4–6**.

18. Resuspend the cells in approximately 300 µL of cold SM containing PI at a final concentration of 1 µg/mL and transfer into a 5-mL round-bottom polystyrene tube.

19. Set up the flow cytometer by using the unstained bone marrow sample and compensations controls (*see* **Note 9**).

20. Acquire at least 5×10^5 events (PI⁻ viable cells) for analysis of subpopulations (*see* **Note 10**).

3.3. Lineage Depletion of Mouse Bone Marrow for Prospective Sorting of Subpopulations (See Note 11)

1. Obtain the bone marrow mononuclear cells from the tibia and femur bones of two adult mice as described in **Subheading 3.1**, to acquire approximately 4×10^7 to 6×10^7 total BMN cells (*see* **Note 12**).

2. Resuspend the cells in 200 µL of cold SM containing 1:40 dilution of each of the purified unconjugated rat antibodies anti-Gr-1, -CD11b, -B220, -Ter119, -CD3ε, -CD4, and -CD8a and transfer to a sterile 5-mL round-bottom polystyrene tube with a cap.

3. Incubate on ice for 30 min.

4. Add 4 mL of cold SM to wash the cells.

5. Pellet the cells by centrifugation at $300 \times g$ for 5 min at 4°C.

6. Aspirate or carefully decant the supernatant.

7. Repeat wash.

8. Resuspend cells in 1.6 mL of cold SM and place on ice until the magnetic beads have been washed (**step 9–13**).

9. Mix the magnetic beads (Dynabeads) well and transfer desired volume of beads (usually ~300 µL of beads for BMN cells from two mice) into a sterile 5-mL round-bottom poly-styrene tube (*see* **Note 13**).

10. Add 2 mL of cold SM to the beads.

11. Place the tube in a MPC-L magnet for 1 min and discard supernatant using a pipette.

12. Remove the tube from the magnet.

13. Repeat **steps 10–12**.

14. Transfer the medium and cells from **step 8** to the washed beads.

15. Incubate at 4°C on a rotating mixer for 30 min.

16. Add 2 mL of SM to cells.

17. Place the tube on to the magnet for 2 min.

18. Transfer the unbound (Lin⁻) cells to a fresh tube.

19. Remove the tube from the magnet, and add 4 mL of cold SM to the magnetic beads and mix.

20. Repeat **step 17**.

21. Transfer the unbound cells and pool with the cells from **step 18**.

22. The cells can be processed as described from **steps 7–18** in **Subheading 3.2**.

23. Specific subpopulations can be isolated using a FACS sorter (e.g., BD FACSVantage DiVa or BD FACSAria). The purity of the sorted populations can be increased if the isolated sub-populations are re-sorted.

3.4. Analysis of Cell Subpopulations in Mouse Bone Marrow (See Note 14)

3.4.1. HSC and Subpopulations

HSCs and early progenitors are found within the lineage$^{-/lo}$ (Lin$^{-/lo}$) fraction as they do not express, or express at a low level, markers of mature cells. The Lin$^{-/lo}$Sca1$^+$c-Kit$^+$(LSK) fraction of the bone marrow contains the HSC compartment and is approximately 3% of the Lin$^{-/lo}$ fraction. This LSK population is heterogeneous and contains LT-HSCs, ST-HSCs and MPPs. Thy1.1 and Flt3 can be used to distinguish between LT-HSC (LSKThy1.1^{lo}Flt3$^-$),

ST-HSC (LSKThyl.1^{lo}Flt3$^-$) and MPPs (LSKThyl.1$^-$Flt3$^+$) in the LSK population *(6)*. However, since many genetically altered mouse strains do not express the Thy1.1 antigen, it is not feasible to distinguish between the ST-HSCs and MPPs using Thy1.1. LT-HSCs are enriched within the LSKFlt3$^-$ fraction, ~40% of LSK cells, whereas the LSKFlt3$^+$ will contain both the ST-HSCs and MPPs, ~60% of LSK cells *(6, 7)* (**Fig. 2** and **Table 1**). Other criteria have been used to identify HSC and progenitor populations based on the expression of other markers, such as the SLAM family markers *(8–11)* (*see* **Note 15**).

Flow cytometric analysis of these populations can give an indication of any perturbations, including both the absolute numbers and proportion of stem or progenitor cells in the mouse bone marrow, but does not indicate any functional defect. This can only be definitively determined by carrying out in vivo transplantation experiments using purified subpopulation of cells in order to determine, for example, whether the sorted HSCs are capable of conferring long-term reconstitution of a lethally-irradiated recipient mice. Certain functional defects, such as self-renewal and proliferative capacity may be assessed using in vitro colony-forming assays.

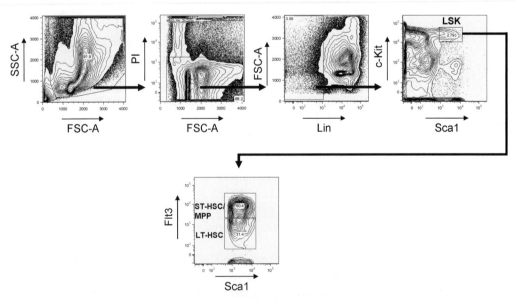

Fig. 2. Identification of subpopulations of HSCs. HSCs are highly enriched in the Lin$^{-/lo}$Sca1$^+$c-Kit$^+$(LSK) fraction of the bone marrow. Firstly, gates are set to remove debris based on forward scatter (FSC-A) and side scatter (SSC-A) and dead cells (PI$^+$) from the analysis. Cells, which were Lin$^{-/lo}$ were analyzed for their expression of Sca1 and c-Kit. LSK cells constitute approximately 0.05–0.1% of total BM. LSK cells can be further subdivided into LT-HSCs and ST-HSCs and MPPs based on Flt3 expression. Bone marrow cells were isolated from a female 8-week-old C57BL/6 mouse.

Table 1
Expected size of HSC and progenitor populations in a normal adult mouse

Population	% Bone marrow	Absolute no.[a]	Reference
LSK (Lin$^{-/lo}$ Sca1$^+$c-Kit$^+$)	0.1%	2.0×10^4	(12–14)
LT-HSC (LSKFlt3$^-$)	0.04%	8.0×10^3	(6, 7)
ST-HSC/MPP (LSKFlt3$^+$)	0.06%	1.2×10^4	(6, 7)
CLP (Lin$^{-/lo}$IL-7Rα^+Sca1^{lo}c-Kit^{lo})	0.02%	4.0×10^3	(1)
CMP (Lin$^{-/lo}$Sca1$^-$c-Kit$^+$CD34$^+$CD16/32^{lo})	0.2%	4.0×10^4	(2)
GMP (Lin$^{-/lo}$Sca1$^-$c-Kit$^+$CD34$^+$CD16/32^{hi})	0.4%	8.0×10^4	(2)
MEP (Lin$^{-/lo}$Sca1$^-$c-Kit$^+$CD34$^-$CD16/32^{lo})	0.1%	2.0×10^4	(2)

[a] Based on 2.0×10^7 BMN cells from a normal adult mouse

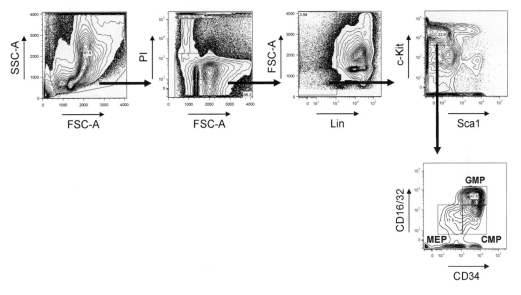

Fig. 3. Identification of myeloid progenitor populations. After exclusion of cellular debris and dead cells, CMPs, GMPs and MEPs are found within the Lin$^{-/lo}$Sca1$^-$c-Kit$^+$ fraction of the bone marrow. These three myeloid progenitor populations are identified on the basis of CD34 and CD16/32 expression. CMPs, GMPs and MEPs constitute 0.2, 0.4, and 0.1% of the total BMN cells, respectively. Bone marrow cells were isolated from a female 8-week-old C57BL/6 mouse.

3.4.2. Common Myeloid Progenitors and Sub-populations

CMPs give rise to either megakaryocyte/erythrocyte progenitors (MEPs) or granulocyte/macrophage progenitors (GMPs) (2). These cells are contained within the Lin$^{-/lo}$Sca1$^-$c-Kit$^+$ compartment (~20% of Lin$^{-/lo}$ cells) of the mouse bone marrow (**Fig. 3** and **Table 1**). Within this compartment, these myeloid progenitors can be identified by their expression of the markers CD34 and CD16/32 (also called F$_c$γR). CMPs are Lin$^{-/lo}$Sca1$^-$c-Kit$^+$CD34$^+$CD16/32^{lo},

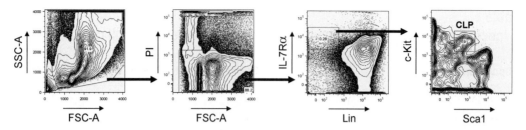

Fig. 4. Identification of common lymphoid progenitors. After exclusion of cell debris and dead cells, CLPs can be identified as Lin$^{-/lo}$ IL-7Rα^+Sca1^{lo}c-Kit^{lo} cells and constitute 0.02% of the bone marrow. Bone marrow cells were isolated from a female 8-week-old C57BL/6 mouse.

GMPs are Lin$^{-/lo}$Sca1$^-$c-Kit$^+$CD34$^+$CD16/32^{hi} and MEPs are Lin$^{-/lo}$Sca1$^-$c-Kit$^+$CD34$^-$CD16/32^{lo} cells. CMPs, GMPs and MEPs constitute 0.2, 0.4, and 0.1% of the bone marrow cells, respectively.

In vitro colony-forming assays show that FACS sorted CMPs can generate colonies consisting of macrophages, granulocytes, megakaryocytes, and erythrocytes. However, GMPs form colonies consisting of macrophages and/or granulocytes, whereas MEPs generate colonies consisting of only megakaryocytes or erthyrocytes *(2)*. Defects in these progenitors that lead to alteration of myeloid development in the bone marrow or peripheral organs can be assessed by flow cytometry using antibodies against various mature myeloid cell markers.

3.4.3. Common Lymphoid Progenitors

CLPs have been shown to generate lymphoid-restricted reconstitution in irradiated animals *(1)*. CLPs are found within the Lin$^{-/lo}$IL-7Rα^+ fraction of the bone marrow (0.28% of bone marrow). CLPs expressing low levels of Sca1 and c-Kit are defined as Lin$^{-/lo}$IL-7Rα^+Sca1^{lo}c-Kit^{lo} cells and constitute about 0.02% of the bone marrow (**Fig. 4** and **Table 1**). The lymphocyte subpopulations in bone marrow, spleen, and thymus can be analyzed by flow cytometry in order to assess functional consequences of any changes in CLP proportion or numbers.

4. Notes

1. Antibody-fluorochrome conjugates for flow cytometry are available from numerous suppliers, e.g., BD, E-Biosciences, Biolegend, etc. Several antibodies may be available for the same antigen. The antibody clones used in this protocol were selected based on the original publications describing their use in identifying the different bone marrow HSC

and progenitor populations. We find this panel of antibody-fluorochrome combination is optimal for our purposes as it can obtain the most information about the bone marrow populations using a single reaction/staining tube. This is particularly useful for analyzing precious samples, that have very limited number of cells, such as those derived from mice that have severe hematopoietic defects. Other antibody-fluorochrome combinations can be used and will have to be optimized for each laboratory. It will ultimately depend on the configuration of the flow cytometer and on the availability of the different antibody formats (as not all are commercially available).

2. Alternatively, to prepare a single-cell suspension without using a cell strainer, gently draw the medium and cells up and down a syringe and 21-guage needle 3–4 times. The preferred method of preparing a single-cell suspension from bone marrow varies between laboratories and even between operators. Whichever method is used, ensure that all the bone marrow cells are recovered and a cell count is made so that the absolute number of each population can be calculated later on.

3. This step will lyse the majority of the erythrocytes to leave the BMN cells. As hemolysis proceeds, the color of the sample will change from an initial red color to a red/orange color and the sample will become slightly clearer as it will have fewer cells. Occasionally, erythrocyte lysis may be much less efficient even when using the same batch of lysis buffer. Repeat the erythrocyte lysis again with 1 mL of erythrocyte lysis buffer and incubate at room temperature for between 5 and 10 min at room temperature, depending on how inefficient the previous lysis step was. Then proceed to the wash step, continuing with the remainder of the protocol. The lysis can also be done at 4°C or on ice with longer incubation time, which may be more gentle on cells.

4. Most of the cells within the bone marrow are maturing or differentiated cells that have committed to a specific lineage (Lin$^+$). HSC and progenitor fractions do not express these antigens (or express them at a low level) and will be detected as a Lin$^{-/lo}$ population by flow cytometry. The lineage antibody cocktail contains antibodies that recognize the lineage-restricted antigens on maturing/mature myeloid cells (Gr-1, CD11b), B cells (B220), T cells (CD3, CD4, CD8), and residual erythrocytes (Ter119), that were not removed by the erythrocyte lysis step. Unconjugated purified antibodies are used to label the Lin$^+$ cells. These cells are subsequently labeled with a fluorochrome in a step using a goat F(ab')$_2$ anti-Rat IgG (H + L)-Tri-Color® antibody. Alternatively, antibodies directly conjugated to a fluorochrome can be used

to label the Lin⁺ cells. This would reduce the time required to process the samples, but is much less cost-effective as these reagents are available in much smaller quantities and are more expensive. The additional benefit of the use of these unconjugated purified antibodies is that they can also be used for the preparation of Lin⁻ bone marrow cells via depletion using MACS (cell sorting using antibody-labeled magnetic particles).

5. Cell staining can be carried out in 5-mL round-bottom polystyrene "FACS" tubes, but care must be taken to minimize cell loss during wash steps. The wash steps are more convenient when 5-mL tubes are used compared to plates, as there is no need for a prior centrifugation step before the wash buffer is added. However, 96-well V-bottom plates are convenient for processing numerous samples and ensure minimal cell loss. They are particularly convenient for processing samples which contain less than the recommended minimum number required for the staining procedure e.g., cells from mice which have severe hematopoietic defects and have greatly reduced numbers of total bone marrow cells. Always ensure that the cells have been pelleted before decanting the supernatant. Occasionally, after centrifugation, the cells do not form a tight pellet at the bottom of the well, but have instead formed a thin layer along the sides of the well, so that it appears as if the sample has been lost. If this occurs, continue with the subsequent steps in the protocol, as described, as the cells will eventually pellet.

6. This step blocks undesirable binding between the residual goat anti-rat IgG and the fluorochrome-conjugated antibodies used in the subsequent steps.

7. Using these antibody dilutions in a 200 μL volume, we use the equivalent of 4 μg of anti-CD34-FITC, 0.8 μg of anti-Flt3-PE, 0.5 μg anti-CD16/32-APC, 0.4 μg of anti-c-Kit-PE-Cy7, 2 μg anti-Sca1-Pacific Blue, and 1 μg anti-IL-7Rα. The antibody concentration may need to be optimized for each lab and different batches of antibodies may require testing prior to use.

8. There is intrinsic spectral overlap when different fluorochromes are used. If this is not corrected (i.e., compensated), then this will result in misinterpretation of data from false-positive and artefactual populations. Compensation for spectral overlap can be accomplished by electronic subtraction of unwanted signal by using appropriate single stained controls. Compensation cannot be carried out accurately if cells express antigen at low levels. This can be overcome by using two populations of microparticles, e.g., BD anti-rat Ig, k BD™ CompBead Set. One is a negative control and the other one binds any rat k light chain-bearing antibody. Together they generate distinct

negative and positive populations, which are used to set the compensations levels either manually, or automatically using instrument set-up software. As the same fluorochrome-conjugated antibodies are used to set up the compensation settings and for labeling the cells, the compensation corrections for spectral overlap can be established more accurately. An additional advantage is that it avoids the need to use up valuable/limited cells for the sole purpose of setting up the compensation, particularly when using numerous fluorochromes. We use the unstained bone marrow sample to adjust the photomultiplier tube (PMT) for the negative populations.

9. We do not find it necessary to compensate for PI as all analysis is carried out in viable, PI$^-$ cells. All non-viable PI$^+$ cells are excluded from analysis and therefore any spectral overlap with other fluorochromes does not affect the results.

10. Aim to acquire the data for at least 5×10^5 viable cells. This will ensure that there are a sufficient number of events for rare subpopulations for further analysis. The cell populations are expressed as a proportion of total bone marrow, but this is based on the cell count after erythrocyte lysis and should probably be referred to as a proportion of the BMN cells. If the total number of BMN cells is known, then the absolute number of each of the cell populations can be determined for each mouse.

11. This depletion step reduces the time required for cell sorting as the target cell populations are greatly enriched by removing the majority of the Lin$^+$ cells and it also helps to increase purity of the sorted populations. This procedure involves labeling the Lin$^+$ cells with unconjugated rat antibodies specific for lineage markers and subsequent incubation with magnetic particles coated with anti-rat Ig antibody. This enables the labeled cells to be physically separated from the unlabeled (Lin$^{-/lo}$) cells by use of a strong magnet. Approximately 10% of the starting population is recovered after the lineage depletion step with a significant enrichment of the desired sort population. Other magnetic separation reagents and apparatus that are available from other suppliers can also be used for lineage depletion, e.g., Miltenyi. It is possible to reduce the sample process time by e.g., using biotinylated antibodies and anti-biotin beads for the lineage depletion step, but this will need to be optimized. It may be less cost-effective as the same lineage antibodies have to be purchased again in another format. Volumes of the reagents can be scaled-up if more mice are used as starting material.

12. Carry out all steps in a microbiological safety cabinet and use aseptic techniques where possible if the cells are to be used in downstream in vitro or in vivo studies.

13. Usually ~200 µL beads per mouse (~2 × 10⁷ total BMN cells) to give at least four beads per Lin⁺ target cell. 25 µL of the stock of beads contains 1 × 10⁷ beads.

14. There are a number of commercial, readily available software programs that can be used for analysis of flow cytometry data. We use FlowJo™ software for all subsequent analyses after data acquisition. To visualize the data we use high-resolution contour plots set to 5% probability and show outliers. These contour plots are particularly useful when analyzing rare populations of cells.

15. A simple combination of the SLAM family markers, CD150, CD244, and CD48, have been used to isolate and purify HSCs and identify them within tissue sections *(11)*. LT-HSCs are enriched within the CD150⁺CD244⁻CD48⁻ fractions of the bone marrow. MPPs are CD150⁻CD244⁺CD48⁻, and most restricted progenitors are CD150⁻CD244⁺CD48⁺. The SLAM family markers, CD150 and CD48, can also be used in combination with Sca1 and c-Kit to greatly increase the purity of prospectively sorted HSCs.

Acknowledgments

The authors thank Ian Titley and members of the So's lab for constructive advice. The Association for International Cancer Research (AICR), Cancer Research UK, the Kay Kendall Leukaemia Fund, Medical Research Council, Wellcome Trust, and Leukaemia Research Fund supported this work. Eric So is an AICR fellow and an EMBO young investigator.

References

1. Kondo M, Weissman IL, Akashi K. (1997). Identifi-cation of clonogenic common lymphoid progenitors in mouse bone marrow. *Cell*; **91**(5): 661–72.

2. Akashi K, Traver D, Miyamoto T, Weissman IL. (2000). A clonogenic common myeloid progenitor that gives rise to all myeloid lineages. *Nature*; **404**(6774): 193–7.

3. So CW, Karsunky H, Wong P, Weissman IL, Cleary ML. (2004). Leukemic transformation of hematopoietic progenitors by MLL-GAS7 in the absence of Hoxa7 or Hoxa9. *Blood*; **103**(8): 3192–9.

4. So CW, Karsunky H, Passegue E, Cozzio A, Weissman IL, Cleary ML. (2003). MLL-GAS7 transforms multipotent hematopoietic progenitors and induces mixed lineage leukemias in mice. *Cancer Cell*; **3**(2): 161–71.

5. Cozzio A, Passegue E, Ayton PM, Karsunky H, Cleary ML, Weissman IL. (2003). Similar MLL-associated leukemias arising from self-renewing stem cells and short-lived myeloid progenitors. *Genes Dev*; **17**(24): 3029–35.

6. Christensen JL, Weissman IL. (2001). Flk-2 is a marker in hematopoietic stem cell differentiation: a simple method to isolate long-term stem cells. *Proc Natl Acad Sci U S A*; **98**(25): 14541–6.

7. Adolfsson J, Borge OJ, Bryder D, et al. (2001). Upregulation of Flt3 expression within the bone marrow Lin(−)Sca1(+)c-kit(+) stem cell compartment is accompanied by loss of self-renewal capacity. *Immunity*; **15**(4): 659–69.

8. Yang L, Bryder D, Adolfsson J, et al. (2005). Identification of Lin-Sca1+kit+CD34+Flt3-short-term hematopoietic stem cells capable

of rapidly reconstituting and rescuing myelo-ablated transplant recipients. *Blood*; **105**(7): 2717–23.

9. Morrison SJ, Weissman IL. (1994). The long-term repopulating subset of hematopoietic stem cells is deterministic and isolatable by phenotype. *Immunity*, **1**(8): 661–73.

10. Morrison SJ, Wandycz AM, Hemmati HD, Wright DE, Weissman IL. (1997). Identification of a lineage of multipotent hematopoietic progenitors. *Development*; **124**(10): 1929–39.

11. Kiel MJ, Yilmaz OH, Iwashita T, Yilmaz OH, Terhorst C, Morrison SJ. (2005). SLAM family receptors distinguish hematopoietic stem and progenitor cells and reveal endothelial niches for stem cells. *Cell*; **121**(7): 1109.

12. Ikuta K, Weissman IL. (1992). Evidence that hematopoietic stem cells express mouse c-kit but do not depend on steel factor for their generation. *Proc Natl Acad Sci*; **89**(4): 1502–6.

13. Spangrude GJ, Heimfeld S, Weissman IL. (1988). Purification and characterization of mouse hematopoietic stem cells. *Science*; **241**(4861): 58–62.

14. Li CL, Johnson GR. (1995). Murine hematopoietic stem and progenitor cells: I. Enrichment and biologic characterization. *Blood*; **85**(6): 1472–9.

Chapter 16

In Vitro Differentiation of Mouse Embryonic Stem Cells as a Model of Early Hematopoietic Development

Patrycja Sroczynska, Christophe Lancrin, Stella Pearson, Valerie Kouskoff, and Georges Lacaud

Summary

Embryonic Stem (ES) are pluripotent cells derived from the inner cell mass of blastocysts. ES cells differentiate in vitro into all kind of cells and the development of endothelial and hematopoietic cells from mouse ES cells has been especially established. As such, the in vitro differentiation of ES cells provides a powerful experimental model to study and determine the role of specific genes in the development of the hematopoietic system. Using this approach we have demonstrated the critical function of the transcription factor *AML1/Runx1* at the onset of hematopoietic development (Blood 100:458–466, 2002; Blood 103:886–889, 2004). In this chapter, we will describe our protocols and methods for the culture of healthy ES cells, their effective differentiation toward hematopoiesis, and the quantitative analysis of their hematopoietic potential by replating or gene expression analyses.

Key words: ES cells, Hematopoietic development, AML1/Runx1, In vitro differentiation, Embryoid bodies, Hemangioblast, Transcription factor, Gene expression

1. Introduction

Embryonic stem (ES) cells spontaneously differentiate and generate 3D structures known as embryoid bodies (EBs) that contain precursors of multiple lineages, including those of the hematopoietic system (*1–6*). Several studies have demonstrated that the early cellular and molecular events leading to hematopoietic commitment in vitro in EBs parallel those found in vivo (*7–13*). The earliest site of hematopoiesis in the mouse embryo is the yolk sac where blood islands consisting of primitive erythroid cells surrounded by a layer of angioblasts develop around day 7.5 of gestation

C.W.E. So (ed.), Leukemia, *Methods in Molecular Biology, vol. 538*
© Humana Press, a part of Springer Science + Business Media, LLC 2009
DOI: 10.1007/978-1-59745-418-6_16

(14–16). The parallel development of blood and endothelium lineages in close association provided the basis for the hypothesis that they arise from a common precursor, a cell called the hemangioblast (17, 18). Using the ES cell in vitro differentiation model system, a precursor was identified that generates blast colonies containing precursors of endothelial and hematopoietic lineages (8, 10). The blast colony-forming cells (BL-CFCs) that generate these colonies represent a transient population that appears in the EBs prior to the emergence of any other hematopoietic lineage precursors. The characteristics of the BL-CFC suggest that it represents the in vitro equivalent of the hemangioblast, the earliest stage of hematopoietic development described to date.

These findings highlight the power of the in vitro ES cell differentiation system as a quick and inexpensive model to study the development of the hematopoietic system. In vitro differentiation of genetically altered ES cells provides also a robust and rapid alternative or complementary approach to in vivo mouse model to define the role of a specific gene in the development of the embryonic hematopoietic system. Using this system we have recently demonstrated the critical requirement for the function of the transcription factor *AML1/Runx1* for the development of hemangioblast and the generation of hematopoietic precursors ((19–21) and **Fig. 1**). The ES/EB system is also well suited to gain-of-function studies, as the consequences of sustained expression of specific genes on hematopoietic commitment can be easily determined.

The in vitro differentiation of ES cells involves three subsequent stages (**Fig. 1**). First, healthy ES cells are cultured, amplified, and prepared for EB generation. In the next step, ES cells are differentiated through the formation of EBs. This step is most often performed in presence of serum. In addition to a well-established serum-supplemented culture condition, we also describe here a novel serum-free protocol (22) that supports hematopoietic precursor development during EB formation in a highly reproducible and robust fashion and that does not require the prior identification of an optimal batch of serum for efficient differentiation. The last stage of this in vitro culture system allows the quantitative analysis of the hematopoietic potential. For this step, EBs are disrupted into single cells and replated in semisolid methylcellulose media containing cocktails of cytokines supporting the maturation of hemangioblast or hematopoietic precursors. The resulting colonies are easily identified and quantified, allowing a direct measurement of the type and number of hematopoietic precursors generated at different stages of differentiation by wild-type or genetically modified ES cells.

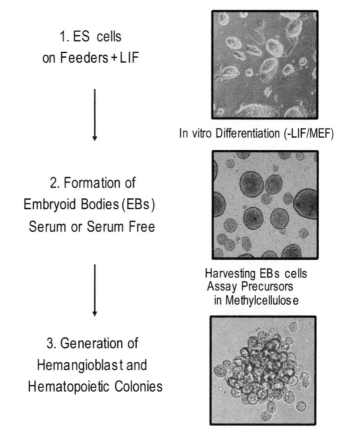

1. ES cells
on Feeders + LIF

In vitro Differentiation (-LIF/MEF)

2. Formation of
Embryoid Bodies (EBs)
Serum or Serum Free

Harvesting EBs cells
Assay Precursors
in Methylcellulose

3. Generation of
Hemangioblast and
Hematopoietic Colonies

Fig. 1. Scheme of in vitro embryonic stem cell differentiation.

2. Materials

2.1. Growth and Maintenance of ES Cells (See Note 1)

1. Penicillin/streptomycin (5,000 U/mL) (Gibco #15070-063).
2. L-Glutamine (200 mM) (Gibco #25030-081).
3. HEPES buffer 1 M (Gibco #15630-056).
4. Tissue culture grade water (Gibco #15230-089).
5. Phosphate buffered saline (PBS) (Oxoid Ltd #BR0014): Dissolve 10 tablets in 1 L of tissue culture grade water to obtain 1× PBS, and filter-sterilize.
6. Alpha-monothioglycerol (MTG) (Sigma #M6145). MTG should be stored frozen in small aliquots (0.5 mL). When the aliquots are thawed, they can be used for several experiments and then discarded. The concentration is 11.56 M and an intermediate stock solution at 0.15 M is extemporarily prepared by diluting 26 μL of MTG in 2 mL of Dulbecco's modified eagle medium (DMEM) or Iscove's modified Dulbecco's medium (IMDM) media (*see* **Note 2**).

7. DMEM: Combine a package of DMEM powder (Gibco #12800-116) with 100 mL penicillin/streptomycin (50 U/mL final), 250 mL HEPES buffer (25 mM final), and 30.25 g NaHCO$_3$ (3.025 g/L final), and add tissue culture grade water to make up to 10 L, and filter-sterilize.

8. IMDM: Add to 500 mL IMDM liquid (Lonza #BE12-726F) 5 mL penicillin/streptomycin (50 U/mL final), 5 mL L-glutamine (2 mM final) and filter-sterilize.

9. TrypLE express, a cell dissociation recombinant enzyme (Gibco #12605-036).

10. Gelatin 0.1% solution: Prepare a 0.2% solution of gelatin (Sigma #G1890) in water, bring to a boil for 5 min, dilute with the same volume of 2× PBS, cool for 1 h at 4°C, and sterilize by filtering.

11. Fetal bovine serum (FBS) pretested for maintenance of ES cells (*see* **Note 3**). We currently use a batch from PAA Ltd. FBS batches selected for growth and maintenance of mouse ES cells are commercially available from many manufacturers.

12. Leukemia Inhibitory Factor (LIF): Can be purchased from different companies. We use LIF from Chemicon/Millipore (ESG1107; use at 10^3 U/mL final) or conditioned medium (CM) from an LIF-producing cell line.

13. DMEM-ES and IMDM-ES media. For 100 mL, combine 84 mL of DMEM or IMDM, 15 mL of FBS, pretested for maintenance of ES cells, 100 μL of a 0.15 M dilution of MTG (1.5×10^{-4} M final), and mouse recombinant LIF (10 ng/mL final) or CM tested to be used at an optimal concentration.

14. Gelatinized flasks and dishes: Gelatin coating is accomplished by covering the surface of a dish or flask (e.g., 2 mL for a well of a 6-well tissue culture plate, 12 mL for a T175 flask) with the gelatin solution for 20 min at room temperature. The gelatin is then aspirated, and the gelatin-coated plates can be stored at room temperature or 4°C for up to 2 weeks provided they remain sterile.

15. Recommended culture dishes: 6-well tissue culture plates (Falcon #353046) and 175 cm^2 flasks (Falcon #353028).

16. X-ray irradiator. Mouse embryonic fibroblasts (MEFs) are mitotically inactivated by irradiation at 3,000 rad with a X-ray or γ irradiator.

2.2. Generation of EBs

1. IMDM-FBS: For 100 mL combine 89.9 mL of IMDM, 10 mL of FBS pretested for ES cells differentiation, and 100 μL of a dilution of MTG at 0.15 M (1.5×10^{-4} M final).

2. Ascorbic acid: l-Ascorbic acid (Sigma #A-4544): Prepare a stock solution of 5 mg/mL in tissue culture grade water and

filter-sterilize. Aliquot and store at –20°C. Use aliquots once and discard.

3. Transferrin (Roche Diagnostics Limited #652-202): 30 mg/mL.

4. FBS pretested for ES cell differentiation (*see* **Note 4**): We currently use FBS from Harlan Sera-lab.

5. EB media with serum: For 10 mL combine 8.2 mL of IMDM, 100 μL of L-glutamine 2 mM, 60 μL of transferrin (180 μg/mL final), 30 μL of a dilution of MTG at 0.15 M (4.5×10^{-4} M final), 100 μL of ascorbic acid at 50 ng/mL, and 1.5 mL of FBS pretested for ES cell differentiation.

6. StemPro-34 Serum Free Media (Gibco #10639-011): Reconstitute according to the manufacturer's instruction (*see* **Note 5**).

7. EB serum-free media: For 10 mL combine 9.6 mL of StemPro-34 SFM, 100 μL of penicillin/streptomycin (50 U/mL final), 100 μL of L-glutamine (2 mM final), 60 μL of transferrin (180 μg/mL final), 100 μL of ascorbic acid at 50 ng/mL, 30 μL of a dilution of MTG at 0.15 M (4.5×10^{-4} M final), and 4 μL of BMP4 at 10 μg/mL (4 ng/mL final).

8. Protein-free hybridoma medium (PFHM-II) (Gibco #12040-093).

9. Recommended culture dishes for EB generation: 60- or 90-mm Petri dishes single vent (Sterilin #123) and (Sterilin #101R20).

10. Cytokines: We use the following from R&D Systems: Activin A: #338-AC, BMP4: #314-BP, VEGF: #293-VE, bFGF: #233-FB.

2.3. Assaying Hematopoietic Development During Embryoid Bodies Differentiation

1. Methylcellulose (VWR #9004-67-5) (500 g).

2. Methylcellulose stock solution (2.0%) (*see* **Note 6**): Weigh a sterile 2-L Erlenmeyer flask, add 450 mL of tissue culture grade water, and bring to boil on a hotplate. Add 20 g of methylcellulose powder, swirl, and bring to boil. Swirl the mixture to disperse the powder and prevent overflow, until the mixture is homogeneous, and then cool to room temperature. Prepare 500 mL of 2× IMDM by combining the IMDM powder for 1 L (Gibco 42200-014), 10 mL of L-glutamine (4 mM final), 10 mL penicillin/streptomycin (100 U/mL final), 2 mL of a 0.15 M dilution of MTG (3×10^{-4} M final), bring to 500 mL with tissue culture grade water, and filter-sterilize. When the methylcellulose solution has cooled to room temperature, add the 2× IMDM and swirl to mix. Weigh the flask and adjust the weight with sterile water to 1 L (1,000 g) of methylcellulose solution.

Transfer to 4°C, swirl the mixture every 15 min during the first hour, and leave overnight. The following day the cold methylcellulose is much more viscous and is aliquoted and frozen at –20°C before it can be used.

3. Endothelial cell growth supplement (ECGS) (R&D Systems #231-BC-025).

4. Cytokines: We use the following cytokines from R&D Systems or medium conditioned by cell lines producing some of these cytokines. R&D Systems G-CSF: #415-CS, TPO: #488-TO, GM-CSF: #415-ML, EPO: #287-TC, M-CSF: #416-ML, KL: #455-MC, IL-3: #403-ML, IL-6: #406-ML, IGF-1: #291-61, IL-11: #418-ML.

5. D4T endothelial cell conditioned medium: Medium conditioned by the embryonic endothelial cell line D4T is used together with vascular endothelial growth factor (VEGF) and IL-6 to support the growth of EB-derived hemangioblast colonies (7). D4T cells are grown on gelatinized flasks in IMDM with 10% FBS, 50 U/mL final penicillin/streptomycin, and 2 mM final L-glutamine. When the cells reach confluency, replace medium and add ECGS at 50 ng/mL. Allow the new medium to condition for 72 h. Conditioning can be repeated 4–5 times with the same cell population. The conditioned medium is pooled, filtered, and tested for its ability to stimulate EB-derived blast cell colonies in cultures containing VEGF and IL-6. Most batches of D4T-conditioned medium are used at 15–25%. Once tested, the conditioned medium should be aliquoted and stored frozen at –20°C.

6. Fetal bovine plasma-derived serum platelet poor (PDS) (Antech).

7. Methylcellulose for hemangioblast colony-forming assay: For 10 mL, combine 5.5 mL of methylcellulose stock (1.1% final, see **Note** 7), 1 mL of FBS pretested for ES cell differentiation (10% final), 0.1 mL of L-glutamine stock (2 mM final), 0.6 mL of transferrin stock (180 µg/mL final), 30 µL of a dilution of monothioglycerol at 0.15 M (4.5×10^{-4} M final), 0.5 mL of ascorbic acid stock (50 ng/mL final), 2 mL of D4T-conditioned medium (20% final), 10 µL of VEGF at 5 µg/mL (5 ng/mL final), and 20 µL of IL-6 at 5 µg/mL (10 ng/mL final). Bring to 10 mL with IMDM and mix thoroughly.

8. Methylcellulose for hematopoietic colony-forming assay (see **Note** 8): For 10 mL, combine 5.5 mL of methylcellulose stock (1.1% final), 1.5 mL of PDS (15% final), 1 mL of PFHM-II (10% final), 0.1 mL of L-glutamine stock (2 mM final), 0.6 mL of transferrin stock (180 µg/mL final), 30 µL of a dilution of MTG at 0.15 M (4.5×10^{-4} M final), 0.5 mL of ascorbic acid stock (50 ng/mL final), 0.1 mL of Kit

Ligand (KL) at 10 μg/mL (100 ng/mL final), 0.01 mL of IL-3 at 1 μg/mL (1 ng/mL final), 0.03 mL of G-CSF at 10 μg/mL (30 ng/mL final), 0.01 mL of IL-11 at 5 μg/mL (5 ng/mL final), 0.02 mL of erythropoietin at 2,000 U/mL (4 U/mL final), 0.02 mL of IL-6 at 5 μg/mL (10 ng/mL final), 0.01 mL of TPO at 5 μg/mL (5 ng/mL final), and 0.01 mL of M-CSF at 10 μg/mL (10 ng/mL final). Bring to 10 mL with IMDM and mix thoroughly.

9. Recommended culture dishes: 35-mm Petri dish (Falcon #1008).

10. Blunt-end needles: Becton Dickinson #300149.

11. Gene expression analysis. RNeasy Plus Micro Kit (50) (Qiagen #74034), Omniscript RT Kit (Qiagen #205111), Random primers (Roche #1034731), GoTaq mastermix (Promega #M7112).

12. Polymerase chain reaction (PCR) primers:

REX1   5′CCGCATCGCTGTGGGCATTAGA3′   and 5′GGGCCGCCTGCAAGTAATGAGC3′

FGF5 5′FGTGTCTCAGGGGATTGTAGGAATACG3′ and 5′GTGAAGGAAAGTTCCGGTTGC 3′

BRACHYURY   5′CCACCACGGCTGTATTTATG   3′ and5′GGTCACAATCATCTCGTTAGTTAGC 3′

FLK-1   5′CACCTGGCACTCTCCACCTTC3′   and 5′GATTTCATCCCACTACCGAAAG3′

SCL/TAL-1   5′ATGGAGATTTCTGATGGTCCTCAC 3′ and 5′AAGTGTGCTTGGGTGTTGGCTC 3′ AML1/ RUNX1   5′CCAGCAAGCTGAGGAGCGGCG   and 5′CGGATTTGTAAAGACGGTGA 3′

GATA1 5′CATTGGCCCCTTGTGAGGCCAGAGA 3′ and 5′ACCTGATGGAGCTTGAAATAGAGGC 3′

βH1 GLOBIN 5′AGTCCCCATGGAGTCAAAGA 3′ and 5′CTCAAGGAGACCTTTGCTCA 3′

βACTIN   5′ATGAAGATCCTGACCGAGCG   3′   and 5′TACTTGCGCTCAGGAGGAGC 3′

3. Methods

3.1. Growth and Maintenance of ES Cells and Preparation of ES Cells for In Vitro Differentiation

ES cells are maintained on gelatin-coated plates containing irradiated primary MEFs. The MEFs provide an additional substrate compared to gelatin for the ES cells to grow on and secrete factors necessary for the ES cells to maintain their pluripotency. The combination of gelatin and MEFs is widely considered to be the best culture condition to preserve the potential of ES cells to contribute to the germ line following injection into host blastocysts. ES cells should be passaged before they reach confluence and prior to acidification of the media. In general, ES cells require passaging every other day. Passaging at too high a density promotes differentiation, whereas passaging at too low a density is detrimental to the growth of the cells. The absolute number of cells to be split varies according to each ES cell line but a density between 1×10^5 and 4×10^5 cells per well of a 6-well tissue culture plate (surface of 9.5 cm²) is generally appropriate. ES cells should not be kept for long times (more than 3 weeks) in cultures. It is critical that ES cells are well maintained to retain their ability to differentiate in vitro. We provide below the basic protocols for the culture of ES cells and preparation of irradiated primary MEFs.

3.1.1. Preparation of Primary Embryonic Fibroblasts (See Note 9)

1. Prepare mice timed matings. At 14.5 days post coitus, sacrifice the pregnant females and douse with 70% ethanol for the removal of the embryos under aseptic conditions.

2. Dissect the uterine horns containing the embryos from the animal and wash in sterile PBS. Remove the individual embryos and place them on a sterile Petri dish. Remove the heads and embryonic organs. Wash three times in PBS.

3. Using two large scalpel blades reduce the tissues into a fine slurry in TrypLE express (around 2 mL per embryo). Transfer to a sterile tube and incubate for 5–10 min at 37°C, with inversion every 2 min.

4. After 5–10 min remove the cell suspension from above the tissue slurry.

5. Add 2 mL of the trypsinized tissue (one embryo/flask) to a 175-cm² flask (containing 25 mL DMEM–FBS) and incubate overnight at 37°C, 5% CO_2. The next day change the medium without removing the attached material if possible.

6. When confluent, trypsinize with 10 mL of TrypLE express and freeze the cells at 2×10^6 cells/mL. Freeze as passage 0 (P0) slowly at –80°C and then transfer to liquid nitrogen. The freezing medium is 10% DMSO, 40% FBS, and 50% DMEM.

7. To prepare irradiated feeder cells, thaw one vial of frozen P0 cells in a T175 flask. When confluent, split into twenty T175 flasks (*see* **Note 10**). When confluence is again reached, harvest the cells by trypsinization and irradiate at 3,000 rad (*see* **Note 11**).

8. Freeze the irradiated MEFs at 10^6 cells/mL per vial in the freezing medium (10% DMSO, 40% FBS, 50% DMEM). The 20 flasks should generate between 70 and 100 vials. Freeze

Color Plates

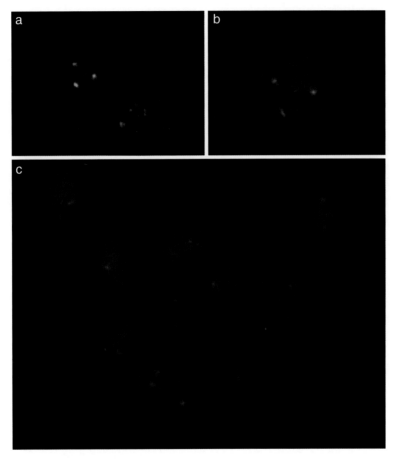

Chapter 12, Fig. 4. Example of FISH analysis of human AML blasts recovered from NOD/SCID mice 12 weeks post-transplant. Dual fusion, dual fluorescent in situ hybridization of a t(8, 21) (AML/ETO) AML-M2 sample. In (**a**), the cell on the left is positive for the rearrangement and exhibits 1 *green*, 1 *red*, and 2 *orange spots* whereas the cell on the right is an example of an inconclusive result and as such is excluded from counts. An example of a cell that is positive for the rearrangement but the resolution of the microscope is sufficient to resolve the co-localised dots as separate *red* and *green dots* rather than a composite *yellow dot* (**b**). A lower power image showing a complete field of view, in which the majority of cells are positive for the t[8,21] rearrangement (**c**).

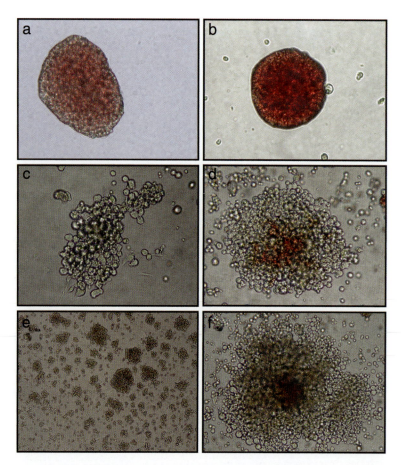

Chapter 16, Fig. 3. Pictures of representative primitive and definitive colonies. Primitive erythroid (ERY/P) colonies are tight and bright red (**a**, **b**). Macrophage colonies contain big granular cells (**c**), whereas bipotential macrophage/erythroid colonies contain erythroid red cells in addition to macrophages (**d**). Mast cell colonies are loose and are composed of small, round, highly refringent cells (**e**), whereas mix colonies are composed of erythroid cells and cells from at least two other myeloid lineages (**f**). Original magnification ×100.

slowly at −80°C. A vial of 10^6 irradiated MEFs should provide enough cells to cover a complete 6-well plate (57 cm^2).

3.1.2. Preparation of Gelatin-Coated Plates with Irradiated MEFs

1. Dispense 2 mL of gelatin per well of a 6-well tissue culture plate. Gently swirl to ensure that the surface of each well is completely coated.

2. Incubate for at least 20 min at room temperature.

3. Aspirate the gelatin solution.

4. Thaw the irradiated MEFs and plate in DMEM-ES cells on the gelatinized wells. Culture in a humidified incubator at 37°C and 5% CO_2.

3.1.3. Thawing ES Cells

Remove vial from liquid nitrogen and thaw rapidly by immersing in a 37°C water bath.

1. Transfer the cells to a 15-mL tube containing 10 mL of warmed DMEM-ES media.

2. Centrifuge at 1,200 rpm (300g) for 5 min.

3. Resuspend the pellet in 2 mL of DMEM-ES and transfer to a well containing gelatin and irradiated MEFs. Culture in a humidified incubator at 37°C and 5% CO_2.

4. Tiny clusters of adherent cells corresponding to the start of ES cell colonies should be visible the following day. If dead cells are present, remove the media and replace with 2 mL of fresh DMEM-ES.

3.1.4. Freezing ES Cells

1. Aspirate the medium from the wells containing ES cells at 50–70% confluence. One half-confluent well should yield between 1 and 2×10^6 cells.

2. Add 1.5 mL of warmed TrypLE express per well and incubate for 3 min in an incubator at 37°C. When observed under a microscope, the ES colonies should have detached from the plate, and single cells should be clearly visible. If not, incubate for one additional minute at 37°C.

3. Complete the dissociation by pipetting, add 3 mL of DMEM-ES media, and transfer into a 15-mL tube. An aliquot of the cells is counted. Ideally the cells should be frozen at a concentration between 1×10^6 and 3×10^6 cells/mL. The presence of a few MEFs is not detrimental.

4. Centrifuge for 5 min at 1,200 rpm (300g). Prepare labeled cryovials.

5. Resuspend the pellet in an appropriate volume of cold freezing medium (10% DMSO, 40% heat-inactivated FBS, 50% DMEM-ES). Dispense 1 mL per labeled cryovials, place in a freezing chamber that lowers the temperature slowly, and

store at –80°C overnight. If a freezing chamber is not available, cells can be placed in well-insulated polystyrene box.

6. Transfer to liquid nitrogen for long-term storage.

3.1.5. Splitting ES Cells

1. Aspirate the medium from 50–70% confluent ES cells.

2. Add 1.5 mL of warmed TrypLE express per well, and incubate for 3 min in an incubator at 37°C.

3. Dissociate homogeneously the cells by repeated pipetting, add 3 mL of DMEM-ES media, and transfer into a 15-mL tube. It is essential to have a good single-cell suspension.

4. Centrifuge for 5 min at 1,200 rpm (300g).

5. Resuspend the cells in DMEM-ES and dispense at the chosen dilution (in general between 1×10^5 and 4×10^5 cells per well) onto new gelatinized wells with MEFs. Gently disperse the cells by moving the plate back and forth; never swirl in a circular manner as this will cause the cells to accumulate in the middle on the wells.

3.1.6. Preparation of ES Cells for In Vitro Differentiation

Prior to differentiation, ES cells must be passaged two times at 24-h intervals on gelatin-coated plates to remove the MEF cells which may affect the efficient differentiation of the ES cells. The second passage is done in IMDM-ES media to promote a better hematopoietic differentiation. The number of cells to be passaged depends on the ES cell line, and several dilutions should be tested. The ES cells should be passaged at relatively high density to avoid spontaneous differentiation and should retain typical ES cell colony morphology.

1. When the ES cells grown on MEFs are 50–80% confluent, trypsinize with TrypLE express. The incubation time of the cells with TrypLE can be reduced to 2 min at 37°C to reduce the carry-over of MEFs which are less prone than ES cells to a quick release by trypsinization.

2. Plate the cells in DMEM-ES media at several dilutions on gelatin-coated wells of a 6-well plate. Absolute number of cells to be split varies between each ES cell line; for example, for E14-based ES cell lines a density of 3×10^5 cells per gelatin-coated well is generally appropriate.

3. The following day, passage again the ES cells and plate them in IMDM-ES media at various dilutions in each gelatin-coated well. For E14-based ES cell lines a density of 2×10^5 cells per gelatin-coated well is appropriate.

3.2. Generation of EBs

EBs are generated by culturing ES cells in the absence of LIF and MEFs. Petri-grade dishes should be used to avoid adherence of the EBs, and several batches/brands should be tested to select the ones with the least adhesiveness for the developing EBs. The number of input ES cells should be determined for each ES cell line, as each one generates EBs at a different efficiency. The numbers of input cells per milliliter will vary also as a function of the number of days of culture necessary to reach the stage of hematopoietic development to be evaluated. Similarly, the components of the EB culture will vary depending on the stages of hematopoietic development to be reached. We describe below a method to generate embryoid bodies in presence of serum, and a new protocol to generate EBs in serum-free condition *(11)*. This latter method does not require the availability of a pretested serum supporting EB development, and is extremely robust and easily amenable to different ES cell lines.

3.2.1. Harvesting ES Cells

Choose wells containing ES cells with the best morphology and density. ES cells are harvested by trypsinization and washed two times in IMDM-FBS to remove all traces of LIF.

3.2.2. Generation of EBs

Generation of EBs in Presence of Serum

1. ES cells resuspended in IMDM-FBS are counted.

2. Dispense the cells in EB media with serum at the adequate density. For the E14 ES cell line, prepare media with 30,000 cells/mL for differentiation until day 3.5, and with 10,000 cells/mL for cultures until day 6–7 of differentiation. For EBs generated to test the development of primitive and definitive hematopoietic precursors (day 4–9), the cultures are supplemented with 5% PFHM-II.

3. Distribute in 60-mm (5 mL cultures) or 90-mm (10 mL cultures) Petri dishes and place in an incubator at 37°C, 5% CO_2.

4. EB culture maintained for more than 7 days should be supplemented at day 7 with IL-3 (1 ng/mL final), IL-11 (25 ng/mL final), and Kit Ligand/Stem Cell Factor (KL/SCF, 100 ng/mL).

Generation of EBs in Serum Free Conditions

1. Resuspend the cells at 25,000 cells/mL of EB serum-free media.

2. Distribute in 60-mm (5 mL cultures) or 90-mm (10 mL cultures) Petri dishes and place in an incubator at 37°C, 5% CO_2.

3. At day 2.5, supplement the cultures with basic fibroblast growth factor (bFGF) (5 ng/mL final) and Activin A (5 ng/mL final) to induce the development of hemangioblast progenitors. Alternatively, supplement the cultures at day 2.5 with bFGF (5 ng/mL final), Activin A (5 ng/mL final), and VEGF (5 ng/mL final) to induce and support the development of primitive and definitive hematopoietic precursors.

3.3. Assaying Hematopoietic Development During Embryoid Body Differentiation

Standard colony-forming cell assays are used for quantitative assessment of hematopoietic precursor development. EB-derived cells are cultured in a methylcellulose-containing medium supplemented with hematopoietic cytokines. Precursor numbers and developmental potential are determined from the number and type of hematopoietic colonies that develop.

3.3.1. Harvesting EBs (See Note 2)

1. Transfer EB cultures to 50-mL conical tubes and centrifuge for 5 min at 1,200 rpm ($300g$).
2. Discard supernatant, add 3 mL of warmed TrypLE express, and incubate 3 min in a 37°C waterbath with occasional mixing.
3. Add 7 mL of IMDM-FBS, centrifuge for 5 min at 1,200 rpm ($300g$), and resuspend in IMDM-FBS for counting. Bring to a concentration of 10^6 cells/mL and keep on ice until distribution to methylcellulose cultures. Cells should be >95% viable after this treatment.

3.3.2. Hemangioblast Methylcellulose Colony-Forming Assay

These bipotential progenitors are transiently present in EBs between day 2.5 and 4 of differentiation. They form typical blast colonies after 3–4 days of incubation at 37°C in presence of VEGF, IL-6, and D4T-conditioned medium. These blast colonies contain loose cells and are easily distinguished from the more compact vascular colonies or secondary EBs (**Fig. 2**).

1. Add between 2×10^4 and 10^5 cells from day 2.5 to 4 EBs per milliliter of hemangioblast methylcellulose colony-forming media. The EB cells are assayed in triplicate dishes of 1 mL.

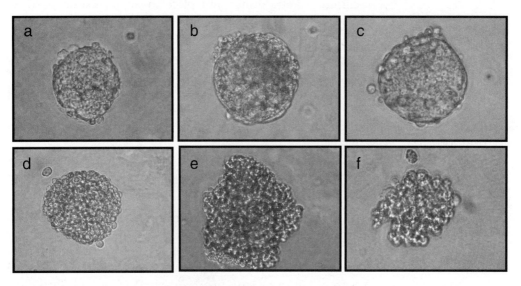

Fig. 2. Pictures of representative secondary embryoid bodies (EBs) and blast colonies. Secondary EBs (**a–c**) are generated from the remaining ES cells in the cultures and are large and smooth. In contrast, blast colonies (**d–f**) are characterized by well-defined individual cells in the colony. Original magnification ×100.

Prepare a volume in excess (at least 3.5 mL), as it is impossible to recover all the methylcellulose solution from the tube. The added volume of cells should not exceed 10% of the final volume.

2. Incubate 5 min in a 37°C waterbath to loosen up the methylcellulose, vortex vigorously to mix, and allow the air bubbles to dissipate before dispensing.

3. Aspirate in a syringe using an 18G blunt-end needle and aliquot as 1 mL culture in 35-mm Petri dishes. Culture in a humidified incubator at 37°C and 5% CO_2 (*see* **Note 13**).

4. After 3–4 days, count the number of blast colonies per dish under a microscope (*see* **Note 14**).

3.3.3. Hematopoietic Methylcellulose Colony-Forming Assay

Primitive erythroid precursors develop within EBs shortly after the hemangioblast, and their number increases dramatically over the next 2–3 days. They produce small, tight, bright red colonies, which are better scored 4–5 days after replating in methylcellulose (**Fig. 3**). The identity of primitive erythroid colonies can be confirmed by demonstrating the expression of the βH1 globin, specific to primitive erythrocytes, and the observation of cells with a large nucleated morphology following May–Grunwald/Giemsa staining. All the hematopoietic precursors other than primitive erythroid are defined as definitive hematopoietic progenitors. Precursors of the macrophage lineage develop shortly after the onset of primitive erythropoiesis. Bipotent (macrophage/erythrocytes, megakaryocyte/erythrocytes) and multipotent precursors are found in day 4–9 EBs. Restricted neutrophil, megakaryocyte, definitive erythroid, and mast cell precursors are mostly generated later (from day 7) in EBs. Definitive erythroid colonies are distinguished from primitive erythroid colonies by the fact that they are less red and more brownish, contain small cells, are often larger, and do not express βH1 globin. Colonies with red erythroid cells and at least two other myeloid lineage cells are scored as mix colonies. A typical count of primitive erythroid, macrophage and mix colonies generated by day 5 Runx1[+/+], Runx1[+/−], and Runx1[−/−] EBs is shown in **Fig. 4**.

1. Add between 2×10^4 and 10^5 cells for day 4 to day 8 EBs per milliliter of hematopoietic methylcellulose colony-forming media. The EB cells are assayed in triplicate dishes of 1 mL. Prepare a volume in excess (at least 3.5 mL), as it is impossible to recover all the methylcellulose solution from the tube. The added volume of cells should not exceed 10% of the final volume.

2. Incubate for 5 min in a 37°C waterbath to loosen up the methylcellulose, vortex vigorously to mix, and allow the air bubbles to dissipate before dispensing.

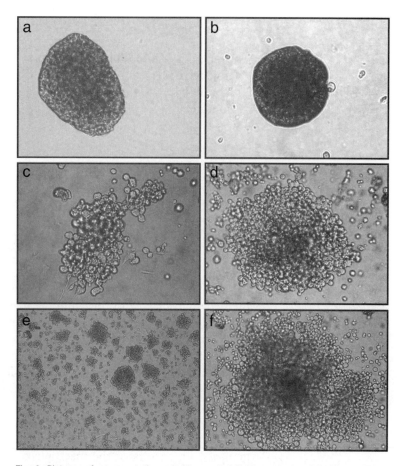

Fig. 3. Pictures of representative primitive and definitive colonies. Primitive erythroid (ERY/P) colonies are tight and bright red (**a**, **b**). Macrophage colonies contain big granular cells (**c**), whereas bipotential macrophage/erythroid colonies contain erythroid red cells in addition to macrophages (**d**). Mast cell colonies are loose and are composed of small, round, highly refringent cells (**e**), whereas mix colonies are composed of erythroid cells and cells from at least two other myeloid lineages (**f**). Original magnification ×100. (*see* Color Plates)

Colonies per 10^5 day 5 EB cells

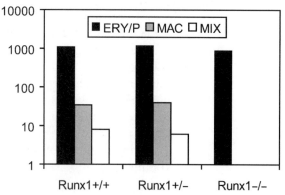

Fig. 4. Myeloid and erythroid potential of *Runx1*[+/+], *Runx1*[+/−], and *Runx1*[−/−] ES cells. 10^5 EB cells of day 5 were replated in hematopoietic methylcellulose colony-forming assay. Primitive erythroid (ERY/P), macrophage (MAC), and multilineage (MIX) colonies were scored after 7 days.

3. Aspirate in a syringe using an 18G blunt-end needle and aliquot as 1 mL culture in 35-mm Petri dishes. Culture in a humidified incubator at 37°C and 5% CO_2.

4. Primitive erythroid colonies are mature after 5 days, whereas most definitive colonies are easier to score after 7–10 days of culture.

3.3.4. Gene Expression Analysis

The development of the hematopoietic system upon in vitro ES cell differentiation can be also followed and evaluated by gene expression analysis. As shown in **Fig. 5**, when ES cells are differentiated in serum-free conditions, the expression of the stem cell marker *Rex1* is rapidly downregulated during differentiation. Expression of *FGF5* between day 1 and 3 and expression of *Brachyury* between day 2 and 4 are indicative of the successive commitment to epiblast and mesodermal fate, respectively. *Flk-1* expression marks the onset of endothelial and hematopoietic development. The expression of the transcription factors *Scl/Tal-1* and *AML1/Runx1*, frequently found translocated in leukemia, indicates the generation of the first hematopoietic precursors. This is further confirmed by the subsequent detection of the expression of the transcription factor *Gata1*, predominantly expressed in erythroid cells, and of *βH1 globin*, expressed specifically in primitive erythroid cells. The gene expression analysis is complementary to the replating assays in methylcellulose to detect and characterize any alterations of hematopoietic development induced following sustained expression or knock down of a candidate regulator of early hematopoietic development.

1. Harvest between 5×10^5 and 10×10^5 cells each day of EB development. Pelletize the cells in an RNAse-free Eppendorf tube by centrifugation (5 min at 400*g*), aspirate the supernatant, and freeze the pellet at –80°C.

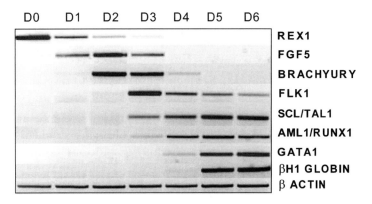

Fig. 5. Pattern of gene expression observed upon 6-day in vitro differentiation of wild-type ES cells.

2. Extract total RNA from each sample with an Rneasy plus mini kit following the manufacturer's instructions. Quantify the amount of RNA obtained.

3. Reverse-transcribe 2 µg into cDNA with random hexamer using an Omniscript reverse transcriptase (RT) kit.

4. Perform PCR using GoTaq and 0.2 µM of each primer. Cycle conditions are as follows: 94°C for 5 min followed by 30 cycles of amplification (94°C denaturation for 30 s, 60°C annealing for 30 s, 72°C elongation for 60 s) with a final incubation at 72°C for 10 min. The PCR products are normalized for β-actin expression.

4. Notes

1. ES cells are extremely sensitive to traces of detergent. To avoid the potential presence of remaining detergent on glassware after washing, all tissue culture media and reagents should be prepared and stored in plastic bottles and tubes.

2. MTG is extremely thick, so the 26 µL should be pipetted slowly to ensure that the whole volume is aspirated in the tip.

3. To select a FBS serum for ES cells, passage the ES cells five times in the different test lots and monitor the cultures for cell viability, growth, and maintenance of undifferentiated morphology.

4. The FBS optimal for ES cell differentiation is likely to be different from the one selected for ES cell maintenance. Several batches of FBS should be tested for their potential to support the development of embryoid bodies and the generation of hematopoietic precursors in these EBs. Alternatively, generation of EBs in serum-free conditions alleviate the need of selection of an appropriate serum for EB development.

5. Once reconstituted, store at +4°C in the dark.

6. Already prepared methylcellulose stock solutions are commercially available from several manufacturers such as R&D Systems or Stem Cell Technologies Inc.

7. Syringes must be used to dispense methylcellulose solution, as the viscosity makes pipetting impossible.

8. This methylcellulose solution supports the growth of a broad range of myeloid and erythroid precursors. Ready-made methylcellulose solutions containing cocktails of cytokines supporting the development of a broad range or subset of hematopoietic precursors are also commercially available from Stem Cell Technologies Inc.

9. Frozen stocks of early passage primary embryonic fibroblasts (MEFs) are commercially available from several companies such as Stem Cell Technologies Inc., Globalstem, or Open Biosystems. Irradiated MEFs are available from R&D Systems or Globalstem.

10. The growth of MEFs is more efficient in low oxygen conditions. We culture MEFs in a humidified incubator at 37°C, 5% CO_2 and 5% O_2.

11. As an alternative to irradiation, MEFs can be mitotically inactivated by treatment with mitomycin C. The cells in the 20 near-confluent T175 flasks are then incubated for 3 h in presence of mitomycin C at 10 μg/mL and washed three times with PBS before harvesting and freezing (**Subheading 3.1.1, step 8**).

12. For EBs that are more than 8 days old, collagenase instead of TrypLE express should be used to obtain a single-cell suspension. Resuspend pelletized EBs in a solution of collagenase (2.5 mg/mL, Sigma #C0310), DNAse (10 mg/mL, Merck#260912), and 20% FBS in PBS and incubate at 37°C for 1–2 h. The suspension should be vortexed every 30 min. Disrupt EBs by passing three times through a 21G needle on a 5-mL syringe.

13. To avoid drying of the methylcellulose media, the dishes are placed in a large Petri dish with an open 35-mm dish containing 3 mL of water.

14. Blast colonies are easier to recognize and score if the dishes are brought to room temperature 30 min before scoring.

Acknowledgments

This work was supported by Cancer Research UK.

References

1. Doetschman T.C., Eistetter H., Katz M., Schmidt W., Kemler R. (1985). The *in vitro* development of blastocyst-derived embryonic stem cell lines: formation of visceral yolk sac, blood islands and myocardium. *J Embryol Exp Morphol* **87**, 27–45.

2. Wiles M., Keller G. (1991). Multiple hematopoietic lineages develop from embryonic stem (ES) cells in culture. *Development* **111**, 259–267.

3. Schmitt R., Bruyns E., Snodgrass H. (1991). Hematopoietic development of embryonic stem cells *in vitro*: cytokine and receptor gene expression. *Genes Dev* **5**, 728–740.

4. Burkert U., von Ruden T., Wagner E.F. (1991). Early fetal haematopoietic development from *in vitro* differentiated embryonic stem cells. *New Biol* **3**, 698–708.

5. Keller G., Kennedy M., Papayannopoulou T., Wiles M. (1993). Hematopoietic commitment

during embryonic stem cell differentiation in culture. *Mol Cell Biol* **13**, 473–486.

6. Nakano T., Kodama H., Honjo T. (1994). Generation of lymphohematopoietic cells from embryonic stem cells in culture. *Science* **265**, 1098–1101.

7. Keller G. (1995). *In vitro* differentiation of embryonic stem cells. *Curr Opin Cell Biol* **7**, 862–869.

8. Kennedy M., Firpo M., Choi K., Wall C., Robertson S., Kabrun N., Keller G. (1997). A common precursor for primitive erythropoiesis and definitive haematopoiesis. *Nature* **386**, 488–493.

9. Kabrun N., Buhring H.J., Choi K., Ullrich A., Risau W., Keller G. (1997). Flk-1 expression defines a population of early embryonic hematopoietic precursors. *Development* **124**, 2039–2048.

10. Choi K., Kennedy M., Kazarov A., Papadimitriou J.C., Keller G. (1998). A common precursor for hematopoietic and endothelial cells. *Development* **125**, 725–732.

11. Nishikawa S.I., Nishikawa S., Hirashima M., Matsuyoshi N., Kodama H. (1998). Progressive lineage analysis by cell sorting and culture identifies FLK1+ VE-cadherin+ cells at a diverging point of endothelial and hemopoietic lineages. *Development* **125**, 1747–1757.

12. Fehling H.J., Lacaud G., Kubo A., Kennedy M., Robertson S., Keller G., Kouskoff V. (2003). Tracking mesoderm induction and its specification to the hemangioblast during embryonic stem cell differentiation. *Development* **130**, 4217–4227.

13. Lacaud G., Keller G., Kouskoff V. (2004). Tracking mesoderm formation and specification to the hemangioblast *in vitro*. *Trends Cardiovasc Med* **14**, 314–317.

14. Russel E. (1979). Hereditary anemias of the mouse: a review for geneticists. *Adv Genet* **20**, 357–459.

15. Moore M., Metcalf D. (1970). Ontogeny of the hematopoietic system: yolk sac origin of in vivo and in vitro colony forming cells in the developing mouse embryo. *Br J Hematol* **18**, 279–296.

16. Haar J.L., Ackerman G.A. (1971). Ultrastructural changes in mouse yolk sac associated with the initiation of vitelline circulation. *Anat Rec* **170**, 437–456.

17. Sabin F.R. (1920). Studies on the origin of blood vessels and of red corpuscles as seen in the living blastoderm of the chick during the second day of incubation. *Contrib Embryol* **9**, 213–262.

18. Murray P.D.F. (1932). The development in vitro of the blood of the early chick embryo. *Proc R Soc London* **11**, 497–521.

19. Lacaud G., Gore L., Kennedy M., Kouskoff V., Kingsley P., Hogan C., Carlsson L., Speck N., Palis J., Keller G. (2002). Runx1 is essential for hematopoietic commitment at the hemangioblast stage of development *in vitro*. *Blood* **100**, 458–466.

20. Lacaud G., Kouskoff V., Trumble A., Schwantz S., Keller G. (2004). Haploinsufficiency of Runx1 results in the acceleration of mesodermal development and hemangioblast specification upon *in vitro* differentiation of ES cells. *Blood* **103**, 886–889.

21. Lacaud G., Robertson S., Palis J., Kennedy M., Keller G. (2001). Regulation of hemangioblast development. *Ann N Y Acad Sci* **938**, 96–107.

22. Pearson S., Sroczynska P., Lacaud G., Kouskoff V. (2008). The step-wise specification of embryonic stem cells to hematopoietic fate is driven by sequential exposure to BMP4, Activin A, FGF and VEGF. *Development* **135**, 1525–1535.

Chapter 17

Analysis of the Mouse Placenta as a Hematopoietic Stem Cell Niche

Katrin Ottersbach and Elaine Dzierzak

Summary

Hematopoietic stem cells are at the foundation of the blood system. Their study is not only relevant to the understanding of the basic cellular mechanisms of self-renewal, lineage commitment, and differentiation, but they have also been the target of intense clinical research into the causes of leukemia and the exploitation of these cells for cell replacement therapies. The basic mechanisms of hematopoietic stem cell regulation become evident in the way these cells are first generated and expanded during development. Isolating and analyzing hematopoietic stem cells from the embryo is therefore of direct clinical importance.

Key words: Placenta, Hematopoietic stem cells, Embryo, Transplantation, Flow cytometry

1. Introduction

The murine midgestation placenta has recently been identified as an additional rich source for hematopoietic stem cells (HSCs) during embryo development *(1, 2)*. Although it is currently unknown whether the placenta can generate HSCs de novo, it was demonstrated that it can very efficiently expand these rare cells *in vivo*. Therefore, identifying the molecular mechanisms underlying this expansion capacity will deliver new strategies for the *ex vivo* expansion of HSCs for cell replacement therapies.

Studying HSCs in the placenta may also be relevant to leukemia etiology, as there is growing evidence that links the occurrence of acute infant leukemia to transplacental chemical agents

C.W.E. So (ed.), Leukemia, *Methods in Molecular Biology, vol. 538*
© Humana Press, a part of Springer Science + Business Media, LLC 2009
DOI: 10.1007/978-1-59745-418-6_17

(reviewed in *(3)*). It could therefore be argued that placental HSCs present the initial target for these transforming agents. In fact, infantile hemangioma was recently shown to be of placental origin *(4)*.

The isolation and analysis of HSCs from other embryonic tissues have already been described in detail *(5, 6)*. As the placenta is substantially larger and contains a different cellular composition than other hemogenic tissues in the embryo, many techniques had to be adapted to allow analysis of this challenging tissue. These techniques are described in detail in the following sub-headings.

2. Materials

2.1. Isolation and Dissection of Placentas

1. Dissection tools: Watchmaker Precision Forceps (no. 5 and no. 5/45°), 1-ml insulin needles (BD, Cat. No. U-100).
2. Dissection microscope.
3. 60-mm plastic tissue culture plates.
4. Dissection medium: Phosphate-buffered saline (PBS; without calcium and magnesium) with 10% fetal calf serum (*see* **Note 1**), penicillin (100 U/ml), and streptomycin (100 µg/ml).

2.2. Organ Explant Culture

1. 0.65-µm DV Durapore membrane filters (Millipore) are washed at least five times with boiling tissue culture water (Sigma, Cat. No. W3500) and dried on a nylon membrane in a tissue culture hood.
2. Stainless-steel mesh supports: Stainless-steel wire mesh is bent to produce a 12×12 mm^2 supportive platform that stands 5 mm high. Grids are passivated by soaking them in nitric acid (HNO_3) overnight and then washed five times with autoclaved MilliQ water. They are then sterilized in 70% ethanol, washed twice with tissue culture water, and dried in a tissue culture hood.
3. 6-well tissue culture plates.
4. Myeloid long-term culture (M-LTC) medium (StemCell Technologies, Cat. No. M5300).
5. Hydrocortisone succinate (Sigma, Cat. No. H-2270; final concentration 10^{-6} M).

2.3. Preparation of Single-Cell Suspensions

1. Type I Collagenase (Sigma, Cat. No. C0130): Prepare a 2.5% stock in PBS, filter using a 0.45-µm filter, and store at −20°C in aliquots. Use at 1:20 in dissection medium (*see* **Note 1**).
2. 14-ml round-bottom plastic tubes.

2.4. Enrichment for HSCs by Ficoll Gradients

1. 40 μm Cell strainers (BD, Cat. No. 352340).
2. Lymphoprep™ (Axis-shield).
3. 50-ml plastic tubes.

2.5. Cell Staining for Flow Cytometry and Cell Sorting

1. 5-ml round-bottom tubes.
2. 5-ml round-bottom tubes with cell strainer cap (BD Falcon, Cat. No. 352235).
3. 7-Aminoactinomycin D (stock: 1 mg/ml in PBS; 7AAD; molecular probes).
4. Hoechst 33258 (stock: 0.1 mg/ml in water; Molecular Probes).
5. Fluorescent-labeled antibodies suitable for flow cytometry, e.g., anti-CD31-PE (clone MEC 13.3), anti-Ter119-PE (clone TER-119), anti-CD45-PE (clone 30-F11), anti-CD34-PE (clone RAM34), anti-c-kit-PE (clone 2B8), anti-c-kit-APC (clone 2B8), and anti-CD41-PE (clone MwReg30) all from BD Biosciences Pharmingen (*see* **Note 2**).

2.6. Transplantation

1. Recipient mice of the same strain as the donor mice.
2. Gamma radiation source.
3. Hydrochloric acid (0.037% in sterile water).
4. Neomycin sulfate (Sigma, Cat. No. N1876; 0.16% in sterile water).
5. 1-ml injection syringes.
6. Needles for injection (25G × 5/8″).
7. Heating lamp.
8. Mouse restraining apparatus.

2.7. Genomic DNA Extraction and Analysis by PCR

1. 1.5-ml Safe-lock Eppendorf tubes.
2. Blood Mix (*see* **Note 3**): 0.05 M Tris–HCl, pH 7.8, 0.1 M EDTA, 0.1 M NaCl, 1% SDS, 0.2 mg/ml proteinase K.
3. RNase A: 10 mg/ml stock solution.
4. Phenol:chloroform:isoamyl alcohol (25:24:1, v/v).
5. 2 M Sodium acetate, pH 5.6.
6. Isopropanol.
7. 70% Ethanol.
8. Primers specific to the donor genetic marker.

2.8. Multilineage Analysis

Lineage-specific antibodies: B220-FITC (clone RA3-6B2), Ly6C-FITC (clone AL-21), CD4-PE (clone GK1.5), CD8a-PE (clone 53-6.7), CD31-PE (clone MEC 13.3), anti-Gr-1-PE (clone RB6-8C5), and anti-Mac1-PE (clone M1/70) all from BD Biosciences Pharmingen (*see* **Note 4**).

3. Methods

3.1. Isolation and Dissection of Placentas

1. Formation of the placenta initiates at embryonic day (E) 8.5 with the fusion of the allantois with the chorion, and functional placentas can be isolated starting from E9 (reviewed in *(7)*). To obtain embryos from different stages, timed matings are set up between male and female adult mice in the late afternoon and the female checked for a vaginal plug the following morning. The morning of vaginal plug detection is considered E0. For the analysis of placental HSCs in transplantation assays, it is especially important that the genetic marker that is used to detect donor cell contribution in the recipient is transmitted through the male line. Therefore, to avoid contribution from maternal blood cells present in the placenta, wild-type females should be used for the timed matings.

2. Pregnant females are sacrificed on the chosen day of development and their uteri removed into a 60-mm dish containing dissection medium.

3. Embryos inside the yolk sac and with the placenta attached are taken out of the uterus, using a dissection microscope and two pairs of watchmaker precision forceps to open up the muscular wall of the uterus.

4. The embryo inside the yolk sac can then be separated from the placenta by inserting the two pairs of forceps between the two and forcing them apart. Alternatively, the yolk sac can be opened up, the embryo removed, and the yolk sac then separated from the placenta by grasping it in a tight bundle near the point where it is attached to the placenta and by pulling it away. In either case, care should be taken that the chorionic plate is not peeled away with the yolk sac and that all of the yolk sac tissue and the umbilical vessels are removed, as these are known to also contain HSCs *(8, 9)*.

5. At this point, the placenta still has the maternal decidua attached. Although embryonic cells of the trophoblastic lineage are known to invade the decidua (reviewed in *(10)*), the majority of the cells are maternally derived. Embryo-derived HSCs are not detected in the decidua. The decidua should therefore be removed. At the edge of the placenta, the embryonic part can easily be distinguished from the maternal decidua, as it is vascularized and therefore redder in appearance than the white tissue of the decidua (*see* **Note 5**). Using the two pairs of forceps and working one's way around the edge of the placenta, the two parts can be separated and the embryonic part peeled away in one piece. Dissection needles are then used to trim the edge of the placenta (*see* **Fig. 1**).

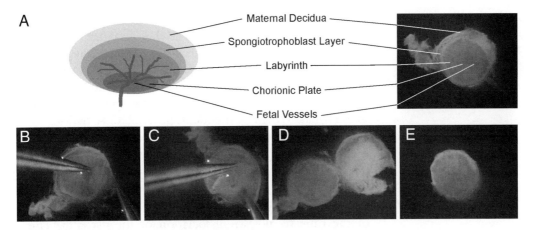

Fig. 1. Dissection of an E12 mouse placenta. (**A**) Schematic diagram and photograph of an E12 mouse placenta explaining the different components. (**B–E**) The dissection of an E12 placenta. After the removal of the embryo and the yolk sac, the maternal decidua and the fetal part of the placenta are pulled apart, starting from the edge of the placenta (**B**, **C**). (**D**) The separated placenta (*left*) and the decidua (*right*). The edges of the placenta are then trimmed (**E**).

3.2. Organ Explant Culture

1. Unlike what has been observed for HSCs from the aorta-gonad-mesonephros region, HSCs in the placenta appear not to be expanded during an explant culture step *(2)*. They are, however, maintained during the culture step. This additional step is therefore useful if the genotype of the embryos needs to be determined prior to transplantation or if soluble reagents added to the explant culture medium are to be tested for their effect on HSCs *(11)*. For direct transplantations, one should omit this culture step and proceed directly to the preparation of single-cell suspensions of the dissected placentas (**Subheading 3.3**).

2. The following steps should be performed in a tissue culture hood.

3. The stainless-steel grids are placed in the middle of each well in a 6-well plate and covered with 5 ml of M-LTC medium supplemented with 10^{-6} M hydrocortisone.

4. Filters are carefully laid on top of the grids without getting their top surface wet, but allowing medium absorption from the bottom surface.

5. Because of the large size of an E12 placenta, it has to be cut into six pieces in order to allow adequate permeability to medium. The six pieces of the placenta can be placed close to each other, with a maximum of four placentas per filter.

6. Any unused wells should be filled with sterile PBS or water to maintain humidity.

7. Plates are then incubated at 37°C/5% CO_2 for 3 days.

8. At the end of the culture period, placentas are removed from the filters using a sterile scalpel and single-cell suspensions obtained as described in **Subheading 3.3**.

3.3. Preparation of Single-Cell Suspensions

1. HSC numbers in the placenta peak at E12 *(1, 2)*. At this stage, because of the large size of the placentas, they should be treated individually in 1 ml of dissection medium with 50 µl of 2.5% collagenase in a 14-ml round-bottom tube. Unless the placentas are placed into explant culture, they should not be cut into pieces, but treated with collagenase as a whole, as this makes their subsequent physical dissociation easier. The tubes are placed in a 37°C water bath for 1.5 h.

2. A 1-ml "blue" disposable tip on a P1000 Gilson pipette set to the maximum volume is used for the physical dissociation of placental cells. The tip is placed in the center of the placenta and the plunger released while rubbing the tip to the bottom of the tube to aid the dissociation of the placenta. This is repeated with larger pieces of the placenta, until all of the placental cells can be sucked into the pipette tip. The cells are then vigorously pipetted up and down for 35 times and placed on ice. Cold dissection medium (2.5 ml) is then added to each tube, the cells centrifuged at $250 \times g$ for 5 min, the supernatant removed, and the cells resuspended in cold dissection medium.

3.4. Enrichment for HSCs by Ficoll Gradients

1. As the placenta is a relatively large tissue, enriching for HSCs by Ficoll gradients should be considered if more than one placenta equivalent is to be injected directly or if cell populations are to be isolated by fluorescence-activated cell sorting. Prior to the Ficoll gradient enrichment, dissociated placental cells are passed through a 40-µm cell strainer over a 50-ml tube to remove any larger cell clumps or debris. The strainer is washed with dissection medium.

2. Dissociated cells of up to five E12 placentas can be pooled and the total volume is adjusted to 20 ml with dissection medium.

3. The Ficoll gradient should be set up at room temperature as follows. Twenty milliliters of Lymphoprep™ are placed into a 50-ml plastic tube and overlaid by 20 ml of cell suspension (*see* **Note 6**). It is important to pipette the cell suspension very slowly down the side of the tube in order to avoid mixing with the layer of Ficoll.

4. The tubes are then centrifuged for 15 min at $850 \times g$ with an acceleration of 9 and a deceleration of 1 (i.e., no brakes applied).

5. Following centrifugation, a ring of cells is visible at the interface between the Lymphoprep™ and the dissection medium. Erythrocytes will settle in the bottom of the tube. About two-thirds of dissection medium are removed from the top. Now use a blue tip on a P1000 Gilson pipette to collect the cells from the ring and transfer them into 20 ml of fresh, cold

dissection medium. Cell clumps and debris are visible near the ring of cells and also within the Lymphoprep™ layer underneath. These should be avoided. The cells collected from the ring are centrifuged for 5 min at $250 \times g$.

3.5. Cell Staining for Flow Cytometry and Cell Sorting

1. If sorting for the stem cell population, enrichment by Ficoll gradient should be performed prior to cell sorting (*see* **Subheading 3.4**) to reduce sorting time.

2. Dissociated placental cells are filtered through a cell strainer into a 5-ml round-bottom tube and the staining with fluorescently labeled antibodies performed on ice in a small volume of dissection medium for 20–30 min.

3. Tubes are then filled with dissection medium, centrifuged at 250 $\times g$ for 5 min and cells resuspended in dissection medium.

4. For live–dead discrimination, 1 µl of Hoechst 33258 is used for cell suspensions that are to be sorted. As most analyzers lack the laser required for the use of Hoechst 33258, 1 µl of 7AAD is added to each milliliter of cell suspension for flow cytometric analysis. Cell suspensions should be checked for cell clumps and filtered again, if necessary, as placental cells tend to reaggregate.

5. As there is usually debris in total placental cell preparations, we have routinely decreased the voltage of the forward scatter to exclude this from the final picture (*see* **Fig. 2**).

6. Cells are sorted into 50% fetal calf serum/50% PBS. For transplantations, cells should be centrifuged and resuspended in PBS only.

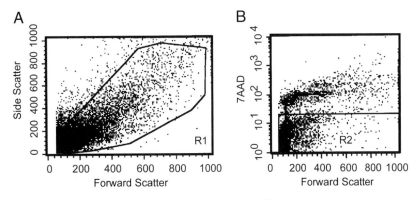

Fig. 2. FACS profile of unfractionated E12 placental cells. E12 placentas were dissociated as described in **Subheading 3.3** and prepared for flow cytometric analysis (**Subheading 3.5**). (**A**) The forward and side scatter profile of unfractionated E12 placental cells. The voltage of the forward scatter was reduced to exclude cell debris. (**B**) Live–dead discrimination by 7AAD staining (dead cells are 7AAD$^+$). Further analysis of cell surface marker expression by specific antibody staining was performed on cells gated for their morphology (R1) and for their exclusion of 7AAD (R2).

3.6. Transplantation

1. As recipients, we use mice that are between 2 and 6 months of age and that are of the same background strain as the donor mice. These mice are housed in filter-top microisolator cages and are maintained on 0.037% HCl water up to 2 weeks prior transplantation.

2. On the day of transplantation, recipient mice receive a total irradiation dose of 900 rad from a gamma source, as two split doses of 450 rad with a 2–3-h interval.

3. Dissociated total or sorted placental cells are resuspended in PBS and supplemented with 2×10^5 spleen cells (of the same strain as the recipients) per injected mouse.

4. The mice are warmed under a heating lamp to dilate the blood vessels and then restrained in a transparent plastic container that leaves the tail accessible for injection. The tail is cleaned with 70% ethanol.

5. Cells are normally injected in a volume of 0.2–0.5 ml. Total placental cells, however, should be injected in a volume of 0.5 ml to decrease the cell concentration per milliliter, as this will reduce the formation of cell aggregates. Nevertheless, syringes should be kept upright for 2–3 min before injection to allow cell aggregates to sink to the bottom. These should not be injected. If the recipients are young females or if more than one E12 placenta equivalent is injected per mouse (*see* **Note 7**), a Ficoll gradient should be performed to reduce the injected cell dose per mouse.

6. After transplantation, mice are maintained on antibiotic water containing 0.16% neomycin for at least 1 month.

3.7. Genomic DNA Extraction and Analysis by PCR

1. At 1 month (to test for short-term repopulation) and at 4 months (to test for long-term repopulation), 100–200 µl of peripheral blood are collected by orbital puncture or from the tail vein and placed directly into individual safe-lock Eppendorf tubes containing 500 µl Blood Mix. Tubes are shaken immediately and then incubated overnight at 55°C (*see* **Note 8**).

2. On the next day, tubes are given a quick spin to remove any liquid from the lids. Fifteen microliters of RNase A (at 100 µg/ml) are added to each tube and the samples incubated at 37°C for 30–60 min.

3. Five hundred microliters of phenol:chloroform:isoamyl alcohol (25:24:1) are added and the tubes placed in a shaker for 15 min.

4. After a 15-min centrifugation at $16,000 \times g$ in a bench-top centrifuge, the top, aqueous phase is transferred to a fresh tube containing 400 µl isopropanol and 50 µl 2 M NaAc. The tubes are inverted and stored at –20°C for 2 h.

5. The precipitated DNA is pelleted by centrifugation for 15 min at $16,000 \times g$ and the pellets washed by adding 700 μl of 70% ethanol, followed by a brief vortex.

6. The tubes are centrifuged again at $16,000 \times g$ for 8 min, the supernatant removed, and the pellets dried for 5–10 min at 37°C.

7. Fifty microliters of TE is added to each pellet and the DNA is dissolved by shaking the tubes at 55°C for 1 h.

8. The samples are kept at 4°C until after successful analysis, but should be moved to –20°C for long-term storage.

9. To estimate levels of reconstitution, genomic standards should be prepared by mixing genomic DNA from mice that carry the donor marker in their genome with DNA from wild-type mice of the same strain to give ratios of 100, 60, 30, 10, 6, 3, 1, and 0% (i.e., wild type). These standards are included with the samples in PCR experiments for the detection of the donor marker. A PCR for a housekeeping gene such as myogenin is also performed to allow accurate quantification.

10. The PCR products are run on an ethidium bromide-containing 1.5% agarose gel and images obtained by scanning the gel on a confocal Imager (e.g., Typhoon™, GE Healthcare), using green (532 nm) excitation and a 610 BP 30 emission filter.

11. Bands are quantified using appropriate software (e.g., Image-Quant). Ratios between the donor marker and the housekeeping gene are calculated in Excel and percentages of repopulation for each sample obtained from a standard curve that has been constructed from the genomic standards.

3.8. Multilineage Analysis

1. After 4 months posttransplantation, repopulated mice are sacrificed for multilineage analysis (*see* **Note 9**). Peripheral blood, lymph nodes, thymus, spleen, and bone marrow are isolated and are directly placed (only part of the spleen and bone marrow cells) in 500 μl Blood Mix and incubated overnight at 55°C. Genomic DNA is isolated and analyzed for donor marker contribution as described in **Subheading 3.7**.

2. $2–3 \times 10^6$ total bone marrow cells (without added spleen cells) are used for secondary transplantations. Repopulation of secondary recipients after 4 months confirms self-renewal potential of the injected donor cells.

3. 5×10^6 bone marrow cells are stained with Ly6C-FITC and CD31-PE, as described in **Subheading 3.5**. Ly6C$^+$ cells represent the myeloid compartment, Ly6C$^-$ CD31^{intermediate} cells the lymphoid compartment, and Ly6C$^-$ CD31$^-$ the

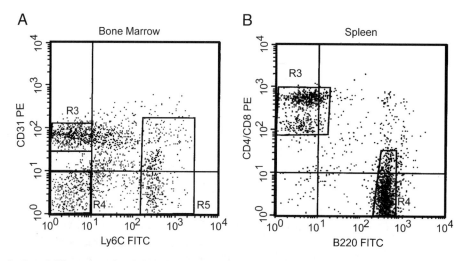

Fig. 3. Sorting of different hematopoietic cell subsets for multilineage analysis. Reconstituted recipients were analyzed for multilineage repopulation as described in **Subheading 3.8**. (**A**) Bone marrow cells were stained for CD31 and Ly6C expression, and live cells gated for the following cell subsets: R3, lymphoid cells; R4, erythroid cells, and R5, myeloid cells. (**B**) Spleen cells were stained for CD4/CD8 and B220 expression, and live cells gated for T lymphoid cells (R3) and B lymphoid cells (R4).

erythroid compartment of the bone marrow (*see* **Fig. 3A**). $2-4 \times 10^5$ cells are sorted for each subset. These are centrifuged, resuspended in 100 µl PBS, and then added to 500 µl Blood Mix for genomic DNA isolation. The donor contribution to each population is then determined as described in **Subheading 3.7**.

4. 5×10^6 spleen cells are stained with B220-FITC and CD4-PE/ CD8-PE. CD4$^+$CD8$^+$ cells (T cells) and B220$^+$ cells (B cells) are sorted (*see* **Fig. 3B**), their genomic DNA isolated and donor contribution determined as described earlier (*see* **Note 4**).

4. Notes

1. Because of the variability in different batches of fetal calf serum and collagenase preparations, it is important to request samples of different batches that can be tested for their efficiency before purchasing large amounts of a particular batch. If testing a lot of different batches, colony-forming-unit spleen (CFU-S) assays (which are described in detail elsewhere *(5)*) can be carried out on cultured tissues as a fast alternative to long-term transplantations in order to do a first quick screen. Ultimately, the batches chosen from those pre-screens have to be tested in long-term transplantations before firmly deciding on a particular batch.

2. When we analyzed LacZ expression in transgenic placentas by using fluorescein di-β-D-galactopyranoside (FDG), a fluorescent substrate for β-galactosidase, we found very high levels of background staining (up to 60%) in wild-type placentas. Inhibitors of endogenous β-galactosidase activity, such as chloroquine, should therefore be included.

3. If placentas are isolated from embryos whose genotype needs to be determined, the same Blood Mix can also be used to isolate genomic DNA from any part of the embryo that would normally be discarded. We routinely use half of the head for DNA extraction. The method is essentially the same, although the RNase treatment can be omitted, and the pellets should be resuspended in 200 µl of TE as they will be larger.

4. If the donor marker encodes a fluorescent protein that will be detected in the same channel as either PE or FITC, a different combination of antibodies must be used for sorting the different cell populations from the spleen and bone marrow for the multilineage analysis. In our case, when we injected Ly6A-GFP⁺ donor cells from the placenta *(2)*, we used CD4-PE/CD8-PE, B220-PE, and Ter119-PE to sort T cells, B cells, and erythroid cells, respectively, from the spleen in three separate sorts. A combination of Mac-1-PE and Gr-1-PE was used to isolate myeloid cells from the bone marrow in a single sort.

5. The ratio in size between the fetal placenta and the maternal decidua can vary quite substantially depending on the age of the embryo. At early stages of placenta development, the decidua is substantially larger than the placenta, with the placenta being a small, flat disc within the decidua. This ratio then changes with every day of development and is eventually reversed after about E13–E14. However, the method of separating the two layers stays essentially the same.

6. There are other types of Ficoll gradients available. We have also tested a discontinuous Ficoll gradient according to the Schneider protocol *(12)*, but do not recommend this one for the enrichment of HSCs from the placenta. In a normal scenario, HSCs should accumulate at the interface between the 19 and 22% Ficoll layer. However, we also detected placental HSCs on top of the 19% layer when we transplanted the different cell layers.

7. Injecting different cell doses (expressed as embryo equivalent [ee], i.e., within the indicated number of embryos/specific tissues, the number of equivalent cells) allows for the estimation of the number of HSCs per tissue, using Poisson statistics *(2)*.

8. After the overnight incubation at 55°C, the blood samples can be stored at –20°C for extended periods of time. Before continuing the DNA extraction, samples should be allowed to defrost at 55°C.

9. The degree of repopulation by donor cells in the different organs of the recipient can also be determined by flow cytometry. If the hematopoietic cells of the donor and the recipient express different isoforms of a specific cell surface marker (e.g., Ly5.1/Ly5.2), they can be distinguished by allele-specific antibodies. However, if HSCs from different transgenic or gene-targeted mouse models are to be analyzed that have not been backcrossed into a different isoform strain, then the PCR-based method for analyzing repopulation levels, as described here, should be employed.

Acknowledgements

We acknowledge the technical assistance of Fredrik Wallberg, Kam-Wing Ling, and Catherine Robin. This work was supported by Wellcome International Prize Travelling Fellowship GR063331MA (K.O.), Netherlands VICI ZonMW 916.36.6001 (E.D.), and Netherlands BSIK 03038 SCDD Award (E.D.). K.O. is currently supported by a Kay Kendall Leukaemia Fund Intermediate Fellowship (KKL276).

References

1. Gekas C, Dieterlen-Lievre F, Orkin SH, Mikkola HK. (2005). The placenta is a niche for hematopoietic stem cells. *Dev Cell*;8(3): 365–75.

2. Ottersbach K, Dzierzak E. (2005). The murine placenta contains hematopoietic stem cells within the vascular labyrinth region. *Dev Cell*;8(3):377–87.

3. Greaves M. (2006). Infection, immune responses and the aetiology of childhood leukaemia. *Nat Rev Cancer*;6(3):193–203.

4. Barnes CM, Huang S, Kaipainen A, et al. (2005). Evidence by molecular profiling for a placental origin of infantile hemangioma. *Proc Natl Acad Sci U S A*;102(52):19097–102.

5. de Bruijn M, Dzierzak E. (2002). Isolation and analysis of hematopoietic stem cells from mouse embryos. *Methods Mol Med*;63:1–14.

6. Robin C, Dzierzak E. (2005). Hematopoietic stem cell enrichment from the AGM region of the mouse embryo. *Methods Mol Med*;105:257–72.

7. Rossant J, Cross JC. (2001). Placental development: lessons from mouse mutants. *Nat Rev Genet*;2(7):538–48.

8. de Bruijn MF, Speck NA, Peeters MC, Dzierzak E. (2000). Definitive hematopoietic stem cells first develop within the major arterial regions of the mouse embryo. *EMBO J*;19(11): 2465–74.

9. Muller AM, Medvinsky A, Strouboulis J, Grosveld F, Dzierzak E. (1994). Development of hematopoietic stem cell activity in the mouse embryo. *Immunity*;1(4):291–301.

10. Cross JC. (2005). How to make a placenta: mechanisms of trophoblast cell differentiation in mice – a review. *Placenta*;26 Suppl A:S3–9.

11. Robin C, Ottersbach K, Durand C, et al. (2006). An unexpected role for IL-3 in the embryonic development of hematopoietic stem cells. *Dev Cell*;11(2):171–80.

12. Schneider E, Pollard H, Lepault F, Guy-Grand D, Minkowski M, Dy M. (1987). Histamine-producing cell-stimulating activity. Interleukin 3 and granulocyte-macrophage colony-stimulating factor induce de novo synthesis of histidine decarboxylase in hemopoietic progenitor cells. *J Immunol*;139 (11):3710–7.

Chapter 18

Identification of Protein Interaction Partners by the Yeast Two-Hybrid System

Maria-Paz Garcia-Cuellar, Deniz Mederer, and Robert K. Slany

Summary

The two-hybrid system is a genetic method to search for and to identify direct interaction partners of a protein of interest. This method is instrumental to elucidate the transformation mechanism of several oncogenes that play a role in childhood leukaemia. With respect to mixed lineage leukaemia gene (*MLL*) fusions, two-hybrid screening was applied to discover proteins that bind to various MLL fusion partners. Here we describe a streamlined protocol that enables any average molecular biology laboratory to conduct and evaluate a standard two-hybrid screen. Starting with a general explanation of the biological background of the two-hybrid method, this chapter covers the construction of bait vectors and two comprehensive protocols for screening either by yeast mating or yeast transformation. In addition, it also gives guidelines for the evaluation of two-hybrid results.

Key words: Two-hybrid screening, Protein–protein interaction, MLL fusion partner

---

1. Introduction

Since the first description of the two-hybrid system by Fields and Song 20 years ago *(1)*, the method has seen changing fates. Initially it was considered a complicated tool apt only for the most skilful yeast geneticist. The mid-1990s brought two-hybrid screening into the reach of the "common" lab. This was made possible by dedicated biosupply companies that standardized and simplified many procedures by offering specially adapted reagents and yeast strains. This created a real two-hybrid bonanza culminating in genomewide interaction screens *(2)*. Lately, with the advent of sensitive mass spectrometry, two-hybrid screening has started to drift out of the mainstream again. Still it has undoubted benefits

C.W.E. So (ed.), Leukemia, *Methods in Molecular Biology*, vol. 538
© Humana Press, a part of Springer Science + Business Media, LLC 2009
DOI: 10.1007/978-1-59745-418-6_18

that make it a valuable tool to study protein–protein interactions and to search for novel protein binding partners. With respect to mixed lineage leukaemia gene (MLL) fusions, the two-hybrid technique has been used widely to discover proteins interacting with the ENL, AF9, AF4, AF6, EEN, and ELL fusion partners *(3–14)*.

The basic principle of the two-hybrid system is very straightforward and relies on the fact that the DNA binding domain and the transactivation domain of the *Saccharomyces cerevisiae* GAL4 transcription factor are two physically separable units *(15)*. **Figure 1** gives a schematic overview of the two-hybrid mechanism.

The DNA binding domain of the yeast transactivator GAL4 is fused to a protein of interest to form the so-called "bait." Bait constructs are expressed in suitable yeast reporter strains, where they bind to natural GAL4-responsive "upstream activation sequences" that contain the cognate GAL4 DNA recognition sites. However, this binding does not lead to gene activation because the GAL4 DNA binding domain lacks a functional activation moiety. Subsequently, a library of fusion proteins consisting of potential interaction targets joined to the GAL4 activation domain is introduced into the reporter strain. If bait and target proteins form a productive interaction, the GAL4 transcription factor will be reconstituted, thereby leading to an activation of the gene under control of the GAL4 UAS. Skilful engineering has placed different reporters under control of the GAL4 UAS sequence. Activation of a reporter allows the selection of yeast clones that harbor an interacting pair of proteins. This is mostly done by reporter genes that complement nutritional auxotrophies allowing overcoming a block, e.g., in histidine or adenine biosynthesis (auxotrophy is the need for an exogenously supplied nutrient). In addition, reporter genes such as *lacZ* are available that allow a quantitative assessment

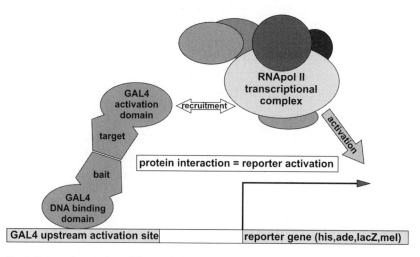

Fig. 1. Schematic overview of the two-hybrid mechanism.

of the interaction strength because the amount of reporter produced will be proportional (within limits) to the dissociation constant of the bait–target couple.

The elegant molecular mechanism behind the two-hybrid system also defines the two major limitations of the method:

1. Normally, only proteins that interact directly will be detected; therefore the method is not suitable to determine the composition of macromolecular complexes in which many proteins are held together by indirect associations. Also, protein interactions that require post-translational modifications will be likely missed because the participating proteins very often are not modified in a heterologous yeast system.

2. Bait and interaction targets are compulsorily imported to the nucleus by the nuclear localization sequences contained in the GAL4 portions. In particular, hydrophobic proteins or gene fragments coding for hydrophobic portions of proteins that are normally locked away in the protein interior will become "sticky" once expressed as GAL4 fusions, and therefore the two-hybrid system will always create false-positive results which must be carefully weeded out.

Still a properly conducted two-hybrid screen is a valuable tool to investigate the function of a protein by determining the interaction partners. All protein interactions of the MLL fusion partner ENL that were discovered in our lab by two-hybrid screens could be later confirmed with biochemical methods. Therefore conducting a two-hybrid screen is a highly recommendable option especially if biochemical purification of the protein in question is not feasible or if there is no access to the sophisticated mass spectrometry necessary to identify the minute quantities of proteins obtained after the purification procedure.

An exhaustive description of all modifications and adaptations of the basic two-hybrid procedure that have been published during the last two-decades is clearly out of the scope of this protocol series. The instructions given here will allow a scientist with some basic experience in molecular biology to conduct a screen in approximately 2–3 months' time. For further information one should consult the abundant literature covering that topic *(16)*.

2. Materials

2.1. Yeast Media

1. Peptone, a crude enzymatic digestion product of meat proteins (*see* **Note 1**).

2. Yeast extract, a water-soluble extract of autolyzed yeast cells (*see* **Note 2**).

3. Glucose (reagent grade is sufficient).

4. Adenine hydrochloride 100× stock solution: Prepare a 2 mg/ml solution in water; sterilize by filtration (*see* **Note 3**).

5. Kanamycine 10 mg/ml in water stock solution; sterilize by filtration.

6. Agar-agar, microbiology grade.

7. Yeast nitrogen base without amino acids (YNB) as a nitrogen source.

8. To prepare a homemade nutrient drop-out mix lacking uracil, adenine, leucine, histidine, and tryptophane, mix the following substances (*see* **Note 4**):

Alanine	7.6 g
Arginine hydrochloride	7.6 g
Asparagine monohydrate	7.6 g
Aspartic acid	7.6 g
Cysteinehydrochloride monohydrate 0	7.6 g
Glutamic acid monosodium salt	7.6 g
Glutamine	7.6 g
Glycine	7.6 g
myo-Inositol	7.6 g
Isoleucine	7.6 g
Lysine monohydrochloride	7.6 g
Methionine	7.6 g
p-Aminobenzoic acid potassium salt	0.8 g
Phenylalanine	7.6 g
Proline	7.6 g
Serine	7.6 g
Threonine	7.6 g
Tyrosine disodium salt	7.6 g
Valine	7.6 g

Mix thoroughly and store in a tightly closed container. The powder is highly hygroscopic and tends to clump.

9. The following aqueous solutions should be prepared to be added to the minimal drop-out medium when necessary. All solutions are 100× concentrated: histidine 2 mg/ml, leucine 12 mg/ml, tryptophane 8 mg/ml, uracil 2 mg/ml. Sterilize by filtration except uracil which should be autoclaved to aid dissolution.

10. Full medium (yeast/peptone/adenine (YPAD)):

   – Dissolve 20 g of glucose in 200 ml water.

   – Dissolve 10 g yeast extract and 20 g peptone in 800 ml water.

– Autoclave separately (*see* **Note 5**) and mix after the components have cooled to below 80°C. Then add 13 ml/l of 100× adenine solution. Yeast extract does not contain sufficient adenine to support optimal growth.

– Optional: Supplement YPAD with 1 mg/l kanamycine before use to avoid contamination with bacteria.

Media are solidified by 20 g/l agar-agar. Autoclave separately with part of the necessary water in a vessel that contains a magnetic stirring bar. This allows easier mixing with glucose and yeast extract/peptone after sterilization.

11. Drop-out medium (minimal medium):

Culture in a defined minimal medium is necessary for the selection of nutritional mutants. The most frequently used selection markers are auxotrophies for the amino acids leucine, tryptophane, histidine, and/or for the nucleobases adenine and uracil.

– Dissolve 20 g glucose in 200 ml water.

– Dissolve 6.7 g yeast nitrogen base and 1.4 g drop-out mix in 800 ml water.

– Important: Adjust the pH of YNB/drop-out mix with NaOH to approximately pH 7 (*see* **Note 6**).

– Autoclave separately, cool to approximately 60°C, and mix (*see* **Note 7**).

– This basal medium can be supplemented with 100× stock solutions of amino acids/nucleobases as appropriate.

For solid media, include 20 g/l agar-agar. Again, add a magnetic stirring bar before sterilization (*see* **Note 8**).

12. Glycerol, autoclaved for preparation of freezer stocks.

2.2. Preparation and Analysis of Bait Constructs

2.2.1. Yeast Electroporation

1. 1 M sorbitol in water: autoclave.

2. 1 M HEPES: adjust to pH 7.4 with HCl and autoclave.

3. Sorbitol/HEPES: Mix 49 ml 1 M sorbitol with 1 ml 1 M HEPES pH 7.4.

4. Electroporation cuvettes, 2 mm gap width.

5. Electroporation apparatus, with settings adjusted to 1.66 kV for electroporation voltage, 200 Ω for resistance, and 25 μF capacitance.

2.2.2. Testing of Bait Constructs for Autonomous Transactivation

Solution of 1 M 3-amino-1,2,4-triazole (3-AT). Dissolve in water and sterilize by filtration.

2.2.3. Lacz Filter Assay

1. Z buffer: 16.1 g/l $Na_2HPO_4 \cdot 7H_2O$, 5.50 g/l $NaH_2PO_4 \cdot H_2O$, 0.75 g/l KCl, 0.246 g/l $MgSO_4 \cdot 7H_2O$; Adjust to pH 7.0. Sterilize by autoclaving and store at room temperature.

2. X-GAL stock solution: Dissolve 5-bromo-4-chloro-3-indolyl-b-D-galactopyranoside (X-GAL) at 20 mg/ml in N,N-dimethylformamide; store in the dark at –20°C.

3. Z buffer/X-GAL solution: 50 ml Z buffer, 130 μl β-mercaptoethanol, 830 μl X-GAL stock solution (*see* **Note 9**).

4. Sterile filter paper circles, also known as "Whatman paper."

2.2.4. Yeast Cracking for Western Blotting

1. Cracking buffer: 8 M urea, 0.1 mM ethylenediaminetetraacetic acid (EDTA), 5% sodium dodecyl sulfate (SDS), 40 mM Tris–HCl (pH 6.8), 0.4 mg/l bromphenol blue.

2. 100 mM phenylmethylsulphonyl fluoride (PMSF): prepare in isopropanol (*see* **Note 10**).

3. Immediately before use add 10 μl 100 mM PMSF and 10 μl β-mercaptoethanol per milliliter of cracking buffer.

4. Supplement the solution with the appropriate amount of a protease inhibitor solution adapted for yeast proteases (e.g., Sigma # P8215).

5. Glass beads (425–600 μm) (*see* **Note 11**).

2.3. Library Screening

1. Selective plates that test for the activation of two-hybrid reporter genes should be prepared in advance. Start with 50 plates of 150 mm diameter to accommodate a sufficient number of clones that is necessary for effective screening (*see* **Note 12**).

2. 2×YPAD: 40 g/l glucose, 20 g/l yeast extract, 40 g/l peptone. Supplement with 1 mg/l kanamycine after sterilization to inhibit bacterial contamination.

3. LiTE: 100 mM lithium acetate, 10 mM Tris–HCl (pH 8.0), 1 mM EDTA (pH 8.0). Autoclave and store at room temperature.

4. 40% PEG/LiTE: Dissolve 10 g poly(ethylenglycol), MW 3350 (*see* **Note 13**), in 25 ml LiTE, add a magnetic bar and stir well at room temperature or with slight heating if necessary to help the PEG dissolve. Autoclave and store at room temperature for a maximum of 2 months.

5. Sonicated salmon sperm DNA (10 mg/ml) as carrier. It can be obtained commercially. If sonication equipment is available, it can be easily prepared from dried salmon sperm DNA. Dissolve salmon sperm DNA in 10 mM Tris–HCl, pH 8.0, and 0.5 mM EDTA (TE) to a concentration of 10 mg/ml. This will take several days at 4°C. Sonicate until DNA fragment length is in the range of 1 kb. Control shearing by agarose-gel electrophoresis, and add more sonication time if necessary. Phenol-extract the sonicated DNA twice and precipitate with ethanol. Redissolve in TE at 10 mg/ml concentration.

2.4. Analysis of Two-Hybrid Positive Clones

1. Blasting buffer: 10 mM Tris–HCl (pH 8.0), 1 mM EDTA, 2% Triton X100, 1% SDS, 100 mM NaCl; can be stored at room temperature.
2. TE-saturated phenol.
3. Chloroform/isoamylalcohol 24:1.
4. Glass beads (0.5 mm).
5. TE buffer: 10 mM Tris–HCl (pH 7.5), 1 mM EDTA.
6. 3 M sodium acetate pH 5.5.
7. 100% Ethanol.
8. 70% Ethanol.

3. Methods

3.1. Growing and Freezing Yeast Strains

3.1.1. Growing Yeast in Liquid and on Solid Media

Saccharomyces cerevisiae is a haploid, unicellular eukaryote. Therefore yeast is not sensitive to most of the commonly used antibiotics. Selection, e.g., for plasmid maintenance is usually done by complementation. Most laboratory yeast strains depend on the exogenous supply of nutritional compounds (usually amino acids or nucleotide precursors) because they carry mutations in genes that code for key enzymes in the respective biosynthetic pathways (auxotrophy). Therefore culture media will have to be supplemented with the respective molecules. Alternatively, a complementing gene can be introduced on a plasmid, or it can be activated as a reporter gene. Two general types of yeast media are commonly used: full media and selective (drop-out) media.

The temperature optimum for *S. cerevisiae* is 30°C. Starting from single cells, visible colonies usually will appear on YPAD plates after 24–36 h. Colonies grown on drop-out media can be expected after 2–3 days if complementation is efficient (e.g., as plasmid selection marker). Under stringent selection conditions, however, it may take up to 1 week before colonies are detectable (*see* **Note 14**). In liquid YPAD medium a stationary culture can be expected (starting from a single colony inoculum) after approximately 24–36 h. Liquid cultures are incubated in a shaker at 180 rpm to aid aeration.

3.1.2. Freezing Yeast Stocks

S. cerevisiae strains can be stored indefinitely in a mixture of 50% glycerol and 50% YPAD at –70°C and below. To establish a stock culture, disperse several large colonies with a sterile pipette tip into a 1:1 mixture of sterile glycerol and YPAD. Freeze immediately at –70°C. To recover the cells, directly scrape a small amount of frozen stock from a vial and streak on YPAD plates (*see* **Note 15**). Avoid thawing the stock completely.

3.2. Preparation and Analysis of Bait Constructs

3.2.1. General Considerations

The first critical question during the setup of a two-hybrid screen is the choice of the bait. If possible the GAL4 DNA binding domain should always be fused with the complete protein of interest. Unfortunately, sometimes the inherent limitations of the two-hybrid method do not allow such a straightforward approach. Three frequently encountered problems may necessitate modification or, in the worst case, may even preclude a two-hybrid screen altogether.

1. Quite a number of bait proteins contain domains that transactivate the reporter promoters also in the absence of an interacting target protein. This is especially true for the nuclear MLL fusion partners. Most of these proteins contain intrinsic transactivation domains that may also work in yeast. It is absolutely mandatory to control for this possibility before one embarks on a larger screening project. In some cases, changing the screening strain may alleviate the problem, as different strains use distinct upstream activating sequences (UASs) to drive the same reporter genes. Not all UASs will be equally sensitive to the activation by heterologous proteins. A prime example for such a situation is the ENL fusion partner which transactivates the lacZ but not the adenine or histidine reporters in the two-hybrid screening strain AH109. More frequently, however, one will have to conduct a structure–function analysis to try to delete the interfering activation domains. While it is likely that natural interaction partners will still recognize the altered bait, one has to keep in mind that a mutated protein was used for screening and more care has to be applied to verify the interactions by other means.

2. Not all baits will be expressed in yeast. In particular, large proteins with an unusual codon usage outside of the yeast repertoire may be problematic. Bait expression can be easily monitored by western blotting. Sometimes, expression can be re-established with shorter fragments of the bait. As mentioned above, care should be taken to verify the interactions obtained with isolated protein domains. As a rule of the thumb and in our experience, a stable protein domain retaining its function as a separate module will normally consist of at least 60–90 amino acids.

3. An often overlooked problem is that all available bait vectors fuse the protein of interest at the C-terminus of the GAL4 DNA binding domain. Therefore an N-terminal interaction might become sterically impossible. If a suspected protein–protein interaction domain is close to the N-terminus, the insertion of a glycin–serin linker between the GAL4 DNA binding domain and the protein of interest sometimes resolves the problem.

3.2.2. Choice of Vectors

Several companies offer two-hybrid vectors. In our lab, the pGBTK7 of Clontech is the vector of choice. The major difference between different vector formats is the strength of the promoter that drives bait expression. We prefer to use vectors that ensure a maximum expression level. Once the bait protein has been cloned, expression and potential autonomous activation capability can be tested. For this purpose, the bait vector has to be introduced into the screening strain. Small-scale transformation of yeast with plasmids is best done by electroporation. Compared to chemical transformation procedures, electroporation yields moderate transformation efficiencies. However, the simplicity of the procedure makes it the method of choice if optimal efficiency is not required.

3.2.3. Yeast Electro-poration

1. Grow the yeast strain to be transformed on YPAD (or the appropriate selective medium if necessary) plates for 2–4 days at 30°C. Streak broadly to create a "lawn" of cells. Use only "fresh" cells (*see* **Note 16**).

2. Scrape a "glob" of cells from the patch with a sterile yellow tip, and resuspend it in 1 ml of ice-cold sorbitol/HEPES (*see* **Note 17**).

3. Wash the cells twice in 1 ml of ice-cold sorbitol/HEPES (*see* **Note 18**).

4. Use 40 µl ice-cold sorbitol/HEPES per electroporation to resuspend the cells.

5. Add 1 µg plasmid DNA and transfer the cell/DNA mixture to a sterile 2-mm cuvette (*see* **Note 19**).

6. Electroporate once (*see* **Note 20**).

7. Immediately add 250 µl of ice-cold 1 M sorbitol and remove the cells from the cuvette to a centrifuge tube.

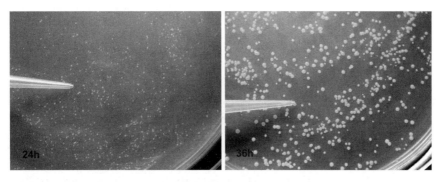

Fig. 2. Yeast colonies 24 and 36 h after electroporation. After electroporation with a plasmid carrying a complementing leucine gene, the yeast cells were plated on drop-out medium lacking leucine and incubated at 30°C. Pictures were taken 24 and 36 h after electroporation. Pipette tip is shown for size comparison.

8. Incubate cells for 30 min at 30°C and plate all of them on appropriate selective medium (*see* **Note 21**).

9. Incubate plates for 2–4 days at 30°C (**Fig. 2**). Freezer stocks can be easily prepared from transformed yeast.

3.2.4. Control for Autonomous Activation Capacity

To exclude the possibility that the bait protein contains an inherent transactivation domain, bait-transformed yeast has to be tested under the same conditions that will be applied for the actual screening process. Procedures for the three most frequent reporter genes are detailed here.

His-Reporter Gene

1. Pour several minimal medium plates lacking histidine and the appropriate amino acid that allows selection for the bait plasmid.

2. Supplement the medium by spreading 1 M 3-AT solution evenly on the agar, preparing at least five plates with different final 3-AT concentrations. For a start use final concentrations of 0.5, 1, 2, 5, and 10 mM 3-AT (*see* **Note 22**).

3. Streak out yeast transformed with empty vector (negative control), yeast transformed with the bait construct, and a positive control containing the complete GAL4 transcription factor sequence (*see* **Note 23**).

4. Incubate at 30°C for 8 days. At the optimal 3-AT concentration, no growth should be visible for the negative control and the bait construct. The positive control should yield visible colonies after approximately 36–48 h.

Ade-Reporter Gene

Screening for adenine complementation is easy because the mutation is "tight." No growth will occur without activation of the reporter. In addition, many strains will turn brownish-red under adenine-deficient conditions because an adenine precursor product accumulates. Therefore the strength of reporter activation can be semiquantitatively estimated by the color of the colony. A strong transactivation will produce whitish colonies.

1. Pour selective plates without adenine and streak the reporter strain transformed with empty vector, bait, and a positive control vector.

2. Judge growth after 2–8 days of incubation as indicated in **Fig. 3** (*see* **Note 24**).

lacZ-Reporter Gene

There are different methods to detect lacZ activity in yeast cells. One of the more sensitive methods involves reaction of the lacZ enzyme with X-GAL to produce a blue indigo dye. In contrast to bacterial blue-white screening, lacZ activity in GAL4-based two-hybrid strains is too weak to be detected directly by incorporation of X-GAL into the yeast plates (*see* **Note 25**). In this procedure a freeze–thaw cycle is used to effectively lyse the yeast cells.

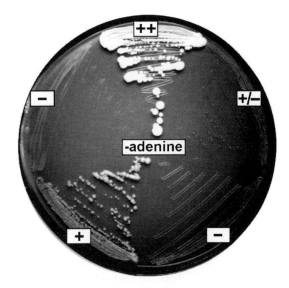

Fig. 3. Selection of yeast on adenine drop-out medium. The yeast strain AH109 was transformed with different bait/target pairs, allowing a graded activation of the adenine reporter. The cells were streaked on the drop-out medium lacking adenine and incubated for 4 days at 30°C. Different levels of adenine deficiency are indicated by the growth rate (colony size) and colony color. (++) very strong interaction, (+) strong interaction, (+/−) weak interaction, (−) no interaction (*Note:* some remainings of the yeast inoculum will normally be visible also in the negative control streaks).

1. Streak the yeast strains to be tested including positive and negative controls on plates selecting for the presence of the plasmid.

2. Wrap small sheets of filter paper in aluminium foil and autoclave (*see* **Note 26**).

3. Prepare a dish with sterile Z-buffer/X-GAL solution and soak a Whatman filter paper completely with this solution.

4. Put a sterile filter paper circle on top of the colonies, and push gently with forceps to allow good contact between paper and colony surface. Pull off the filter carefully and submerse completely (colony side up) in liquid nitrogen. Freeze completely.

5. Take out filter, thaw at room temperature, and place (colonies up again) on filter soaked with Z-buffer/X-GAL.

6. Incubate at room temperature and observe color formation. Positive control colonies should become blue after approximately 30 min to 1 h. Do not incubate for more than 4 h, as false-positive results may appear.

3.2.5. Control of Bait Expression by Western Blotting

The successful expression of the bait construct needs to be verified by western blotting. Because yeast has a very strong cell wall, a special procedure has to be applied to liberate sufficient protein for western blotting. This method is known as "cracking."

1. Inoculate a fresh colony of the bait-transformed yeast in 10 ml minimal medium supplemented with the appropriate amino acids to allow selection of the bait plasmid. Shake overnight at 30°C with good aeration.

2. After approximate 16 h of incubation, determine the OD_{600} of the overnight culture. Dilute with YPAD to an OD_{600} of 0.4 in a final volume of 15 ml (*see* **Note 27**). Grow until OD_{600} = 1.

3. Harvest cells and wash once with 10 ml ice-cold water.

4. Resuspend the pellet in 200 µl of fully supplemented cracking buffer (add PMSF and ß-mercaptoethanol) preheated to 70°C, add 160 µl glass beads, and incubate 10 min at 70°C.

5. Vortex for 1 min, spin down, and store the supernatant on ice.

6. Re-extract the remaining pellet in 100 µl cracking buffer and boil for 5 min. Spin the beads down and combine the supernatants.

7. The protein extract can be stored at –20°C. Run 20 µl per lane for western blotting.

8. Immunodetection of bait proteins is best done using anti-GAL4 DNA binding domain antibodies. Some bait vectors also contain epitope tags.

3.3. Library Screening

If the bait protein shows proper expression, and autonomous transactivation is absent or very weak, one can embark on the actual screening procedure. Although there are only approximately 25,000 different genes in a mammalian cell, in our experience it is necessary to screen 1×10^6 and more independent clones of an expression library to cover potential interactions with rare proteins. Many good two-hybrid libraries are commercially available. If possible, one should use a library that was developed from the tissue where the bait protein is expressed. For example, a bait normally present in haematopoietic cells (like many MLL fusion partners) should be screened with a bone marrow library. Alternatively, foetal brain and testis libraries may be used because, for unknown reasons, these tissues transcribe almost all genes. There are two principal methods to search a library for interaction partners.

3.3.1. Screening by Mating

This is the preferable strategy because a complex library can be searched with high efficiency, thereby minimizing hands-on time and material expenses. The natural life cycle of yeast includes a sexual phase where two cells of opposite "sex" or mating type (designated either "a" or "α") conjugate to form a diploid cell. If the bait was introduced into an "a" strain, it can be mated with a library pretransformed into an "α" strain and vice versa. The resulting diploids will contain the bait and the interaction target plasmids and therefore, if the encoded proteins will interact, the diploid cells will have the GAL4-sensitive reporters activated. Mating is easy and straightforward. However, it is not advisable to prepare a "homemade" mating library since the transfection and control procedures necessary to ensure a homogenous library representation among the yeast transformants are cumbersome. Therefore, we recommend mating strategies only if pretransformed libraries are available from trustworthy commercial vendors.

1. A commercial strain suitable for screening by mating is AH109, which can be obtained from Clontech (now TaKaRa). The genotype of AH109 is MATa, trp1-901, leu2-3, 112, ura3-52, his3-200, gal4Δ, gal80Δ, LYS2:: GAL1$_{UAS}$-GAL-1$_{TATA}$-HIS3, ade2-101::GAL2$_{UAS}$-GAL2$_{TATA}$-ADE2, URA3:: MEL1$_{UAS}$-MEL1$_{TATA}$-lacZ (*see* **Note 28**).

2. Pick a colony of AH109 pretransformed with the bait plasmid and grow an overnight culture at 30°C in 50 ml of selective minimal medium. Grow till the culture reaches an OD$_{600}$ of 0.8.

3. Harvest the cells for 5 min at 2,500g and 4°C.

4. Discard the supernatant and resuspend cell pellet in the remaining liquid.

5. Mix the cell pellet with 1 ml of the MATα strain pretransformed with the interaction library.

6. Add the mixture of "a"/"α" strains to 45 ml of 2 x YPAD/Kan in a large, sterile (e.g. 2 l) Erlenmeyer flask. Shake yeast culture slowly (30–50 rpm) for 20–24 h at 30°C. (*see* **Note 29**).

7. Transfer the cell suspension to a centrifuge tube and rescue residual cells in the shaking flask by flushing with 2×YPAD/Kan.

8. Harvest the cells for 5 min at 2,500g and 4°C.

9. Resuspend the cell pellet in 10 ml 0.5×YPAD/Kan.

10. To determine the mating efficiency, plate 100 μl of a 1:10; 1:100; 1:1,000, and 1:10,000 dilution on three individual 100-mm plates. On plate number 1 select for the presence of the bait plasmid only. Plate number 2 should allow growth of library clones and plate number 3 should be double selective to restrict growth to diploid cells. By this procedure the number of successful mating events can be calculated (*see* **Note 30**).

11. Plate 200 μl of the mating mixture on 15-cm plates initially selecting *for the histidine reporter only*. Do not forget 3-AT! One mating will yield 50 plates (*see* **Note 31**).

12. Spot a tiny amount (approximately a drop of 5 μl) of a positive two-hybrid control on each plate (*see* **Note 32**).

13. Incubate for 8–10 days at 30°C. Check for contaminations frequently and remove them from plates by "punching out" the unwanted colonies with an inverted, sterile blue pipette tip.

14. Pick positive clones at day 4, day 7, and day 10. Restreak on medium lacking histidine, adenine, or both amino acids. Optionally perform X-GAL filter tests for activation of the lacZ gene (*see* **Note 33**).

15. Keep positive clones for further analysis as described in **Subheading 3.4**.

3.3.2. Screening by Transformation

An alternative to mating is a direct transformation of the screening library into the bait-bearing strain. Since the whole library needs to be covered and because transformation efficiencies are variable, screening of a large number (>100) of 15-cm plates may be necessary to achieve a satisfactory coverage. For a screen with ENL as bait we use a total of 175 plates.

The most crucial parameter for this procedure is transformation efficiency. Depending on the strain, the bait protein, and the experimental parameters, the number of transformants per microgram of DNA can vary widely. Adjustment of the standard procedure may be necessary to achieve optimal transformation rates. In general at least 10^4 cfu/µg DNA (cfu = colony forming units) should be reached. This allows a library with 10^6 independent clones to be screened on 100 plates. The most essential condition for good transformation efficiency is vigorous growth of the strain to be transformed. In some cases it may be helpful to record a growth curve in a pilot experiment to determine the OD values of a culture that is in early to mid-log phase. This protocol will yield competent cells for approximately 10 transformations and can be scaled up.

1. Inoculate 50 ml of the appropriate selective medium with 2–3 colonies of the bait-transformed strain picked from a freshly prepared selective plate (*see* **Note 34**). Grow for 24 h at 180 rpm and 30°C.

2. Dilute the preculture to an OD_{600} of approximately 0.4 in 250 ml YPAD (*see* **Note 35**). Shake at 30°C and 180 rpm till the culture reaches an OD_{600} = 0.8–1.2. This will usually take anywhere from 4 to 8 h depending on the strain and bait protein.

3. Harvest the cells by centrifugation for 5 min at 2,500g and wash with 100 ml of ice-cold sterile water. Use sterile equipment. From now on, work with cold solutions and keep everything on ice.

4. Wash the cells in 20 ml ice-cold sterile LiTE and spin down for 2 min at 4°C and 600g.

5. Resuspend the cell pellet in 1 ml ice-cold sterile LiTE, transfer to a 2-ml microfuge tube, and incubate 30 min on ice (*see* **Note 36**).

6. Denature sonicated salmon sperm DNA (10 µl per transformation) for 5 min at 96°C and place immediately on ice.

7. For a single transformation, mix 150 µl competent yeast with 1 µg appropriate (library) plasmid DNA, 10 µl denatured salmon sperm carrier DNA, and 600 µl 40% PEG/LiTE. Mix gently and incubate for 30 min at 30°C (water bath).

8. Heat-shock the cells for 5 min at 42°C in a water bath and place on ice for another 5 min (*see* **Note 37**).

9. Harvest the cells by a quick spin (5 s) at room temperature in minifuge (14,000*g*). Do not exceed the spinning time to avoid damage to the cells.

10. Resuspend the cell pellet in 500 µl sterile water and plate the mixture on a large (15 cm) selective plate for screening. Initially select *for the histidine reporter only.* Do not forget 3-AT! Follow up like **steps 12–15** of **Subheading 3.3.1** as described for "screening by mating." Important: In order to determine the overall efficiency of the transformation procedure, streak 10 µl of the transformed cells (dilute with sterile water to 100 µl to aid spreading) on two control plates (100-mm dishes are sufficient) containing medium selecting (a) for the presence of bait plasmid only (which allows calculation of the total number of viable competent cells) and (b) medium selecting for the presence of bait and library plasmid (number of cotransformants) (*see* **Note 38**).

3.4. Analysis of Two-Hybrid-Positive Clones

Since the initial selection is done using the less stringent histidine reporter gene, a substantial number of colonies arising on the screening plates will be false positives. However, this strategy has the advantage that no potential interaction partners with weaker binding capacity will be lost. Although it is impossible to predict exactly how many colonies will be found in a screening, any given standard bait should yield at least some clones. In our hands, even empty vector expressing the GAL4 DNA binding domain will cause a few colonies to grow. This necessitates a follow-up strategy that weeds out as many false positives as possible. The following procedures are suggested.

3.4.1. Validation by Drop-Out Culture

Restreak all positive clones on medium without adenine (if adenine is available as second reporter) and on double selective plates omitting histidine and adenine. An efficiently interacting clone should grow on double selective medium. If available, test for lacZ activation. Restrict your further analysis initially to these strong interactors. Depending on the bait, the majority of all clones might be eliminated in this first step.

3.4.2. Extraction of Plasmid DNA from Yeast Cells

Isolate the library plasmid from yeast, and transform again together with the bait into the reporter strain to reconfirm the protein–protein interaction (*see* **Note 39**). A protocol for isolation of plasmids from yeast cells is given below:

1. Grow an overnight culture in 10 ml of the appropriate selective medium.

2. Harvest cells for 5 min at 3,000g at 4°C, wash once with 1 ml water, and resuspend the cell pellet in 200 µl blasting buffer.

3. Add 200 µl of TE-saturated phenol/chloroform/isoamyl alcohol and approximately 100 µl glass beads.

4. Vortex the mixture for 3 min at room temperature.

5. Add 200 µl TE buffer and vortex again for another 30 s.

6. Centrifuge for 5 min at 10,000g to 14,000g in a minifuge at room temperature.

7. Transfer the supernatant into a new tube and re-extract once more with 200 µl phenol/chloroform/isoamyl alcohol.

8. Transfer the supernatant into a new tube and precipitate the plasmid DNA by adding 2.5× vol of 100% ethanol and 1/10× vol of 3 M sodium acetate, pH 5.5. Incubate for 5 min on ice, centrifuge 15 min at 14,000 rpm, and wash the pellet once with 70% ethanol. Dissolve in 20 µl TE and use 1 µl to electroporate/transform to competent *E. coli* (*see* **Note 40**). Isolate the plasmid from *E. coli* by standard procedures and sequence.

3.4.3. General Considerations for the Evaluation of Positive Two-Hybrid Clones

The most frequently encountered false-positive clones arise from random sequences fused to the GAL4-activation domain outside of their cognate reading frame. The production of a random peptide with many hydrophobic amino acids can lead to a "sticky" protein that will be able to interact nonspecifically with some baits. Be aware that interaction targets containing partial coding sequences might also expose hydrophobic amino acids that would be normally hidden in the interior of a correctly folded full-length protein. This type of construct is prone to unspecific interactions. For similar reasons, membrane proteins will be encountered frequently as false positives. As a rule of the thumb, a protein will interact most likely with another protein of the same compartment (e.g., a nuclear protein with another nuclear protein). Of course, many proteins reside in more than one compartment and therefore these "cross-compartment" interactions may be real. This has to be decided individually with the biological background in mind. For MLL fusion proteins, one should remember that all fusions will be normally imported into the nucleus owing to the strong nuclear localization sequences contained in MLL.

In any case, it is mandatory that any two-hybrid interaction is confirmed by other methods like co-immunoprecipitation, pull-down experiments, and colocalization. In our experience, all sufficiently stringent two-hybrid interactions could be confirmed later also by other methods. When performed diligently, two-hybrid screening is a very reliable method.

4. Notes

1. Peptone is sold under different, sometimes confusing, names. Sometimes, peptone is called Bactopeptone. Do not confuse with Tryptone, an enzymatic digestion product from caseine used for bacterial media. Yeast cells will grow considerably more slowly in Tryptone.

2. Identical with yeast extract for bacterial culture media.

3. Use adenine hydrochloride for better solubility in water.

4. The given composition covers the requirements of most yeast strains. If tests for other auxotrophies are necessary, the drop-out mix needs to be adjusted by omission of the respective amino acid. Several companies also sell premixed drop-out reagents.

5. If glucose is autoclaved together with the other ingredients, excessive caramelization will occur and growth will be retarded.

6. The mixture of amino acids reacts acidic, and therefore it is advisable to adjust to neutral pH. After sterilization the medium will be slightly acidic again, an environment that is optimal for yeast.

7. The amino acids in the drop-out mix are sufficiently stable to survive a single autoclave cycle.

8. The minimal drop-out agar can be prepared in advance and stored at room temperature. To prepare single plates, the agar can be melted in a microwave (avoid boiling over) and supplemented with 100× amino acid/nucleobase stock solutions just before use. Let all plates dry for 48 h at room temperature before use. Yeast plates can be stored wrapped in plastic at 4°C for several months; however, they are very prone to fungal growth. Check frequently, and discard contaminated plates. Liquid media can be kept at room temperature for at least 6 months.

9. Once Z-buffer is supplemented with β-mercaptoethanol, it has to be used within 48 h to avoid oxidation.

10. In aqueous solutions PMSF has a half-life of a few minutes. From our experience, isopropanol solutions of PMSF can be stored at room temperature for at least 6 months without loss of activity.

11. New glass beads are contaminated with a variety of impurities that might influence downstream applications. Therefore wash glass beads before use once with 1N HCl for 10 min and rinse thoroughly in water till the runoff is not acidic any more. Dry at 180°C.

12. For plates testing histidine autotrophy add 3-AT. Use the minimum concentration determined in **step 3.2.4** that inhibits background growth of negative controls.

13. Do not use polyethylenglycol of different molecular weights, as this will decrease transfection efficiency.

14. Prolonged incubation at 30°C makes the media very vulnerable to contaminations. Exercise due care to avoid introduction of aerial fungal spores. Always use open flame protection and avoid air drafts. If possible, work in a flow cabinet. Bacterial contamination can be suppressed by addition of 1 mg/l kanamycin.

15. Yeast from freezer stocks should be allowed to recover in complete medium. Direct plating in selective conditions sometimes results in loss of viability.

16. After prolonged storage of plates at 4°C, transformation efficiency drops considerably. Cells can be "rescued" by restreaking them onto new plates before electroporation.

17. The exact amount of cells is not critical. For a single electroporation use a "glob," approximately the size of a drop of water (20 μl). Avoid introducing too many cells.

18. Use a common table-top microfuge at full speed (approximately 10,000–14,000g) for 10 s to pelletize cells.

19. DNA concentrations should be at least 0.2 μg/μl to avoid dilution of sorbitol/HEPES. For double transformations with two plasmids, use 0.5 μg DNA for each plasmid.

20. Electroporation conditions given are for a BIO-RAD micropulser and may vary slightly with other equipment. Consult the manual of your electroporation apparatus.

21. With most bait vectors selection will be either for leucine or tryptophan. Prepare the corresponding drop-out plates in advance. Keep in mind that the reporter genes will not be activated by the bait alone.

22. The "His"-mutation in most reporter strains is leaky. Therefore these strains will grow on medium without histidine, albeit usually at much lower rate. To get a clean screening result, the residual activity of the HIS3 enzyme has to be blocked by the synthetic inhibitor 3-AT. Different reporter strains will require different 3-AT concentrations. For example, AH109 needs 0.5 mM 3-AT, and Y190 approximately 1.5 mM 3-AT. It is absolutely mandatory that a dilution series of 3-AT is tested to determine the minimal concentration necessary to suppress background growth. Too much of 3-AT will also inhibit a positive readout of the his-reporter.

23. A universal positive control for two-hybrid systems can be prepared by fusing the GAL4 transactivation domain (can be released from the target vector) directly to the GAL4 DNA binding domain of the bait vector. This will give the strongest possible reporter readout. Keep in mind that almost all protein–protein interaction pairs will induce a weaker response!

24. Selection for adenine autotrophy usually is more stringent than selection for histidine complementation. It is quite common to observe growth on medium lacking histidine, but the cells will not grow on medium lacking adenine. Even more stringent screening can be achieved by double selection in medium without histidine and adenine.

25. In contrast to bacterial growth substrates, media for yeast are suboptimal for X-GAL-based lacZ tests, precluding direct addition of X-GAL to the plate.

26. Use normal filter paper. Nitrocellulose filters may be used, but they become very brittle during the procedure.

27. Some bait constructs are driven by an alcohol dehydrogenase promoter which will be repressed by the accumulating ethanol in the late log phase. Therefore it is advisable to harvest the cells in the mid-log phase. The main culture is prepared in YPAD full medium to allow for faster growth. The cells will not lose the plasmid during this short time.

28. The mating type "a" of this strain allows mating with any "α" strain. Yeast genotypes are usually noted as follows: any gene symbol in small letters indicates a loss of function; capital letters signify a change in the gene structure that does not disrupt gene function. "::" means an integration event. Consequently, AH109 is auxotroph for Trp, Leu, His, and Ade. It does not require lysine, and the ura mutation was complemented by integration of the lacZ-reporter. Mel1 is a naturally occurring gene for an α-galactosidase that is under control of a GAL4 regulated promoter. The product is secreted and can be detected by direct addition of X-α-GAL to the screening plates (available from Clontech).

29. Higher rpm values will reduce the mating efficiency.

30. The total number of diploid cells plated should at least equal the number of independent clones contained in the library. Several mating procedures might be necessary.

31. Screening for histidine autotrophy will allow also the growth of diploids containing weakly interacting proteins. The number of positives will be reduced in subsequent, more stringent screening rounds.

32. A good positive control is a yeast strain transformed with two plasmids encoding known interacting proteins. Examples

are SNF1 and SNF4 from yeast or p53 and largeT antigen. Positive control plasmids are available from vendors of two-hybrid libraries.

33. There is a correlation between growth rate and interaction strength. Colonies appearing early usually contain the most promising interaction pairs. Screening only for histidine autotroph cells will yield many false positives. For further analysis we advise selection of clones that show strong growth also on plates without adenine. Normally, a true protein–protein interaction will allow growth on drop-out medium lacking both selective agents adenine and histidine. Therefore we recommend concentrating initially on the clones that show robust activation of both reporters. After 10 days, the false-positive rate increases dramatically, and colonies appearing thereafter should be discarded. LacZ filter assays with X-GAL can be used additionally to confirm positive clones. However, in our experience all clones growing on minus adenine and minus histidine will also be lacZ positive. A semiquantitative assessment of interaction strength can be obtained by the color of the yeast colonies on medium lacking adenine. Yeast cells with a strong activation of the ade reporter will appear white, whereas weaker interactions cause a certain degree of adenine deficiency that will induce a more brown-reddish colony.

34. Storage of the plated yeast cell at 4°C will decrease transformation rates.

35. The short time in full medium will not cause a substantial loss of plasmid.

36. For best results, use fresh competent cells. In case transformation efficiency is not crucial, the cells can be stored on ice for several hours.

37. In some cases the addition of 75 µl DMSO before heat shock increases the transformation efficiency. Heat-shock times depend on the geometry and the thickness of the microfuge tubes used. Heat-shock times typically are in the range from 5 to 15 min and should be tested empirically.

38. It is advisable to start with a smaller pilot transformation experiment (10 plates) to determine transformation efficacy. From these result it can be estimated how many further transformations are necessary to cover the library.

39. Watch out for different colony morphologies/sizes on the screening plates to spot contaminants, which can be frequent especially in warm and humid conditions.

40. The amounts of plasmid DNA isolated from yeast are minute. Only a few *E. coli* transformants can be expected.

Acknowledgments

Work in the authors' laboratory is funded by DFG, Deutsche Krebshilfe, and the EU.

References

1. Fields S, Song O. (1989). A novel genetic system to detect protein–protein interactions. *Nature*;**340**:245–246.

2. Legrain P, Selig L. (2000). Genome-wide protein interaction maps using two-hybrid systems. *FEBS Lett*;**480**:32–36.

3. Zeisig DT, Bittner CB, Zeisig BB, Garcia-Cuellar MP, Hess JL, Slany RK. (2005). The eleven-nineteen-leukemia protein ENL connects nuclear MLL fusion partners with chromatin. *Oncogene*;**24**:5525–5532.

4. Erfurth F, Hemenway CS, de Erkenez AC, Domer PH. (2004). MLL fusion partners AF4 and AF9 interact at subnuclear foci. *Leukemia*; **18**:92–102.

5. Bursen A, Moritz S, Gaussmann A, Moritz S, Dingermann T, Marschalek R. (2004). Interaction of AF4 wild-type and AF4.MLL fusion protein with SIAH proteins: indication for t(4;11) pathobiology? *Oncogene*;**23**:6237–6249.

6. Srinivasan RS, de Erkenez AC, Hemenway CS. (2003). The mixed lineage leukemia fusion partner AF9 binds specific isoforms of the BCL-6 corepressor. *Oncogene*;**22**:3395–3406.

7. Begay-Muller V, (2002). Ansieau S, Leutz A. The LIM domain protein Lmo2 binds to AF6, a translocation partner of the MLL oncogene. *FEBS Lett*;**521**:36–38.

8. Hemenway CS, de Erkenez AC, Gould GC. (2001). The polycomb protein MPc3 interacts with AF9, an MLL fusion partner in t(9;11) (p22;q23) acute leukemias. *Oncogene*;**20**: 3798–3805.

9. Garcia-Cuellar MP, Zilles O, Schreiner SA, Birke M, Winkler TH, Slany RK. (2001). The ENL moiety of the childhood leukemia-associated MLL-ENL oncoprotein recruits human Polycomb 3. *Oncogene*;**20**:411–419.

10. Fuchs U, Rehkamp G, Haas OA, et al. (2001). The human formin-binding protein 17 (FBP17) interacts with sorting nexin, SNX2, and is an MLL-fusion partner in acute myelogeneous leukemia. *Proc Natl Acad Sci U S A*;**98**:8756–8761.

11. So CW, So CK, Cheung N, Chew SL, Sham MH, Chan LC. (2000). The interaction between EEN and Abi-1, two MLL fusion partners, and synaptojanin and dynamin: implications for leukaemogenesis. *Leukemia*;**14**: 594–601.

12. Garcia-Cuellar MP, Schreiner SA, Birke M, Hamacher M, Fey GH, Slany RK. (2000). ENL, the MLL fusion partner in t(11;19), binds to the c-Abl interactor protein 1 (ABI1) that is fused to MLL in t(10;11)+. *Oncogene*; **19**:1744–1751.

13. Shinobu N, Maeda T, Aso T, et al. (1999). Physical interaction and functional antagonism between the RNA polymerase II elongation factor ELL and p53. *J Biol Chem*;**274**:17003–17010.

14. Yam JW, Jin DY, So CW, Chan LC. (2004). Identification and characterization of EBP, a novel EEN binding protein that inhibits Ras signaling and is recruited into the nucleus by the MLL-EEN fusion protein. *Blood*;**103**:1445–1453.

15. Ma J, Ptashne M. (1987). Deletion analysis of GAL4 defines two transcriptional activating segments. *Cell*;**48**:847–853.

16. Guthrie C FGR. (2002). Methods in Enzymology, Guide to Yeast Genetics and Molecular and Cellular Biology, Part B., Vol. 350. New York: Academic.

Chapter 19

Complete Array of *HOX* Gene Expression by RQ-PCR

Glenda J. Dickson, Terence R. Lappin, and Alexander Thompson

Summary

In mammals the *HOX* network consists of 39 genes which encode master regulators of developmental processes including hematopoiesis. Many of the chromosomal translocations associated with acute leukemias involve *HOX* genes directly or some of their regulatory factors, e.g., mixed lineage leukaemia (MLL), leading to inappropriate expression of certain subsets of the genes. Evolutionarily, the *HOX* genes are thought to have arisen by duplication and divergence from a primordial gene. Consequently, they exhibit a high degree of sequence similarity, particularly in the homeobox domain. *HOX* gene expression, the *HOXOME*, can be quantified by real-time quantitative PCR (RQ-PCR) using carefully selected reagents. In practice, an RQ-PCR platform based on Taqman probe chemistry has proved valuable for the precise measurement of individual human and murine *HOX* genes with a high degree of specificity, over a wide dynamic range. Defining the roles for HOX in hematopoiesis should help to elucidate the mechanisms of deregulation in leukemia and eventually identify targets for therapeutic intervention.

Key words: *HOX*, RQ-PCR, Hematopoiesis, Leukemia, Gene expression, Transcription factor

1. Introduction

1.1. HOX Genes

The homeobox genes have been highly conserved throughout evolution and are present in many species. In mammals the Class I homeobox (*HOX*) family comprises 39 highly similar members arranged in clusters designated *A–D*, located respectively on four chromosomes 7p15, 17q21, 12q12, and 2q31 in humans and 6p14, 11q21, 15q12, and 2q31in mice. The *HOX* genes have been assigned 13 paralog groups based on homeobox sequence similarity, genetic position in the cluster, and function of the encoded protein *(1)*. All mammalian *HOX* genes comprise two exons, and the homeobox is located in exon 2 proximal to the

C.W.E. So (ed.), Leukemia, *Methods in Molecular Biology, vol. 538*
© Humana Press, a part of Springer Science + Business Media, LLC 2009
DOI: 10.1007/978-1-59745-418-6_19

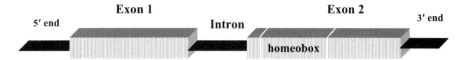

Fig. 1. Diagrammatic representation of the structure of *HOX* genes. The highly conserved homeobox sequence resides in exon 2 of the gene. Adapted from *(2)*.

intron/exon boundary (*see* **Fig. 1**). *HOX* genes encode master regulators of developmental processes, including hematopoiesis. Individual members of the *HOX* gene network have emerged as major targets that are de-regulated in acute leukemia.

Given the interplay and subtle regulation of *HOX* genes, measurement of the entire *HOX* network (*HOXOME*) is required when investigating conditions in which *HOX* expression is altered. The standard polymerase chain reaction (PCR) is a powerful methodology to amplify genetic material (DNA) or expressed genes (RNA) following conversion to complementary DNA (cDNA); however, quantification of this approach has been cumbersome, often involving the incorporation of radionucleotides or labor-intensive approaches. Using TaqMan real-time quantitative PCR (RQ-PCR) the specific analysis of all 39 human or murine genes simultaneously is relatively uncomplicated. Generation or validation of *HOX* gene signatures is rapid and reproducible. The following methodology outlines the protocol for quantifying the *HOXOME* in human and murine cells.

1.2. RQ-PCR Using TaqMan Technology

RQ-PCR has become a core technique used in molecular laboratories worldwide. Various technologies are available such as intercalating dyes SYBR Green, or hybridization probe–based Molecular Beacons. TaqMan probe–based chemistry provides three levels of specificity for each target gene with stringent design of forward, reverse, and probe oligonucleotides. Owing to the high degree of homology within the *HOXOME*, we have selected a TaqMan probe–based approach to measure its expression in human and murine cells. The TaqMan probe is an oligonucleotide modified at the 5′ end with a fluorescent reporter and the 3′ end with a quencher molecule (often also fluorescent). Intact probes emit low-level fluorescence because of energy exchange afforded by the relative proximity of the reporter and quencher molecules (*see* **Fig. 2**). During the PCR reaction, a Y-structure develops at the junction of the extended primer and probe. This structure acts as a substrate for the endogenous exonuclease activity of DNA polymerase, the enzyme that replicates target DNA during PCR. The exonuclease activity digests the intervening DNA molecules between the reporter and quencher, thereby physically removing the quencher and allowing the emitted fluorescence from the reporter to be detected. Importantly, the incorporation

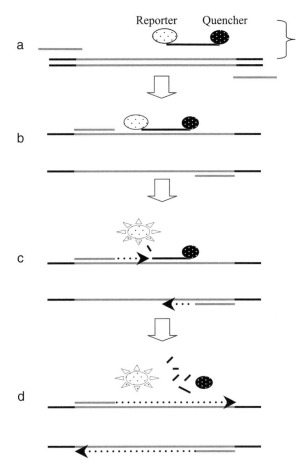

Fig. 2. Schematic representation of the principle of TaqMan RQ-PCR. (**a**) The components of the reaction include DNA template, forward and reverse primers, and probe oligonucleotides. (**b**) Denaturation of the template and annealing of the oligonucleotides. (**c**) Primer extension and probe displacement. (**d**) Cleavage of the probe removing the quencher from the reporter dye allowing measurable fluorescence and faithful completion of the PCR. Adapted from *(3)*.

of the probe does not inhibit the PCR reaction which continues to completion.

New DNA products are generated during the exponential phase (amplification) of the reaction. In ideal conditions, each PCR cycle results in doubling of the quantity of template and the fluorescence increases proportionally (*see* **Fig. 3**). The accumulation of sufficient product to transect a user-defined threshold determines the cycle threshold (C_t) (*see* **Note 1**). To validate specificity of each primer–primer probe (PPP) set for its respective *HOX* gene, amplified target regions between primers (amplicon) were cloned and sequenced. Additionally, RQ-PCR was performed on the cloned amplicons and standard curve values were generated to allow the contribution of the *Hoxome* to be quantified.

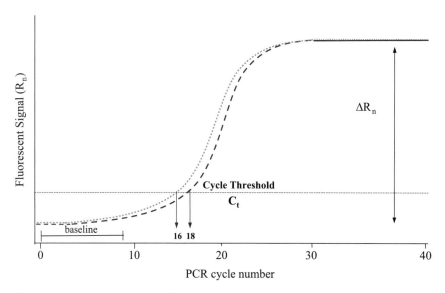

Fig. 3. Graphic representation of a RQ-PCR amplification plot of fluorescence signal against PCR cycle number. The baseline, C_t values, and change in fluorescence (ΔR_n) are shown for two reactions. A lower C_t value is indicative of higher gene expression. The ΔC_t values are used to calculate fold change ($2^{\Delta Ct}$). In the example above, a ΔC_t value of 2 reflects a fourfold (2^2) change in expression.

2. Materials

The culture and collection of cells are outside the scope of this chapter and should be optimized on an individual basis. Materials used are obtainable from various sources and those quoted are for reference purposes only and non-exclusive. Standard benchtop centrifuge and vortex are used throughout to mix and collect solutions.

2.1. Preparation of Template

2.1.1. Extraction, Quantification, and Analysis of Total Cell RNA

1. Murine cells.
2. Sterile 1.5-ml Eppendorf tubes (Eppendorf, Hamburg, Germany) or equivalent.
3. RNase Away solution (Molecular Bioproducts, San Diego, CA).
4. Disposable gloves.
5. TRIzol reagent (Invitrogen, Paisley, UK). Store at 4°C.
6. Chloroform (Sigma, St. Louis, MO). Store at 4°C.
7. Isopropanol (Sigma).
8. Glycogen (Invitrogen). Store at –20°C.
9. Diethylpyrocarbonate (DEPC, Sigma) treated double distilled, deionized water (ddH$_2$O) (0.01%), autoclaved.
10. Ethanol (Sigma) (75% v/v, 0.01% DEPC-treated ddH$_2$O).
11. Agarose (Invitrogen).

12. Tris-acetate–EDTA (TAE) buffer (Sigma).

13. Ethidium bromide (10 mg/ml) (Sigma).

14. Gel tray, combs, and electrophoresis apparatus (e.g., Horizon 11.14, Invitrogen).

15. Bromophenol blue (Sigma).

16. Glycerol (Invitrogen).

17. A spectrophotometer such as the Ultraspec 4300 pro and quartz cuvettes (Amersham Biosciences, Uppsala, Sweden), or a NanoDrop 1000 spectrophotometer (NanoDrop, DE, USA) or Agilent 2100 Bioanalyzer with RNA Nano Chips (Agilent Technologies, CA, USA).

18. Ultraviolet (UV) light transilluminator with optional bioimaging system (Ultra-violet Products, Cambridge, UK), integrated Hamamatsu IEEE 1394 digital camera (Hamamatsu City, Japan), and the associated Labworks Version 4.5 software for Windows.

2.1.2. Deoxyribonuclease I (DNase I) Treatment and Complementary (cDNA) Preparation by RT-PCR

1. Thin-walled 0.2-ml PCR tubes (Ambion, Austin, TX).

2. Ampligrade DNase I (Invitrogen), 10× reaction buffer and 25 mM EDTA. Store all at –20°C.

3. Murine Moloney leukemia virus native reverse transcriptase (MMLV-RT), 0.1 M dithiothreitol (DTT), and 5× First-Strand reaction buffer (Invitrogen). Store all at –20°C.

4. Deoxynucleoside triphosphates (dNTPs) 100 mM (Invitrogen). Store at –20°C.

5. RNase OUT™ recombinant ribonuclease inhibitor (Invitrogen). Store at –20°C.

6. Random hexamer primers (300 ng/µl) (Invitrogen). Store at –20°C.

7. Fetal and adult cDNA libraries isolated from mouse 7-day embryo and adult testis (Clontech, Mountain View, CA). Store at –80°C.

2.2. RQ-PCR Using TaqMan Technology

1. ABI PRISM Sequence Detection System 7700 or similar (Applied Biosystems, Foster City, CA).

2. MicroAmp Optical 96-well reaction plate and lids, or equivalent (Applied Biosystems).

3. 2× TaqMan Universal master mix containing uracil-*N*-glycosylase (UNG) (Applied Biosystems) (*see* **Note 2**), low-retention pipette tips for handling up to 2 and 20 µl volumes (Amgen, Union City, CA).

4. Human *HOX* and murine *Hox* gene-specific RQ-PCR oligonucleotides, *see* **Table 1**, (Applied Biosystems, GENSET Corp, La Jolla, CA or Europins MWG Operon, Ebersberg, Germany). The *HOX* probes are modified at the 5′ end by 6-carboxy-fluorescein (FAM) and at the 3′ end by 6-carboxy-

Table 1
Sequences of PPP sets for HOX gene expression profiling

HOX gene	Forward primer	TaqMan probe (5′ FAM, 3′ TAMRA)	Reverse primer	Accession number
(a) Human *HOX* genes				
HOXA1	ACAGAACTTCAGTGCGCCT-TACA	CCTACGGCGTTAAATCAGGAAGC-AGACCC	GGGAGCGACAGGCTTCTTG	NM_005522*
HOXA2	CACAAAGAATCCCTGGAAATCG	CGCCTGAGAACTGCTTACACC-AACACAC	AAATGAAATTCTTTTC-CAGCTCTAGA	NM_006735*
HOXA3	CCTGGATGAAAGAGTCTCGA-CAA	ACACAAAGCAGAAAACCAGCAGCTC-CAG	GCCAGCGGCAGCTTTCG	NM_030661
HOXA4	TGGTGTACCCCTGGATGAAGA	TCCATGTCAGCGCCGTTAACCCC	CTTAGGCTCCCCTCCGTTATAAC	NM_002141*
HOXA5	TCCCATCGCTTCCCTACCT	ACCCATTGCAAAGTTCAGGGCAT-AAGGT	GCTTTGGAACAGCCTACAGCTT	NM_019102*
HOXA6	AGTACACGAGCCCGGTTTACC	AGCGGATGAACTCCTGCGCGG	CCCATGGCTCCCATACACA	NM_024014
HOXA7	AGCTTGGAAATTCTGCTCA-CT-TCT	ACCCATTGCAAAGTTCAGGGCAT-AAGGT	TCTGATGTCATGGCCAAATTTG	NM_006896*
HOXA9	GCCGGCCTTATGGCATTAA	TGAACCGCTGTCGGCCAGAAGG	CAGGGACAAAGTGTGAGTGTCAA	NM_152739*
HOXA10	AAAGCCTGCGCGGAGAA	AGAGTGGTGGGAAGAAGGGCTGCC	CTCCAGTGTCTGGTGCTTCGT	NM_018951*
HOXA11	TTGAGCATGCGGGACAGTT	AGGCGCTTCTCTTTGTTAATGTA-GACGCTGAA	GTACCAGATCCGAGAGCTGGAA	NM_005523*
HOXA13	TGCCCAACGGCTGGAA	CTGCCCGACGTGGTCTCCCATC	TAAGGCACGGCGTTCTTTCT	NM_000522
HOXB1	GCCATATCCTCCGCAGCAT	CCCCTTATGGGAACGAGCAGACCG	CATAGGCCGGTGCAAAGCT	NM_002144*
HOXB2	GGCCTCTCCCTAGCCTACA	CGACAGCCCGG TCCCTTTTTCC	GGTGAAAAATCCAGCTCTTCCT	NM_002145
HOXB3	TCACCCAGCGATGCAGAA	CCACCTACTACGACAACGCGCGG	CGAGGAATAGCCTCCGAAGA	NM_002146*

HOXB4	CCCTGGATGCGCAAAGTT	AAGCGGCTCTCGGACCGGCTACAC	AATTCCTTCTCCAGCTCCAAGA	NM_024015
HOXB5	TCCTTCCATGCTCCCAACTC	CTTCTGCTTGTCCCAAATCCGCCA	CCACAGACACAAACATTCAGAAAC	NM_002147*
HOXB6	GAAGTGCTCCACTCCGGTCTA	CCGTGGATGCAGCGGGATGAATTC	GCCCAAAGGAGGAACTGTTG	NM_156037*
HOXB7	TCGAGCCGAGTTCCTTCAAC	TGCACTGCGCGCCCTTTGAG	CACACCCGGAGAGGTTCT	NM_004502*
HOXB8	AAGCGGGCGAATGCGAGGTA	CGCACGCCCTGGGACTGACA	GGAACCAGATTTTGACCTGTCTCT	NM_024016*
HOXB9	AACCCCTCCGCCAACTG	CACGCTCGCTCTTCCCGAAAAA	CCAGGCGTCTGGTATTTGGTGTA	NM_024017*
HOXB13	GCTGATGCCTGCTGTCAACTAT	CCTTGGATCTGCCAGGCTCGGC	ATTGCTTTGGCGGCTCC	NM_006361*
HOXC4	CCATAGTCTACCCATGGAT-GAAAAA	TTCACGTTAGCACGGTGAACCCCA	TTGGGTTCCCTCCGTTATAA	NM_014620*
HOXC5	TCTGGCATAGGTACCACAT-AAGGA	CACAGGGAAACAGAGCAGTCCTCTA-GACCA	GACACGGACAGAGCCAGACA	NM_018953*
HOXC6	TCAAACGTGGACCTGAAAGTCA	TCTGGACCCCTCCCTCACCG	GGCGCGTGGAGAAAGAGA	NM_004503*
HOXC8	CGTCTCCCAGCCTCATGTTT	TGGATGAGACCCCACGCTCCG	TCTGATACCGGCTGTAAGTTTGC	NM_022658
HOXC9	TCATCCTTCGATTCTGAAACCA	ATTTTGACCTGCCGCTCGGTGAGAT	GGTGGCCCGGGTTCTC	NM_006897*
HOXC10	GCCCAGACACCTCGGATAAC	AAAGAGGAGGATAAAAGGCAGAAAACAC-CACAGG	GCTCTTTGCTGTCAGCCAATT	NM_017409
HOXC11	GCGGCCGACGAGCTT	TGCACCGGGAGTGCCTGCC	GCCTTCGTTTTTCATGAGGATCT	NM_014212*
HOXC12	GCGAGTTTCTGGTCAACGAGTT	CACACGCCAGCCGCGGAG	AAGATTCAAGCGGTCTGAGAGTTC	NM_173860*
HOXC13	GGCTAGCAAGTTCATCACCAAA	CGCATTCCGCCACCACGAA	GGTTACCTGGCGCTCAGAGA	NM_017410*
HOXD1	TCGAGTGGATGAAAGTGAA-GAGG	ATGCCTCTAAGAAAGG-TAAACTGCCGAGTATG	ATTCGTGCGGATCGCG	NM_024501
HOXD3	CCACGTGATTGGCGAAATAA	AATTCAGCACGTCCCTTAAGAAAC-ACGGAG	CCTTTGCGTGGCAGATTAATG	NM_006898

(continued)

Table 1
(continued)

HOX gene	Forward primer	TaqMan probe (5' FAM, 3' TAMRA)	Reverse primer	Accession number
HOXD4	GAGAGCAGTCTTTGGATGTAC-CATT	AAGGAGCCGCTATCCTTAG-GCAAGTTGG	TTTTAGGAAAGCAGCTTAGCA ACTT	NM_014621*
HOXD8	CTGACCAGGAAAAGAAGA ATCGA	TTCCCACGCCCTAGCCCTCACC	TGGAACCAGATTTTTACCTGTC TCT	NM_019558*
HOXD9	CCCCGAAGCGAACTGGAT	CCCGGAAAAGCGCTGTCCCTACA	GCTCAAGCGTCTGGTATTTGG	NM_014213*
HOXD10	CAGCAGCGGCCAGCATGT	CATGCCACCACCTAGCGGCAGACA	TTCACTTCTCTTTTGGCCAGAGA	NM_002148*
HOXD11	GCTAGCAAGCCTTCGTTCCTT	CAACCGTCGTCCTGCCAGATGACTT	CGGAGCCAGGTTGGAAGAG	NM_021192
HOXD12	AGAAACGCAAGGAATTGTCCAA	CTGAACCTCAGCGACCAGCAAGTCAA	TTCTTCATACGCCTGTTCTGAA	NM_021193
HOXD13	CACTTCGGCAACGGCTACTAC	CCGTATGTCGCAACGGCGTGG	CTTGAGCGCATTCTGCTGTAAG	NM_017410*
(b) Murine Hox genes				
Hoxa1	CCTTGGCAGTGGCGACTCT	CGAGCTTACCCCTGACCATGGGAT	GCGCAGGATTGGAAAGTTGT	NM_010449
Hoxa2	TCGCTGAGTGCCTGACATCT	CCCCTGTCGCTGATACATTTCAAAGT-TCA	AAAGGGTCGAGGTCTTGATTG	NM_010451
Hoxa3	CAATGGGTTCGCTTACAATGC	CAGCCATACGCGCGCGTCCG	AGGCAGGTCGATGGTACTCAAC	NM_010452
Hoxa4	CCGGAGAATGAAGTGGAAGAAA	CACAAACTTCCCAACACCAAGATGCGA	GCCGAGGCAGTGTTGGAA	NM_008265
Hoxa5	TAGTTCCGTGAGCGAACAATTC	CTCGGCGGAGCATGCACTCCG	GCTGAGATCCATGCCATTGTAG	NM_010453
Hoxa6	CCTATTTTGTGAATCCCACT TTCC	CCTGCCCAGCGGCCAGGA	CAGCTGGCCCAAGAAGGA	NM_010454
Hoxa7	ACGGGCTTTTTAGCAAATATACG	CTTCTCTCTTCCAAAATGCCGAGCCG	GGGTGCAAAGGAGCAAGAAG	NM_010455
Hoxa9	CCGAACACCCGACTTCA	TGCAGCTTCCAGTCCAAGGCGG	TTCCACGAGGCACCAAACA	NM_010456

Hoxa10	CACAGGCCACTTCGTGTTCTT	TGCGCAGAACATCAAAGAAGA-GAGCTCC	TTGTTCCGCAGCATCGTAGAG	NM_008263
Hoxa11	AGATTTCTCCAGCCTCCCTTCTT	CCCCAGACCCCGTCTTCGCG	TGGAGGAGTAGGAGTATGTCATTGG	NM_010450
Hoxa13	CCTCCCCACCTCTGGAAGTC	TCTCCCATCCTTCAGACGGCCAGCTC	TAAGGCACGGCGTTCTTTCT	NM_008264
Hoxb1	ACTCTCACTCCCCGGACCTT	AGAGAAACCCACCTAAGACAGCGAAG-GTGTC	CTGGCGCGTGGTGAAGTT	NM_008266
Hoxb2	GCTCGCCGAGTGTCTGACTT	CCCGGCTGTCTTGGAGACATTTCAAA	AATGTCGACTCCTTGATTGATGAA	NM_134032
Hoxb3	TACCAGCGCTCAGCGTGTT	TGCAGTCCCTGGGCAACGCC	TGCCCATTGAGCTCCTTGCT	NM_001079869
Hoxb4	ACTCAAACTATGTCGACCCCAAGT	CACAGAGCGGATTACCTACCCAGCGACC	GGCTGGAAGCCGCTCTCT	NM_010459
Hoxb5	GGGCAGACTCCACAGATATTCC	ATGAGGAAGCTTCACATCAGCCACGATATGA	GGGTCAGGTAGCGATTGAAGTG	NM_008268
Hoxb6	TTCCTATTTCGTGAACTCCACCTT	AGCGGGCAGGAGTCCTTCCTGG	CCGCATAGCCAGACGAGTAGA	NM_008269
Hoxb7	TCTAAATATCCAGCCGGCAAGTTC	TTTCGGCTCCAGGAGCCTTCCCC	CAAAGGCGGCAAGAAGTTTGTT	NM_010460
Hoxb8	AACTCACTGTTCTCCAAATA-CAAAACC	AGTCCCTGGGCCCCAATTATTATGACTG	TTGCGAAGGGTGCTGGAA	NM_010461
Hoxb9	TGTCCATTTCTGGGACGCTTA	ACGCCGAGCACCTGACTTCCC	GAACACCGGCGCTTTGG	NM_008270
Hoxb13	CGCTCGATGCCAACTGTCAAC	CCCCCCTGGATCTGCCAGGC	GACAAGGGTGGCACTGCTTT	NM_008267
Hoxc4	AACCCATAGTCTACCCTTGGATGA	ATTCACGTTAGCACGGTGAACCCCAATTATAA	CGGTTGTAATGAAACTCTT-TCTCTAATTC	NM_013553
Hoxc5	ACCCGTGGATGACCAAACTG	ATGAGCCACGAGACGGATGGCAA	AGGGTCTGGTAGCGCGTGTA	NM_008271
Hoxc6	ACGTCGCCCCTCAATTCCA	CCTATGATCCAGTGAGGCATTTCTC-GACC	CTGAGCTACGGCTGCTCCAT	NM_010465

(continued)

Table 1
(continued)

HOX gene	Forward primer	TaqMan probe (5′ FAM, 3′ TAMRA)	Reverse primer	Accession number
Hoxc8	TCTCCCAGCCTCATGTTTCC	ATGAGACCCCACGCTCCTGGGC	GTCTGATACCGGCTGTAAGT TTGTC	NM_010466
Hoxc9	TGTAGCGGATTTTCCGTCC TGTAG	AGCCGGCTGTATTCAGTACGTC GTGG	CCGTAAGGGTGATAGACCACACAGA	NM_008272
Hoxc10	GGGCCAAGACCGCAGACT	AGTCCAGACACCTCGGATAAC-GAAGCTAAAG	CTGTGGTGTTTCTGCCTTTATCTC	NM_010462
Hoxc11	GCGGCCGACGAGCTTAT	CACCGGGAGTGCCTGCCTCCT	TTTTTCATGAGGATCTCAGT-GACTGT	NM_001024842
Hoxc12	TCTCCTGAATCCTGGGTTT GTG	TGGTGAATATCCACACAGGAGAC AGCTTCTACTT	CCTGACGGCGGCGAAGTT	NM_010463
Hoxc13	GCCACCCTGGGCTATGG	CTACGGCTGCCGCCTGTCGC	TTCTGCTGCAGGTTCACGTT	NM_010464
Hoxd1	CGCCCACAGCACTTTCG	AACGCCCCAAGAAAGCAAACTGTC	GGGCTTGTGGCTCCATATTC	NM_010467
Hoxd3	AAAGAATCCCGACAGAACT CCAA	TGTGCCACTTCAGGAGAACTGT-GAGGA	CACCAGCTGAGCACTCGTGTAC	NM_010468
Hoxd4	GCTGTGGTCTACCCTTGG ATGA	CACGTGAATTCGGTGAACCCCAAC-TACA	AATGAAATTCCTTTCCAGT-TCTAGGA	NM_010469
Hoxd8	GGGAGCCCGCGAAGTT	ACGGATACGATAACTTACAGA-GACAGCCGATTTT	CACTGGACGATTTACAGTCAGGAT	NM_008276
Hoxd9	CGGGCTGCTCGCTGAA	TGACCCAAACAACCCTGCAGCGA	TCCAGCTCTAGCGTCTGGTATTT	NM_013555
Hoxd10	CTGCCTGGCTGAGGTTTCC	AGAAGGAAAGCAAAGAGGAAAT-CAAGTCTGATACTCC	AGCCGTTTGGTGCTTGGTGTAA	NM_013554

Hoxd11	GGAACGCGGAGTTTTTCTT TAATGT	CAACTCTCTCGGATGCTCAACCT CACTGAC	TCCTGGGATTCTGGAACCA	NM_008273
Hoxd12	CCTGTGCCTCCAGCTTCAA	AGACACCAAAGGCCGCTCAACTTG	GCCACTTGCACTGCCATGT	NM_008274
Hoxd13	AGGTGTACTGTGCCAAGG ATCAG	ATCATCCTTTCCAGGAGATGTGGCTT-TAAACC	TGGTGTAAGGCACCCTTTTCTT	NM_008275
Pnx1	CACAGATCAGACAAATCTAC-CACACA	AGCTGGAGAAGTATGAGCAGG CATGCA	TGAATTCACCACCACGTGATGA	NM_183355
Meis1	CCTCGGTCAATGACGCTTTAA	ACACCCCTCTTCCCTCTCTTAG-CACTGA	TTTGAGAAATGTGAATTAGCT ACTTGTACC	NM_010789

The design of the Primer-Primer Probe (PPP) sets of the genes denoted by *asterisk* was carried out by Applied Biosystems.

tetramethylrhodamine (TAMRA). Primers are prepared as 12.5 μM solutions. Probes are prepared as 5 μM solutions. Equal volumes of these working solutions are combined to produce primer–probe mixes and are stored in aliquots at –20°C.

5. Primer-probe set for *18S rRNA* (Applied Biosystems) as an endogenous control gene modified by VIC at the 5′ end and a minor groove binding protein (MGB) at the 3′ end. *18S rRNA* is diluted from 20× to 8.3× in ddH$_2$O and stored in aliquots at –20°C.

2.3. Design of HOX RQ-PCR PPP Sets

1. The online sequence repository database NCBI GenBank available online from http://www.ncbi.nlm.nih.gov/entrez/query.fcgi?db=Nucleotide.

2. Primer Express v1.5 software (Applera Corporation, Norwalk, CT) or similar.

3. BLAST (Basic Local Alignment Search Tool) tool available online from: http://www.ncbi.nlm.nih.gov/BLAST.cgi.

2.4. Validation of RQ-PCR Platform

Cells from various tissues were used to generate a cDNA "pool," which was supplemented with a cDNA library.

2.4.1. Generation of HOX Amplicons by PCR

1. Thin-walled 0.2-ml PCR tubes.

2. Template cDNA.

3. Amplitaq Gold, 10× PCR buffer, and 25 mM MgCl$_2$ (Applied Biosystems).

4. Forward and reverse primers (MWG, Invitrogen, Operon or similar).

5. dNTPs (Invitrogen).

6. Sterile ddH$_2$O.

7. Agarose 1000 (Sigma).

8. DNA ladder (25-bp) (Invitrogen).

9. QIAquick PCR Purification Kit (Qiagen Ltd, Crawley, UK) or equivalent.

2.4.2. Ligation of Amplicons into Cloning Plasmids

1. 1.5-ml Eppendorf tubes.

2. Fresh PCR product.

3. pGEM-T Easy kit (Promega, Madison, WI) or TA-cloning kit (Invitrogen).

2.4.3. Transformation of Plasmids and Selection of Clones

1. 1.5-ml Eppendorf tubes.

2. One Shot TOP10F cells (Invitrogen) stored at –80°C supplied with *pUC19* DNA stored at –80°C and enriched SOC media (Invitrogen) stored at room temperature.

3. Water bath heated to 42°C.

4. Ampicillin (Sigma), filter-sterilized and stored at –20°C.

5. X-Galactose (X-Gal) (Invitrogen).

6. *N,N′*-dimethyl formamide (DMF) (Sigma) sterile filtered and stored at –20°C.

7. Luria–Bertani (LB) agar (Sigma).

8. Petri dishes (35 mm) (Barloworld Scientific, Staffordshire, UK).

9. Incubator/oven heated to 37°C.

10. LB broth powder (Sigma).

11. Sterile 10 ml tubes (Sarstedt, Nümbrecht, Germany).

12. Orbital shaker (Barloworld Scientific) or equivalent heated to 37°C.

2.4.4. Extraction of DNA from Bacterial Clones and Restriction Enzyme Digest

1. 1.5-ml Eppendorf tubes.

2. QIAprep Spin miniprep kit (Qiagen) or similar small-scale DNA extraction kit.

3. Heating block prewarmed to 65°C to warm ddH_2O.

4. *EcoR1* restriction endonuclease (New England Biolabs Inc, Ipswich, MA).

5. Bovine serum albumin (BSA).

6. Water bath heated to 37°C.

7. Agarose 1000 (Invitrogen).

8. TAE buffer.

9. Electrophoresis apparatus and gel combs (Invitrogen).

10. DNA ladder (Invitrogen).

2.4.5. DNA Sequencing of Amplicons

1. 1.5-ml Eppendorf tubes.

2. Sequencing tubes (Applied Biosystems).

3. ABI PRISM 310 Genetic Analyzer (Applied Biosystems).

4. ABI PRISM Big Dye Terminator Cycle Sequencing Ready Reaction Kit (v3.1) (Applied Biosystems) or similar supplied with Terminator Ready reaction mix and buffer.

5. Sequencing Primer (*T7* and *SP6*).

6. DNA template.

7. Sterile ddH_2O.

8. G-50 Sephadex gel filtration cartridges (Edge Bio Systems Performa, Gaithersburg, MD) or similar PCR clean-up kit.

2.4.6. Analysis of Sequences

1. Chromatogram software, e.g., Chromas, which is freely available from: http://www.technelysium.com.au/chromas_lite.html.

2. BLAST (basic local alignment search tool) analysis website: http://www.ncbi.nlm.nih.gov/BLAST.

2.5. Standard Curve Assays

1. 1.5-ml Eppendorf tubes.
2. Sequence-validated plasmid DNA, generated from *HOX* target amplicons.
3. Spectrophotometer, quartz cuvettes, and ddH$_2$O.
4. Water bath heated to 37°C.
5. *Not*I restriction endonuclease enzyme (New England Biolabs).
6. Universal Master Mix (Applied Biosystems), ddH$_2$O, specific oligonucleotides.
7. Plasticware for RQ-PCR as previously mentioned.

3. Methods

3.1. Preparation of Template

Total RNA is extracted from cells by a modified guanidinium isothiocyanate–phenol–chloroform method *(4)* using TRIzol according to the manufacturer's instructions. It is imperative that all surfaces be treated with RNase-Away solution and disposable gloves used throughout to reduce the risk of RNA degradation due to RNase contamination.

3.1.1. Extraction, Quantification, and Analysis of Total Cell RNA

1. For adherent cells, remove culture media by aspiration and directly add TRIzol reagent to the cells (1 ml of TRIzol per 5–10 × 10^6 cells). For suspension cultures collect cells by centrifugation and add 1 ml of TRIzol per 5–10 × 10^6 cells. Homogenize the cell pellet on ice using repetitive pipetting (*see* **Note 3**).
2. Add 200 µl of chloroform to the homogenate and mix by shaking the tubes vigorously for 10 s and cool on ice for 15 min. Centrifuge the samples at 10,000g for 15 min at 4°C. Following centrifugation, RNA molecules reside in the aqueous (upper) phase whereas DNA and proteins are retained in the interphase and phenol phase, respectively.
3. Transfer the aqueous phase to a fresh tube and add 500 µl of isopropanol. Depending on quantity, the RNA sample is precipitated either at room temperature for 5 min or at –20°C for 30 min. RNA samples can be stored at –80°C for up to 6 months.
4. Collect the precipitate by centrifugation (10,000g for 10 min at 4°C) and wash with 75% ethanol v/v 0.01% DEPC- treated ddH$_2$O (*see* **Note 4**). Collect the pellet by centrifugation (10,000g for 10 min at 4°C).
5. Remove the supernatant carefully by vacuum aspiration, and air-dry the pellet for 10–15 min. Dissolve the pellet in 20–50 µl of DEPC-treated ddH$_2$O (depending on pellet size)

by incubation at 55°C for 5 min followed by vortexing and pipetting (*see* **Note 5**).

6. Assess the integrity of the RNA sample (where possible) by electrophoresis through a 1% agarose gel (*see* **Note 6**).

7. Quantify and examine the purity of RNA by diluting 2 μl of the sample in ddH$_2$O and measuring the absorption at 260 (A_{260}) and 280 nm (A_{280}) (*see* **Note 7**). Total RNA is calculated using the following equation:

$$C_{\mathrm{RNA}} = \frac{A_{260} D_{\mathrm{F}} K}{1,000} \tag{1}$$

where C_{RNA} is the concentration of RNA in μg/μl, D_{F} is the dilution factor, and K is a constant of proportionality related to the subject molecule ($K = 40$ for RNA).

3.1.2. DNase I Treatment and cDNA Preparation by RT-PCR

1. Degrade potentially contaminating genomic DNA from the sample by DNase I treatment. For 5 μg of RNA, add, in order, 1 μl of DNase I buffer, 1 μl of DNase I enzyme, and DEPC-treated ddH$_2$O to a final volume of 11 μl. Mix by vortexing and incubate at room temperature for 15 min.

2. Add 1 μl EDTA solution (25 mM) followed by heating at 65°C for 5 min to chelate and inactivate the enzyme.

3. Place the RNA on ice to prevent formation of secondary structures. Store RNA at –80°C until required.

4. Re-analyze 1 μl of the sample by gel electrophoresis to verify degradation of any contaminating DNA previously identified.

5. Generate a 2× RT master mix by adding multiples of the following reagents in order (for standard 20 μl RT reaction) (*see* **Note 8**): 4 μl 5× first-strand buffer, 1 μl random primers (300 ng), 1 μl of dNTP mix (10 mM each), 2 μl dithiothreitol (DTT 0.1 M), 1 μl RNase OUT recombinant ribonuclease inhibitor, 1 μl M-MLV-RT.

6. Combine 10 μl of DNase-treated RNA with 10 μl of 2× RT master mix. Incubate at 37°C for 2 h followed by heat-inactivation of the enzyme at 70°C for 10 min. Include negative control reactions containing all components except the MMLV-RT enzyme.

7. Store cDNA samples at –20°C until required.

3.2. RQ-PCR Design, Validation, and Application

3.2.1. Design of HOX RQ-PCR PPP Sets

1. Obtain the genomic and coding sequence (CD) of each *HOX* gene using database searches such as: http://www.ncbi.nlm. nih.gov/entrez/ to locate appropriate TaqMan PPP sets using Primer Express v1.5 (*see* **Note 9**).

2. Where possible, design cDNA-specific PPP sets which cross the intron–exon boundaries so as to reduce the capability of amplifying genomic DNA.

3. Compare the sequences of each real-time PCR primer, Taq-Man probe, and amplicon to the current NCBI GenBank database to ensure that the PPP designs are specific for the target gene and do not amplify regions of other genes containing similar sequences.

4. If a primer–probe set shows a high degree of similarity to family members (i.e., >80% identity) then it must be redesigned.

3.2.2. Validation of RQ-PCR Platform

Optimize primer and template concentrations by setting up a range of serial dilutions for each component. Reconstitute lyophilized oligonucleotides as per the manufacturer's protocol to a stock concentration of 100 pmol/µl (10^{-4} M) for long-term storage or alter primers to this concentration. Prepare working solutions of oligonucleotides in a concentration range of 1–50 µM. We routinely prepare stocks of the standard forward and reverse primers at 25 µM (1:4 dilution of stock solution) and modified TaqMan probes at a concentration of 5 µM (1:20 dilution of stock solution). RQ-PCR technology is applicable to a large dynamic range of template concentrations (pg to µg). For complete *HOX* gene network quantification, at least 50 ng RNA-equivalents of cDNA template should be provided per reaction. Final concentrations of 1 µM for standard primers and 200 nM for modified probe per RQ-PCR reaction have been deemed optimal in our studies. RQ-PCR reactions are carried out in a volume of 12.5 µl. The *HOX* platform is generated as follows:

1. Carry out a standard PCR reaction (using the same conditions defined for quantification) in the absence of TaqMan probe to validate the specificity of the RQ-PCR oligonucleotide sets.

2. Validate amplicons by PCR-cloning and sequencing using standard protocols. At least five clones per PPP set should be validated in this way to provide an acceptable level of confidence in the specificity.

3.2.3. Generation of HOX Amplicons by PCR

1. Perform standard TaqMan PCR using 500 ng of cDNA (measured as RNA equivalents) with conditions identical to those of RQ-PCR in the absence of the fluorescent probe (*see* **Note 10**).

2. Analyze an aliquot of PCR product (10 µl) by agarose gel electrophoresis in 2% Agarose 1000 alongside a 25-bp DNA ladder to confirm amplification.

3. If large amounts of unincorporated primers are evident, pass the PCR product through a QIAQuick PCR purification column a centrifuging the cartridges at 500g for 2 min. Change the collection tube and elute the amplicons with 30 µl of TE buffer.

4. Confirm the level of expression of the target gene in that mixture by combining 0.25 µl template cDNA (= 0.25 µg total

RNA), 6.25 µl Universal Master Mix, 0.5 µl TaqMan probe, 0.5 µl forward primer, 0.5 µl reverse primer, and 4.5 µl ddH$_2$O.

3.2.4. Ligation of Amplicons into Cloning Plasmids

1. Combine 1.5 µl PCR product, 0.5 µl pGEM-T Easy, 0.5 µl T4 ligase, and 2.5 µl 2× ligation buffer.

2. Our preferred method is to incubate the reactions at 4°C overnight, then place on ice.

3.2.5. Transformation of Plasmids and Selection of Clones

1. Gently mix 2 µl of ligation DNA into freshly thawed aliquots of Top10F competent bacterial cells (50 µl/reaction). Use 1 µl of *pUC19* DNA in a control reaction to assess the transformation efficiency.

2. Incubate the DNA and bacteria on ice for 30 min. Heat-shock the cells at 42°C for 30 s and return the cells to ice for 2 min.

3. Add 450 µl of SOC medium to the cells under sterile conditions, and then incubate the cells with moderate agitation for sufficient aeration at 37°C for 1 h.

4. To enable selection of plasmid-transformed clones, spread 40 µl of X-Gal on to LB agar plates containing ampicillin and allow to dry for 20 min at 37°C.

5. Spread 50 µl of the transformation on to a prewarmed selective plate, invert, and incubate overnight at 37°C.

6. Examine the plates for transformed colonies and select 20 white or light blue bacterial colonies (*see* **Note 11**) with sterile 200 µl pipette tips. Add each to a 10 ml centrifuge tube containing 3 ml of LB broth containing ampicillin. Incubate each colony for 16 h at 37°C with moderate agitation.

3.2.6. Extraction of DNA from Bacterial Clones and Restriction Enzyme Digest

We extract the plasmid DNA from bacterial cells following the microcentrifugation method (5) using the QIAprep Spin miniprep kit according to the manufacturer's instructions.

1. Transfer 1.5 ml of bacterial inoculum to a 1.5-ml Eppendorf tube and centrifuge at 800g for 2 min to pellet the bacteria. Remove the medium.

2. Add 250 µl buffer P1 and homogenize the cells by vortexing. By inverting the capped tube 5 times, gently mix in 250 µl of buffer P2 and incubate the samples at room temperature for 5 min. Add 350 µl of neutralization buffer N3 and immediately mix by inverting the capped tube five times. Centrifuge at room temperature at 10,000g for 10 min.

3. Remove the supernatant and transfer to a Qiagen spin cartridge. Collect DNA in the nitrocellulose membrane by centrifugation for 1 min at 10,000g and discard the flow-through. Wash the

DNA on the column by adding 750 µl of wash buffer PE. Centrifuge as before, discard the supernatant, and spin the cartridge once more to remove residual ethanol.

4. Place spin cartridges into a clean collection tube, and add 50 µl of prewarmed ddH$_2$O to the centre of the cartridge membrane. Soak for 1 min at room temperature. Centrifuge the cartridges for 2 min at 10,000g to collect the DNA.

5. Ascertain the presence of an insert by screening the pGEM-T Easy DNA with the restriction endonuclease *EcoR1* which has sites flanking the insertion site. Combine 10 µl Plasmid miniprep, 2 µl React 3 buffer, 1 µl *EcoR1* enzyme, and 7 µl ddH$_2$O. Incubate at 37°C for 2 h.

6. Separate the reaction on a 2% Agarose 1000 gel by electrophoresis alongside a 25-bp DNA ladder. Select samples containing inserts for DNA sequencing.

3.2.7. DNA Sequencing of Amplicons

1. Follow the Sanger–Coulson (chain terminating nucleotide) method for DNA sequencing by combining the following on ice: 2 µl miniprep DNA, 4 µl Terminator Ready Reaction Mix, 2 µl 5× Sequencing Buffer, 3.2 pmol Primer (*T7* and *SP6* for sequencing forward and reverse strands respectively), and ddH$_2$O to a final volume of 10 µl.

2. Mix and spin the reaction tube. Follow the standard sequence PCR conditions: denature at 96°C for 2 min, then repeat for 30 cycles, denature at 96°C for 10 s, anneal at 50°C for 5 s, and extend at 60°C for 4 min.

3. Prepare a G-50 Sephadex gel column by centrifuging the cartridges at 500g for 5 min. Replace the collection tube and pipette the PCR extension product onto the center of the column to remove contaminating oligonucleotide primers. Centrifuge cartridges again.

4. Transfer the product to sequencing tubes; vortex, centrifuge, and heat the samples to 95°C for 2 min, and then place tubes on ice. Analyze the DNA sequences using the ABI PRISM 310 Genetic Analyzer.

3.2.8. Analysis of Sequences

DNA chromatograms show peaks of fluorescence corresponding to the DNA sequence.

1. Export the data in text format into the NCBI BLAST database for analysis.

2. Identify and compare the sequence obtained for each clone to the predicted amplicon sequence as was designed for each RQ-PCR PPP set.

3.3. Standard Curve Assays

RQ-PCR can provide either 'relative' or 'absolute' quantification of gene expression levels (*see* **Note 12**). Quantification is relative when C_t values for genes of interest are corrected for RNA loading using the expression level of endogenous control gene(s). Quantification is termed 'absolute' when the C_t value that corresponds to amplicon concentrations is known. Levels of each target are corrected for *18S rRNA* loading, and then using the corresponding standard curve values gene copies may be calculated. The protocol presented herein is for standard curve generated. A similar approach may be used for the human PPP sets which have been validated.

3.3.1. Serial Dilution of Plasmids

1. Dilute 50 µl of sequence-validated DNA samples with ddH$_2$O to a total volume of 70 µl.

2. Quantify 50 µl aliquots of 1:10 diluted plasmid using the A$_{260}$ values and determine purity by the A$_{260}$:A$_{280}$ values.

3. Produce a stock solution of 10^9 plasmid copies/µl for each *Hox* plasmid using the formula below, as previously described *(6)*:

$$V = \frac{(S_{\text{plasmid}} + S_{\text{insert}})(309)(1 \times 10^9)}{(1 \times 10^{-6})(6.02 \times 10^{23})C_{\text{plasmid}}} \qquad (2)$$

where *V* is the volume in microliters (µl), C_{plasmid} is the concentration of the plasmid in micrograms/microliters (µg/µl), and (S_{plasmid} + S_{insert}) is the combined size of the plasmid and insert in base pairs.

3.3.2. Linearization and Serial Dilutions of Plasmids

1. Treat plasmid DNA samples (10^9 copies/µl) with *NotI* restriction enzyme (*see* **Note 13**) by combining the following: 95 µl plasmid (10^9 copies/µl), 0.5 µl *NotI* enzyme, 19 µl NE Buffer 3, 0.2 µl BSA (10 mg/ml), 75.4 µl ddH$_2$O. Incubate at 37°C for 2 h.

2. Add 10 µl of this digest to 90 µl of ddH$_2$O to produce a solution with 10^8 template copies/µl.

3. Serially dilute plasmids in ddH$_2$O to provide a range of copy numbers from 10^7 to 10^1 copies/µl.

3.3.3. RQ-PCR

1. For each dilution, produce a master mix consisting of 25 µl of Universal Master Mix, 15 µl of ddH$_2$O, 6 µl of primer and probe mixture, and 4 µl of dilute plasmid.

2. Perform RQ-PCR following standard TaqMan cycling and temperatures (i.e., 50°C for 2 min, 95°C for 10 min, and 40 cycles of 95°C for 15 s and 60°C for 1 min) using 12.5 µl of this master mix in triplicate (*see* **Fig. 4a**).

3. Plot the C_t values obtained from serially diluted plasmids against the copy number to generate standard curves (*see* **Fig. 4b**) using the Sequence Detector System software (*see* **Note 14**).

3.4. Hox Profiling

Reliable results are produced by measuring *Hox* and *18S rRNA* genes in triplicate using 50 ng of cDNA per reaction. Thus 7 µg of cDNA is required per complete profile (40 genes × 3 = 120 reactions (× 50 ng) = 6 µg: additional 1 µg is to allow repeats to be carried out on identical cDNA master mixes). Automation

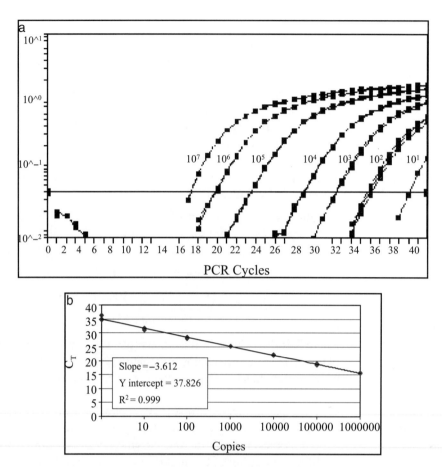

Fig. 4. (**a**) RQ-PCR amplification plots generated in triplicate by serial dilution of the sequence-validated *Hoxa1* amplicon using the *Hoxa1* PPP set. The PCR cycle where amplification plots bisect the threshold (*black horizontal line*) denotes the C_t value. (**b**) A representative standard curve produced from triplicate C_t values generated by RQ-PCR analysis of serially diluted (10^1–10^7 copies/μl) of *Hoxa1* plasmid. The slope, *y*-intercept and correlation coefficient (indicative of the kinetics), sensitivity, and reproducibility, respectively, are shown. C_t values above 35 (~10 copies) are at the limits of sensitivity for the RQ-PCR system.

of small-volume liquid handling and dedicated software for data analysis accelerate the process, enabling interrogation of larger numbers of samples. Manual handling is used for both aspects at present in our laboratory.

3.4.1. Conversion of C_t Values into Copy Number

Each cDNA under investigation is corrected for *18S* loading to produce the corrected C_t (cC_t) for each *Hox* gene as follows:

$$cC_t = 8 + \overline{C}_t - \overline{C}_t^{18S} \tag{3}$$

where $\overline{C}_t$ is the mean C_t for the subject gene and $\overline{C}_t^{18S}$ is the *18S* mean C_t. A change in the expression of a gene can be represented by the change in cC_t (ΔcC_t):

$$\Delta c C_t = c C_{t,2} - c C_{t,1} \tag{4}$$

The cC_t calculated in **Eq. 4** is then used to calculate *Hox* copies by using gradient and *y*-intercept values generated from each *Hox* standard curve (*see* **Note 13**) as follows:

$$\text{Copies} = 10^{\frac{(cC_t - z)}{m}} \tag{5}$$

where z is the *y*-intercept and m is the gradient for the *Hox* gene in question, *see* **Table 2**.

These procedures provide a rapid and convenient approach to generate *HOX* expression signatures.

Table 2
Values obtained from standard curves for each *Hox* PPP set

Gene	Slope	*y*-Inter.	Coeff.	Gene	Slope	*y*-Inter.	Coeff.
Hoxa1	−3.162	37.826	0.999	*Hoxb9*	−3.403	37.759	1.000
Hoxa2	−3.159	37.238	0.999	*Hoxb13*	−3.228	36.841	0.995
Hoxa3	−3.508	38.157	0.999	*Hoxc4*	−3.769	42.527	0.998
Hoxa4	−3.058	37.892	0.999	*Hoxc5*	−3.427	37.836	0.999
Hoxa5	−3.536	38.610	0.999	*Hoxc6*	−3.437	37.627	0.998
Hoxa6	−3.908	41.921	0.992	*Hoxc8*	−3.775	40.368	0.998
Hoxa7	−3.382	37.409	0.999	*Hoxc9*	−3.289	37.903	0.998
Hoxa9	−3.438	37.769	0.999	*Hoxc10*	−3.398	39.201	0.998
Hoxa10	−3.387	39.229	0.998	*Hoxc11*	−3.514	38.529	0.998
Hoxa11	−3.296	38.068	0.998	*Hoxc12*	−3.186	37.565	0.996
Hoxa13	−3.464	39.490	0.998	*Hoxc13*	−3.493	38.209	0.999
Hoxb1	−3.494	38.860	0.996	*Hoxd3*	−3.462	39.308	0.999
Hoxb2	−3.265	38.594	0.999	*Hoxd4*	−3.489	40.183	0.998
Hoxb3	−3.422	38.053	0.999	*Hoxd8*	−3.353	38.190	0.997
Hoxb4	−3.555	39.711	0.996	*Hoxd9*	−3.520	40.317	0.998
Hoxb5	−3.479	40.023	0.998	*Hoxd10*	−3.515	40.941	0.994
Hoxb6	−3.432	38.756	0.996	*Hoxd11*	−3.176	37.467	0.997
Hoxb7	−3.278	37.195	0.998	*Hoxd12*	−3.313	37.118	0.998
Hoxb8	−3.401	39.737	0.997	*Hoxd13*	−3.521	39.576	0.995
Pbx1	−3.429	37.87	0.999	*Meis1*	−3.567	41.41	0.999

Note: '*y*-Inter.' refers to the *y*-intercept value and 'Coeff.' is the calculated correlation coefficient for the relevant gene

4. Notes

1. The fluorescence signal threshold that is greater than background fluorescence and within the exponential phase of the RQ-PCR product amplification is defined. On the ABI 7700, the background fluorescence for transcription factors such as *HOX* genes that are expressed at a low level is typically defined by the baseline value between cycles 3 and 15. In our laboratory the threshold value (C_t) is set to 0.04 for murine *Hox* gene expression analysis and 0.02 for human *HOX* genes. For more highly expressed genes such as the *18S rRNA* reference gene the baseline is typically obtained between cycles 1 and 6 and the threshold is set to 0.05 for all applications.

2. A variety of master mixes for various RQ-PCR strategies are now available. We have tested several including Qiagen, Invitrogen, and Sigma and found them to be as reliable as the Universal Master Mix from ABI.

3. Cell samples lysed in TRIzol may be used fresh or stored at –70°C; however, freezing the homogenate improves RNA yield and quality. Where the sample is limited, cell lysis can be performed using 800 µl of TRIzol reagent and glycogen (5 µg) added to the isopropanol as a carrier for the RNA molecules. The aqueous phase is normally ~400 µl and it is convenient to remove ~200 µl of aqueous phase at a time while avoiding potential contamination from other phases.

4. In advance 0.01% DEPC-treated ddH$_2$O is prepared (50 µl DEPC in 500 ml ddH$_2$O) and autoclaved (at 121°C). Seventy-five percent ethanol:DEPC-treated ddH$_2$O is subsequently prepared (for 100 ml; 75 ml ethanol, 25 ml 0.01% DEPC-treated ddH$_2$O).

5. Over-drying of the pellet may reduce the solubility of the RNA. At this stage the RNA should appear glassy and may be difficult to identify, prior to air-drying. It may be helpful to mark the position of the pellet, particularly if the quantity is low.

6. Combine 1 µl of RNA, 1 µl of 10× loading buffer, and 8 µl of 1× TAE buffer and load gently into the agarose gel. Perform electrophoresis at 50 V. Once the samples leave the wells, increase to 150 V for 20 min. Ethidium bromide intercalates with nucleic acids, permitting their visualization under UV. The presence of ribosomal RNA bands (*28S*, *18S*, and *5S*) signifies that the RNA is intact and of adequate quality for use as a template for cDNA synthesis (**Subheading 3.1.2**). Smearing RNA signifies degraded RNA which may not be suitable for producing reliable RQ-PCR data.

7. The A_{260}: A_{280} ratio is used as an approximation of protein contamination in the RNA samples. A ratio of between 1.7 and 2.0 is acceptable for most RNA applications, e.g., the formation of cDNA.

8. Negative control master mix stocks for RT-negative samples contain equimolar quantities of all the reactants except the MMLV-RT enzyme. Each 10 µl of RT-PCR reaction mix (2×) has the capacity to convert 1 ng to 5 µg RNA.

9. Default parameters, as used by Primer Express v1.5, for designing TaqMan PPP should be set as follows:

    (a) The melting temperature (T_m) of the primers should be 58–60°C, and 59°C is optimal.

    (b) The primers should have a minimum of 20% G/C content, and an optimal length of 20 bases; however, primers between 9 and 40 bases are acceptable.

    (c) The amplicon should be between 50 and 150 bp.

    (d) The T_m of the probe should be 10°C higher than the primers and the probe should not begin with a G.

10. The reaction used to clone the amplicons is a variation of standard RQ-PCR. The total reaction volume is larger (25 µl) and includes a high concentration of template, the concentration of primers should be halved in order to reduce the formation of primer dimers, and no probe should be added since the incorporation of probe reduces cloning efficiency. The simultaneous confirmatory reaction using standard RQ-PCR (12.5 µl volume), in addition to agarose gel electrophoresis indicates whether to continue or to use an alternative source of template for cloning the amplicon. Standard TaqMan thermocycling conditions are as follows: 50°C for 2 min, 95°C for 10 min, and then 40 cycles of 95°C for 15 s and 60°C for 1 min.

11. The pGEM-T Easy plasmid, designed for cloning and sequencing of fresh PCR products, has an ampicillin resistance gene (Amp^r) and insertional inactivation of beta galactosidase (LacZ) which allows blue/white selection. Only bacterial cells that take up the plasmid form colonies on the ampicillin-containing Luria–Bertani (LB) agar. Those plasmids without a PCR amplicon have a functioning *LacZ* gene which will convert the colorless X-Gal substrate into a blue product. Those with an insert have no functioning LacZ and these bacterial colonies remain white (or light blue).

12. 'Absolute' quantification (standard curve) requires serial dilutions of a target DNA sequence to be measured, with the resulting *y*-intercept and gradient used to extrapolate gene copies in the samples of interest following their normalization to a reference gene, e.g., *18S*. 'Relative' quantification

(comparative C_t) involves calculating the ΔC_t value by normalizing expression in samples and controls. The $2^{\Delta\Delta Ct}$ value may then be calculated in line with the principle that accumulated PCR products double with each cycle *(3)*.

13. Linearizing the plasmids enhances the reliability and efficiency of standard curve generation. *NotI* enzyme digestion was chosen as the appropriate method for linearization of the plasmids since the enzyme is a unique cutter for pGEM-T, and *NotI* sites are not found in any of the *Hox* amplicons.

14. All standard curves, correlation coefficients, gradient, and intercept values were generated using the ABI 7700 Sequence Detection System and associated software (version 1.7) in accordance with the manufacturer's instructions *(7)*. The log of starting quantity and C_t values are plotted on the *x*- and *y*-axes, respectively. The correlation coefficient value indicates the reproducibility of the TaqMan system over several orders of magnitude. The *y*-intercept value indicates the level of sensitivity of the system for each target (denotes the C_t value equivalent to one copy), and the gradient reflects the robustness of the kinetics of the PCR over a range of template concentrations (indicative of the difference in C_t value that corresponds to one log difference in starting template; the optimal value is –3.3). The limit of sensitivity for TaqMan technology in our hands is ~10^1 gene copies, equivalent to a C_t value of 35–36 in most cases for *Hox* expression.

Acknowledgments

The authors would like to acknowledge Dr David Grier who played a significant role in designing the murine *Hox* RQ-PCR platform, its validation, and generation of standard curve values and Dr Momin Ahmed, Dr Sean Grimes, Dr Claire O'Neill, and Miss Alexandra Kwasniewska for help in generating and validating human *HOX* PPP sets. We are grateful to the R&D Office for Northern Ireland and the Northern Ireland Leukaemia Research Fund for funding this work.

References

1. Boncinelli E, (1994). Mallamaci A, Lavorgna G. Vertebrate homeobox genes. *Genetica*;**94**:127–40.

2. Grier DG, Thompson A, Kwasniewska A, McGonigle GJ, Halliday HL, Lappin TR. (2005). The pathophysiology of HOX genes and their role in cancer. *J Pathol*;**205**:154–71.

3. Bustin SA. (2000). Absolute quantification of mRNA using real-time reverse transcription polymerase chain reaction assays. *J Mol Endocrinol*;**25**:169–93.

4. Chomczynski P, Sacchi N. (1987). Single-step method of RNA isolation by acid guanidinium thiocyanate-phenol-chloroform extraction. *Anal Biochem*;**162**: 156–9.

5. Sambrook J, Fritsch E, Maniatis T. (1989). Plasmid Vectors. In: Molecular Cloning – A laboratory manual: (ed by C. Nolan): 1.21–1.39. Cold Spring Harbor Laboratory Press. NY.

6. Flora R, Grimwade D. (2004). Real-time quantitative RT-PCR to detect fusion gene transcripts associated with AML. *Methods Mol Med*;**91**:151–73.

7. User bulletin number #2 ABI PRISM 7700 sequence Detection System. Relative Quantification of Gene Expression Level. http://www3.applied biosystem.com/cms/groups/mcb_support/ documents/general documents/cms_040980.pdf.

Chapter 20

Genome-Wide Determination of DNA Methylation by *Hpa*II Tiny Fragment Enrichment by Ligation-Mediated PCR (HELP) for the Study of Acute Leukemias

Maria E. Figueroa, Ari Melnick, and John M. Greally

Summary

Aberrant distribution of cytosine methylation in cancer has been linked to deregulation of gene expression and genomic instability. DNA methylation changes in cancer include both hyper and hypomethylation, and the precise localization of these changes is directly related to the impact they have on gene regulation. To determine both the localization and extent of DNA methylation status under different conditions, we have developed the *Hpa*II tiny fragment enrichment by ligation-mediated PCR (HELP) assay, a microarray-based technique that allows the simultaneous interrogation of the methylation status of hundreds of thousands of CpG dinucleotides. The HELP assay allows methylation levels throughout the genome to be accurately determined so that the epigenetic state of leukemia cells can be identified, compared, and contrasted.

Key words: Cytosine methylation, CpG dinucleotide, Microarray, Epigenetic, Epigenome, Acute leukemia

1. Introduction

Epigenetic deregulation is now recognized as a hallmark of cancer *(1)*. Abnormal cytosine methylation in cancer has been linked to aberrant gene expression as well as genomic instability *(2)*. Specific changes in DNA cytosine methylation of gene promoters that alter their regulatory status have been described for a number of genes involved in differentiation and cell cycle regulation, such as $p15^{CDKN2B}$ *(3, 4)*, homeobox protein A5 (*HOXA5*) *(5)*, CCAAT/enhancer binding protein delta (C/EBP delta) *(6)*, and the tumor suppressor deleted in bladder cancer 1 (*DBC1*) *(7)*.

C.W.E. So (ed.), Leukemia, *Methods in Molecular Biology, vol. 538*
© Humana Press, a part of Springer Science + Business Media, LLC 2009
DOI: 10.1007/978-1-59745-418-6_20

Furthermore, the methylation status of $p15^{CDKN2B}$ and the estrogen receptor α ($ER\alpha$) has recently been shown to predict relapse risk in patients with acute myeloid leukemia (AML) *(8)*. The development of methods to study epigenetic marks on a genome-wide basis is therefore crucial for furthering our understanding of epigenetic mechanisms in leukemogenesis. The HELP (*HpaII* tiny fragment enrichment by ligation-mediated PCR) assay is a microarray-based technique, which allows the determination of DNA methylation status at hundreds of thousands of *HpaII* sites simultaneously across the genome *(9)*.

The assay is based on the differential digestion of genomic DNA by the two isoschizomers *HpaII* and *MspI*. These enzymes both recognize the same restriction site (5′-CCGG-3′). The second cytosine is part of a CpG dinucleotide, a target for cytosine methylation in vertebrate genomes. Although *MspI* will always cut between the first and second cytosines, whether the CpG is methylated or not, *HpaII* will only cut when both cytosines are unmethylated. Because

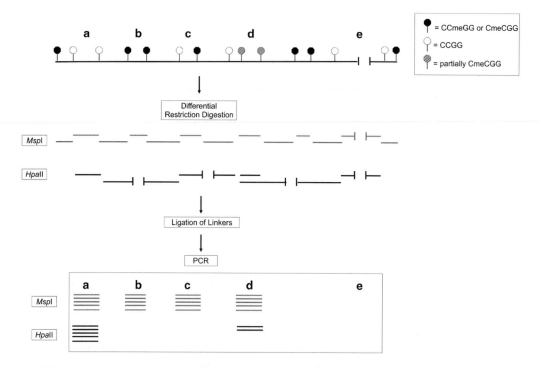

Fig. 1. Schematic representation of the HELP assay. Genomic DNA is digested by either *MspI* or its methylation-sensitive isoschizomer *HpaII*. Specific adapters are ligated onto the fragments generated by both digestions, and then amplified by ligation-mediated PCR. Each fraction is then labeled with a specific dye and co-hybridized onto a microarray designed to cover *HpaII* amplifiable fragments across the genome. The proportional intensity of each signal will reflect the methylation status of the *HpaII* sites interrogated by each fragment. (**a**) When both flanking sites are unmethylated a signal will be obtained with both enzymes. (**b** and **c**) When either one or both flanking sites are methylated, then a signal will be detected only on the *MspI* channel. (**d**) partial methylation will be reflected by an increase in the *HpaII* signal proportional to the amount of hypomethylation present in the samples. (**e**) Fragments greater than 2,000 bp will not be successfully amplified during the PCR and will therefore give no signal on either channel of the microarray.

of the presence of methylated CpG dinucleotides in the genome, *Hpa*II will therefore generate fewer and longer fragments than *Msp*I. DNA adapters of known sequence are then ligated to the sticky ends of the DNA generated by the enzymes, and a primer complimentary to these linkers is subsequently used in a PCR reaction for the amplification of the *Hpa*II and *Msp*I representations, in a ligation-mediated PCR reaction. PCR conditions have been optimized to amplify fragments between 200 and 2,000 bp, thus ensuring the preferential amplification of CpG dinucleotide-dense regions that may be contained within CpG islands and other regulatory sequences. Any given fragment will be present in both the *Msp*I and *Hpa*II fractions only when both of its flanking *Hpa*II sites are unmethylated. If, however, one or both of the flanking *Hpa*II restriction sites are methylated, then *Hpa*II will not be able to cut at that site and the fragment will therefore only appear in the *Msp*I representation of the genome. By determining the relative abundance of any given fragment in both representations we can estimate the proportional cytosine methylation at that region of the genome (**Fig. 1**).

2. Materials

2.1. Genomic DNA Extraction

1. $1\times$ PBS: 137 mM NaCl, 2.7 mM KCl, 4.3 mM Na_2HPO_4 $\cdot 7H_2O$, 1.4 mM KH_sPO_4.

2. 1 M Tris–HCl, pH 8.0: Dissolve 121.14 g Tris-base into about 800 ml of de-ionized ultra-filtered (DIUF) water and adjust pH to 8.0 with HCl. Fill up the solution to 1 L and autoclave.

3. 1 M EDTA: Dissolve 186.12 g EDTA into DIUF water; make up to 1 L and autoclave.

4. 20% SDS: Dissolve 20 g of SDS in autoclaved DIUF water. Bring the solution to a final volume of 100 ml.

5. RNAse A (Sigma, St Louis, MO): Resuspend in water to a final concentration of 10 mg/ml. Aliquot and store at –20°C.

6. Extraction buffer: 10 mM Tris–HCl, pH 8.0, 0.1 M EDTA, pH 8.0, 0.5% SDS, 20 µg/ml RNAse A. Make up fresh each time.

7. Phenol–Chloroform–Isoamyl alcohol (PCI): 25 volumes of phenol: 24 volumes of chloroform: 1 volume of isoamyl alcohol. Make up fresh each time.

8. 3 M Sodium acetate, pH 5.2: Dissolve 123.04 g of sodium acetate in distilled water and fill it up to 500 ml. Use glacial acetic acid to adjust pH to 5.2.

9. 100% Ethanol.

10. 70% Ethanol.

11. Glass Pasteur pipette.

2.2. Amplification of HpaII Tiny Fragments from Genomic DNA

1. *Hpa*II (New England Biolabs, Ipswich, MA).

2. *Msp*I (New England Biolabs).

3. Phenol–chloroform mix: 1 volume of TE-saturated phenol:1 volume of chloroform. Make up fresh each time.

4. Primer JHpaII12 (HPLC purified): 5′-CGGCTGTTCATG-3′
   - Resuspended to a concentration of 6 OD/ml

5. Primer JHpaII24 (HPLC purified): 5′-CGACGTCGAC-TATCCATGAACAGC-3′
   - Resuspended to a concentration of 12 OD/ml

6. Pre-annealing of linkers: Mix equal volumes of the 12-mer and 24-mer linkers (6 OD/ml and 12 OD/ml, respectively) in a screw-top Eppendorf tube. Boil for 5 min and then allow the reaction to cool down to room temperature. The annealed linkers can then be stored at –20°C.

7. 1 M Tris–HCl, pH 8.9: Dissolve 121.14 g Tris-base into about 800 ml of DIUF water and adjust pH to 8.9 with HCl. Fill up the solution to 1 L and autoclave.

8. 1 M Ammonium sulfate: Dissolve 13.21 g of ammonium sulfate in distilled water, make up to 100 ml and autoclave.

9. TE buffer pH 8.0: 10 mM Tris–HCl pH 8.0, 1 mM EDTA pH 8.0

10. 5× RDA buffer: 335 mM Tris–HCl pH 8.9, 20 mM $MgCl_2$, 80 mM $(NH_4)_2SO_4$, 50 mM of β-mercaptoethanol and 0.5 mg/ml of BSA in a final volume of 50 ml with autoclaved DIUF water. Filter-sterilize and aliquot into 1.5-ml tubes and store at 4°C. The buffer is stable for 2 months at 4°C.

11. 4 mM dNTP mix: Dilute from 10 mM stock. Make 200 ml aliquots and store at –20°C.

12. Native Taq polymerase (Invitrogen, Carlsbad, CA).

3. Methods

Identification of hypomethylated regions by the HELP assay depends on the differential digestion and amplification of genomic DNA based on its 5-methylcytosine content. For this difference to become evident, the assay relies on the selective digestion of the DNA at the 5′-CCGG-3′ restriction site recognized by *Hpa*II and

*Msp*I. For this purpose, intact high molecular weight genomic DNA must be used and the restriction digestion reaction must be carried out in such a fashion that digestion to completion is ensured. The protocol as described here has been optimized for such purposes and it is highly recommended that the reader adhere to it in order to ensure the effectiveness and reproducibility of the assay.

3.1. Genomic DNA Extraction

High molecular weight genomic DNA is required for the HELP assay. As the assay is based on selective cutting of the DNA at specific cytosines, genomic DNA used in this assay must appear intact, without any signs of shearing. Although any method for genomic DNA extraction that produces DNA of this quality can be used, we recommend using a standard phenol–chloroform extraction followed by ethanol precipitation and spooling of the DNA with a glass rod as follows (*see* **Note 1**):

1. Pellet down 2–3 million cells (*see* **Note 2**) at room temperature for 5 min at $300 \times g$. Remove supernatant, resuspend the cell pellet in 1 ml of 1× PBS and wash once by spinning 5 min at $300 \times g$. Discard the supernatant.

2. Resuspend the cell pellet in 50 µl of 1× PBS. Pipet up and down until no cell clumps are visible. Add 500 µl of extraction buffer and incubate at 37°C for 1 h in a water bath.

3. Add 2.75 µl of proteinase K (20 µg/µl) to a final concentration of 100 µg/ml and incubate overnight at 50°C in a water bath.

4. Add 1 volume (550 µl) of TE-saturated phenol and mix well by inversion (10 min on the rocker is best); centrifuge for 5 min at room temperature at top speed in micro centrifuge (16,000 $\times g$). Do not mix by vortexing, as this may shear the DNA.

5. Transfer the supernatant into a new tube, leaving behind any impurities and being careful not to disturb the interface. Add an equal volume of PCI (25:24:1) and mix well by rocking for 10 min at room temperature; then centrifuge for 5 min at room temperature at $16,000 \times g$.

6. Transfer the supernatant into a new tube, measure the volume. *If the supernatant is not totally clear, then repeat* **step 5** *until the supernatant becomes completely clear.*

7. Add 1 µl of glycogen (20 mg/µl stock), 1/10 volume of 3 M sodium acetate (pH 5.2), and 2.5 volumes 100% ethanol. Mix gently by inversion. A visible DNA fiber will form. Remove it with the tip of a pipette or with a glass hook (made from heating and twisting the tip of a glass Pasteur pipette). Rinse thoroughly by submerging in 70% ethanol and then transfer into a 2-ml Eppendorf tube (*see* **Note 3**) containing 200 µl of 10 mM Tris–HCl pH 8.0 (*see* **Note 4**).

   - If a DNA fiber does not become clearly visible after adding the 100% ethanol, then proceed to **step 8**.

8. Spin at 4°C for 1 h at 16,000 × *g* and then carefully remove the supernatant without disturbing the DNA pellet. Add 700 μl of 70% ethanol and spin for 30 min at 4°C at 16,000 × *g*. Carefully remove the supernatant without loosening the pellet. Do *not* air dry the pellet as this may significantly reduce its solubility. Dissolve the pellet in 200 μl of 10 mM Tris–HCl pH 8.0. Place on the rocker at room temperature and allow it to dissolve completely over 24 h.

9. On the following day, quantify the DNA using a spectrophotometer and run 1 μl on a 1% agarose gel (**Fig. 2a**). If the DNA is still very sticky, then increase the volume of 10 mM Tris–HCl pH 8.0 and leave another 24 h on the rocker to dissolve.)

10. Do not proceed with digestion or amplification if the DNA does not appears to be intact.

3.2. Amplification of HpaII Tiny Fragments by Ligation-Mediated PCR

1. Set up a restriction digestion of 1 μg genomic DNA with 2 μl of either *Hpa*II or *Msp*I in separate 200 μl reactions, using NEB buffer #1 for *Hpa*II and buffer #2 for *Msp*I as recommended by the manufacturer. Incubate overnight at 37°C (*see* **Note 5**).

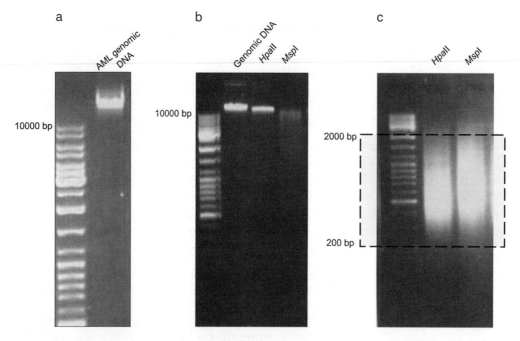

Fig. 2. Genomic DNA electrophoresis. (**a**) High molecular weight genomic DNA from an Acute Myeloid Leukemia (AML) sample. (**b**) Uncut AML high molecular weight genomic DNA (*left lane*) and after digestion with *Hpa*II (*center lane*) and *Msp*I (*right lane*). (**c**) HELP PCR amplification products. A smear spanning from 2,000 to 200 bp can be clearly seen when 10 μL of PCR products are run on a 1.5% agarose gel.

2. Run 15 µl of the digested DNA on a 1% agarose gel. The two digests should appear different: for the *Hpa*II digest, most of the DNA will remain high molecular weight, whereas with *Msp*I there should appear an almost even smear with no remnant of high molecular weight DNA (*see* **Note 6**) (**Fig 2b**).

3. Add 200 µl of TE buffer pH 8.0 to the digested DNA and 400 µl of saturated phenol:chloroform mix (1:1) and vortex briefly. Centrifuge at 16,000 × *g* for 10 min at room temperature.

4. Remove top (aqueous) phase (about 400 µl) from last step and transfer into a clean tube. Add 1 µl of glycogen (20 µg/µl) and 40 µl of 3 M NaOAc pH 5.2 and mix well. Then add 1,000 µl of 100% ethanol, vortex and spin at 16,000 × *g* for 45 min at 4°C.

5. Remove the supernatant and wash the pellet with 70% ethanol. Once you have carefully removed all of the ethanol, resuspend the pellet in 15.5 µl of 10 mM Tris–HCl pH 8.0. Set up the linker ligation on the same day, as the digested DNA will have sticky, single-stranded overhangs that may re-anneal or degrade.

6. Set up ligation reaction in a PCR tube as follows:

5× T4 DNA ligase buffer	6 µl
DNA from last step	15.5 µl
Pre-annealed JHpaII linkers	7.5 µl
T4 DNA ligase	1 µl

Incubate overnight at 16°C in a PCR thermocycler with a heated lid (*see* **Note 7**).

7. On the following day, remove the reactions from the thermocycler and transfer to a clean Eppendorf tube. Dilute each reaction with 970 µl of 10 mM Tris–HCl pH 8.0. The linker-ligated DNA can be stored indefinitely at –20°C.

Set up the PCR reaction as follows in a 1.5-ml tube:

	*Msp*I	*Hpa*II
Diluted ligated DNA from last step (µl)	40	80
JHpaII 24 (12 OD/ml) (µl)	8	8
5× RDA buffer (µl)	80	80
4 mM dNTP mix (µl)	32	32
Native Taq (Invitrogen) (µl)	3	3
Water (µl)	237	197
Total (µl)	400	400

Divide the reaction mix in four PCR tubes and incubate in a thermocycler as follows:

1. 72°C for 10 min

2. 20 cycles of: 30 s at 95°C 3 min at 72°C

3. 10 min at 72°C

4. Hold at 4°C.

8. Run 10 µl of PCR product on a 1.5% agarose gel. A smear of DNA from 200–2,000 bp should be clearly visible (**Fig 2c**).

9. Clean the product using a QIAquick PCR purification kit from Qiagen (Qiagen, Valencia, CA) (*see* **Note 8**), eluting in 50 µl of elution buffer. Quantify the PCR products using a spectrophotometer and run 1 µl on a 1.5% gel to verify that the fragment size range was not altered during the clean-up process.

3.3. Product Labeling and Microarray Hybridization

To determine the proportion of *Hpa*II (unmethylated) to *Msp*I (methylated + unmethylated) representations, HELP PCR products must then be labeled and both fractions co-hybridized onto a microarray. The array must be specifically designed to cover genomic regions contained between two consecutive *Hpa*II restriction sites. These sites occur at different intervals across the genome, but since PCR conditions have been optimized to amplify fragments between 200 and 2,000 bp, only genomic regions contained between *Hpa*II sites located within this distance should be included in the design of the array. These fragments are referred to as "*Hpa*II amplifiable fragments" and 1,016,980 of them can be found in the March 2006 assembly of the human genome (HG18), of which the majority is expected to be unique. The choice of which *Hpa*II amplifiable fragments should be included in the array design is highly dependent on the biological question of interest to the researcher. Both whole genome and focused arrays have been successfully used for DNA methylation studies using HELP by our group and others *(10, 11)*. Similarly, the choice of microarray platform is also something that can be adapted to the needs and resources of each investigator. Any of the currently available technologies that allow the researcher to customize the platform can be used, and the extent of the coverage of each fragment can be adjusted according to the number of fragments to be included and the density of oligonucleotides allowed by the technology of choice.

Our group has chosen to use custom-designed oligonucleotide microarrays from Roche NimbleGen for our studies. The standard microarray has been designed to cover between 1 and 3 *Hpa*II amplifiable fragments per promoter region, using between 10 and 15 probes per *Hpa*II amplifiable fragment. Such designs have been used not only for human studies *(12, 13)*, but also for other species, such as mouse *(9)*, and rat *(14)*. However, current ongoing studies are also using microarrays that have been specifically designed to cover the needs of particular research groups (i.e., covering every single *Hpa*II amplifiable fragment on specific chromosomes or selectively covering promoters known to be regulated by a specific transcription factor)

Roche NimbleGen uses Cy-labeled random primers (9mers) for the labeling of the *Hpa*II and *Msp*I fractions for hybridization. The Cy5-labeled *Hpa*II and Cy3-labeled *Msp*I representations are then co-hybridized onto the corresponding microarray platform and scanned using a GenePix 4000B scanner (Axon Instruments) *(15)*. Specific labeling, hybridization, and scanning protocols will vary according to the microarray platform of choice, and we therefore recommend that the reader refer to the manufacturer's protocols for these steps, as this will help to ensure the highest level of performance in each case.

3.4. Data Analysis and Interpretation

After hybridization and image acquisition, two raw data files are generated for each sample: one for *Hpa*II and one for *Msp*I. The actual steps involved in the analysis will be highly dependent on the microarray platform and assay design chosen by the researcher. However, some general concepts will be common to all designs. As discussed above, proportional methylation at the different *Hpa*II sites can be determined by the relative abundance of the fragment contained between them in the two fractions. Three steps must be followed in order to arrive to that point:

1. *Data summarization:* If more than one oligonucleotide was used to represent each *Hpa*II amplifiable fragment, then the information (i.e., intensity) from all of these oligonucleotides must be summarized as one value per fragment.

2. *Identification of failed fragments:* As *Msp*I represents the total population of possible fragments and therefore the internal control of the method, any fragments that are not generating signal in the *Msp*I representation must be excluded from the analysis. A fragment may be absent in the *Msp*I fraction both for technical and biological reasons. Technical reasons include lack of amplification of the fragment during the PCR step, as well as failure during the labeling or hybridization reactions. Biologically, a given fragment can be absent due to the presence of a genomic deletion, a frequent event in cancer, or the presence of a polymorphism at the restriction site, which prevents it from being recognized by the restriction enzymes.

3. *Computation of Hpa II to Msp I ratios for each fragment:* In a final step, the relative proportion of *Hpa*II to *Msp*I signal must be determined for each fragment. When the distribution of the population of these proportions is studied, a bimodal distribution becomes readily apparent, showing the presence of a methylated fraction of the genome (lacking a *Hpa*II signal) and a hypomethylated fraction, with increasing amounts of *Hpa*II signal (**Fig. 3**).

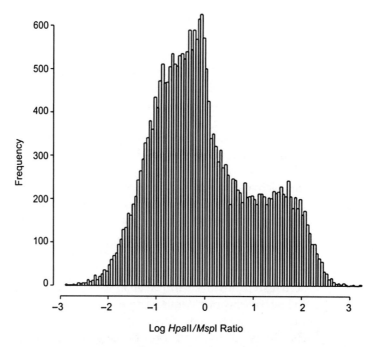

Fig. 3. Frequency histogram of the log *Hpa*II to *Msp*I ratios. In a typical analysis a bimodal distribution will reflect the presence of a methylated fraction of the genome -with no or minimal *Hpa*II signal- (*left peak*), and a hypomethylated fraction -with increasing amounts of *Hpa*II signal- (*right peak*).

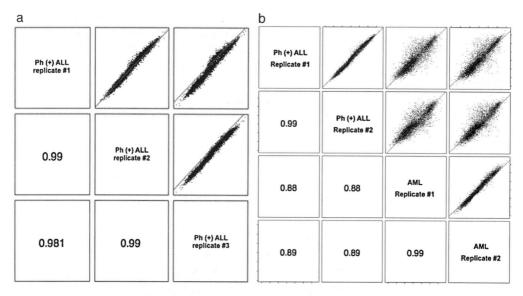

Fig. 4. Correlation between methylation profiles from leukemia patients. Correlation matrix showing scatter plots (*upper panel*) and Pearson correlation value (*lower panel*) for (**a**) three technical replicates from an Acute Lymphoblastic Leukemia (ALL) case, showing high degree of technical reproducibility, and (**b**) an ALL vs. AML comparison, where the lower correlations and broader scatter plots reflect the underlying differences in DNA methylation profiles between the two cases.

When the protocol is followed as described above, we find that technical reproducibility is very high, with Pearson correlation coefficients between replicates greater than 0.96 (**Fig. 4**).

Once the data has been processed as described above, comparisons between different biological samples may be carried out. To identify the methylation differences that naturally separate the samples into different groups, unsupervised clustering analysis may be carried out. A number of different algorithms may be used for this type of analysis, including hierarchical clustering, k-means clustering, principal component analysis, and correspondence analysis. In all these cases the algorithms look for variability in methylation profiles across the different samples, and then segregate them according to their dissimilarities. Unsupervised analysis therefore, permits the unbiased identification of subgroups based on the similarities and differences in their DNA methylation profiles.

If, on the other hand, one wishes to compare the DNA methylation profiles of two previously known groups of samples (e.g., normal hematopoietic progenitors vs. leukemia blasts), then a supervised analysis has to be carried out, in which one group is compared to the other. Several statistical tools have been developed specifically for the supervised analysis of microarray data. Many algorithms have been published that deal with the specific problems and limitations of analysis of complex microarray data, and an extensive review of these exceeds the scope of this chapter. We would like however, to briefly mention the permutation-based method SAM (significance analysis of microarrays) *(16)*, which is widely used and well accepted for the supervised analysis of microarray data. This algorithm, like most of these tools, was initially developed for gene expression microarrays, yet it is likewise useful for the analysis of HELP microarrays.

All of these biological comparisons of HELP data will lead to the identification of differentially methylated *Hpa*II fragments, which are linked to specific genomic regions. Depending on the microarray design chosen by the researcher, these regions may correspond to gene promoters, intergenic regulatory regions and/or even intragenic regions. The known genes as well as the genomic sequences themselves that align with the *Hpa*II amplifiable fragments identified as differentially methylated can then be easily extracted from the microarray design file and used for more complex bioinformatic studies. Currently there are many bioinformatic tools available, such as DAVID *(17)*, GeneMerge, *(18)* TRANSFAC *(19)*, and SOMBRERO *(20)*, among others. These tools can be used for pathway analysis (DAVID), gene ontology analysis (DAVID and GeneMerge), for the identification of common transcription factor binding sites (TRANSFAC) or for the discovery of new sequence motifs (SOMBRERO) that are enriched in the differentially methylated regions identified with HELP.

4. Notes

1. If however, a limited number of cells are available (less than 1 million cells), we then recommend the use of Qiagen's Gentra PureGene kit (Qiagen) according to manufacturer's instructions. This kit has proven useful in recovering sufficient DNA of good quality under these conditions. We strongly advise *against* the use of column-based DNA extraction kits, since these produce DNA that is sheared and difficult to cut with restriction enzymes.

2. This number is adequate when working with frozen samples. If using fresh cell lines, then we recommend using between 1 and 2 million since the yield of DNA is typically higher.

3. A 2-ml tube is recommended since the glass hook may not fit adequately in a smaller tube.

4. The volume of Tris–HCl buffer will depend on starting cell numbers and usual yields for each cell type. Usually volumes between 100 and 1,000 µl are required.

5. Since the success of the assay relies on the comparison of the *Msp*I representation to the *Hpa*II representation, incomplete digestion of the DNA can significantly affect results. For this reason, we strongly recommend adhering to the overnight digestion of DNA by the two isoschizomers, rather than attempting shorter incubations, which may cause incomplete digestion of the genomic DNA.

6. Samples with extreme genome-wide hypomethylation will show only very little high molecular weight remnant with *Hpa*II.

7. To ensure the ligation of the linkers to the vast majority of the genomic DNA fragments, a standard overnight ligation with T4 DNA ligase is recommended instead of a fast ligation reaction. Using a fast ligation might result in only a fraction of the fragments being ligated to the linkers, with the subsequent loss of the remaining fragments during the PCR amplification step.

8. Qiagen recently changed the binding buffer from the previous PB buffer to a version including a pH indicator (PBI buffer). This pH indicator may interfere with subsequent labeling of the PCR products for microarray hybridization, so it is Qiagen's recommendation that for this purpose the old PB buffer be used. The company supplies this buffer at no extra cost when requested.

References

1. Plass C. Cancer epigenomics. (2002) *Hum Mol Genet* **11**(20):2479–88.
2. Herman JG, Baylin SB. (2003) Gene silencing in cancer in association with promoter hypermethylation. *N Engl J Med* **349**(21):2042–54.
3. Tessema M, Langer F, Dingemann J, Ganser A, Kreipe H, Lehmann U. (2003) Aberrant methylation and impaired expression of the p15(INK4b) cell cycle regulatory gene in chronic myelomonocytic leukemia (CMML). *Leukemia* **17**(5):910–8.

4. Melki JR, Vincent PC, Clark SJ. (1999) Concurrent DNA hypermethylation of multiple genes in acute myeloid leukemia. *Cancer Res* **59**(15):3730–40.

5. Strathdee G, Sim A, Soutar R, Holyoake TL, Brown R. 2007 HOXA5 is targeted by cell type specific CpG island methylation in normal cells and during the development of acute myeloid leukaemia. *Carcinogenesis* **28**(2):299–309.

6. Agrawal S, Hofmann WK, Tidow N, et al. 2007 The C/EBP{delta} tumor suppressor is silenced by hypermethylation in acute myeloid leukemia. *Blood* **109**(9):3895–905.

7. San Jose-Eneriz E, Agirre X, Roman-Gomez J, et al. 2006 Downregulation of DBC1 expression in acute lymphoblastic leukaemia is mediated by aberrant methylation of its promoter. *Br J Haematol* **134**(2):137–44.

8. Agrawal S, Unterberg, M, Koschmieder, S, zur Stadt, U, Brunnberg, U, Verbeek, W, Buchner, T, Berdel, WE, Serve, H and Muller-Tidow, C. 2007 DNA methylation of tumor suppressor genes in clinical remission predicts the relapse risk in acute myeloid leukemia. *Cancer Res* **67**(3):1370–7.

9. Khulan B, Thompson R, Ye K, et al. 2006 Comparative isoschizomer profiling of cytosine methylation: the HELP assay. *Genome Res* **16**(8):1046–55.

10. Thompson RF, Figueroa ME, Melnick AM, Greally JM. 2006 Epigenetic dysregulation of candidate cis-regulatory sequences in hematological malignancies. *Blood* **108**(11):631a.

11. Glass J, Thompson R, Khulan B, et al. 2007 CG dinucleotide clustering is a species-specific property of the genome. *Nucleic Acids Res* **35**(20):6798–807.

12. Figueroa ME, Fandy T, McConnell MJ, et al. 2007 Myelodysplastic syndrome (MDS) displays profound and functionally significant epigenetic deregulation compared to acute myeloid leukemia (AML) and normal bone marrow cells. *Blood* **110**:345.

13. Figueroa ME, Wouters BJ, Li Y, et al. 2007 Genetic vs. epigenetic disruption of the CEBPA locus yields epigenomically and biologically distinct leukemia phenotypes. *Blood* **110**:2117.

14. Thompson RF, Simmons RA, Greally JM, Barzilai N. 2007 Experimental intrauterine growth retardation (IUGR) induces global epigenetic changes in rats. Proceedings of the 67th Annual Scientific Sessions of the American Diabetes Association 0390-OR.

15. Selzer RR, Richmond TA, Pofahl NJ, et al. 2005 Analysis of chromosome breakpoints in neuroblastoma at sub-kilobase resolution using fine-tiling oligonucleotide array CGH. *Genes Chromosomes Cancer* **44**(3):305–19.

16. Tusher VG, Tibshirani R, Chu G. 2001 Significance analysis of microarrays applied to the ionizing radiation response. *Proc Natl Acad Sci U S A* **98**(9):5116–21.

17. Dennis G, Jr., Sherman BT, Hosack DA, et al. 2003 DAVID: Database for annotation, visualization, and integrated discovery. *Genome Biol* **4**(5):P3.

18. Castillo-Davis CI HD. GeneMerge – postgenomic analysis, data mining, and hypothesis testing. *Bioinformatics* 2003;**19**(7):891–2.

19. Wingender E, Chen X, Hehl R, et al. 2000 TRANSFAC: an integrated system for gene expression regulation. *Nucleic Acids Res* **28**(1):316–9.

20. Mahony S, Golden A, Smith TJ, Benos PV. 2005 Improved detection of DNA motifs using a self-organized clustering of familial binding profiles. *Bioinformatics* **21** Suppl 1:i283–91.

21. Genome-Wide Determination of DNA Methylation by *Hpa*II Tiny Fragment Enrichment

22. Genome-Wide Determination of DNA Methylation by *Hpa*II Tiny Fragment Enrichment

Chapter 21

Chromatin Immunoprecipitation (ChIP) for Analysis of Histone Modifications and Chromatin-Associated Proteins

Thomas A. Milne, Keji Zhao, and Jay L. Hess

Summary

Disruption of epigenetic regulators of transcription is a central mechanism of oncogenesis. Many of the advances in the understanding of these mechanisms are attributable to the successful development of chromatin immunoprecipitation (ChIP) for in vivo detection of histone modifications as well as chromatin binding regulatory proteins. This is a powerful technique for analyzing histone modifications as well as binding sites for proteins that bind either directly or indirectly to DNA. Here we present two ChIP protocols. The first is particularly useful for identifying histone modifications or binding at specific, known genomic sites. The second, employing serial analysis of gene expression, is particularly powerful for the discovery of previously unidentified sites of modification or binding.

Key words: Chromatin immunoprecipitation, ChIP, Histone modification, Acetylation, Methylation, Quantitative PCR, SAGE

---

1. Introduction

Chromatin immunoprecipitation (ChIP) is a powerful technique for analyzing histone modifications as well as binding sites for proteins that bind either directly or indirectly to DNA [1, 2] (**Fig. 1**). These techniques are based on the ability of formaldehyde to form protein–protein and protein–DNA Schiff's base cross-linkages that can be reversed by acid or increased temperature. The immunoprecipitated DNA can then be detected by a variety of ways, including Southern blotting, conventional PCR, quantitative PCR, hybridization to arrays ("Chip-on-chip"), or cloning and sequencing (ChIP-serial analysis of gene expression – "ChIP-SAGE"). Although straightforward in principle, the ChIP

C.W.E. So (ed.), Leukemia, *Methods in Molecular Biology, vol. 538*
© Humana Press, a part of Springer Science + Business Media, LLC 2009
DOI: 10.1007/978-1-59745-418-6_21

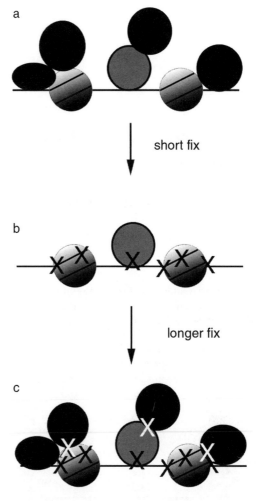

Fig. 1. (a) Nucleosomes (*gray shaded circles*) are intimately associated with DNA at multiple contact points. A transcription factor (*grey circle*) can bind DNA directly but may have only a single interaction point. Other proteins (*black circles*) may interact with DNA only indirectly through interactions with DNA bound proteins. (b) A short fixation efficiently crosslink's (*black "X"*) histones and transcription factors to DNA, but the indirectly bound proteins are less likely to be efficiently cross-linked (c). Longer fixation efficiently cross-links (*white "X"*) the indirectly bound proteins, but histone proteins may become masked by excessive cross-linking to other proteins or by alterations of lysine residues.

technique is dependent on many variables, such as the specific antibody, cross-linking conditions, and sonication conditions that must be empirically determined. Here we present protocols for ChIP with PCR or Q-PCR detection as well as ChIP-SAGE approaches. A number of reviews have been published on ChIP-on-chip (*3, 4*) and a number of companies now offer ChIP-on-chip solutions. One excellent source for protocols and an overview of this approach is given in www.chiponchip.org.

2. Materials

2.1. ChIP with PCR Detection

Most buffers and reagents used are from the Upstate Chromatin Immunoprecipitation (ChIP) kit (Cat No. 17-295) or EZ ChIP™ (Cat No.17-371) kit (Upstate Biotechnology, Charlottesville, VA).

1. Sterile PBS.

2. 10% Paraformaldehyde stock: Microwave 18 mL of PBS in a 50-mL tube placed in a beaker with water until water starts to boil (leave lid of tube slightly ajar). Do the subsequent steps in a hood. Add 2 g of paraformaldehyde (wear a mask when weighing out) and 140 µL of 1 M KOH. Vortex carefully until the paraformaldehyde dissolves. Add additional PBS to 20 mL (about 500 µL). Cool to 37°C before use. Can be stored as frozen aliquots indefinitely.

3. DMP/DMSO/PBS: 20 mM DMP solution in 25% dimethyl sulfoxide (DMSO)/PBS (77.75 mg DMP + 3.75 mL DMSO + 11.25 mL PBS).

4. Dimethyl pimelimidate dihydrochloride (DMP, Sigma D8388).

5. Elution buffer prepared fresh either from EZ kit™ components or by dissolving 0.5 g SDS and 0.42 g $NaHCO_3$ (1% SDS, 0.1 M $NaHCO_3$)in 50 mL sterile Milli-Q™ water.

6. Protease inhibitors (generally use 1:100 dilution of protease inhibitor cocktail (Sigma No. P8340).

7. DNAse-free Proteinase K.

8. Qiagen QIAquick™ PCR purification kit (cat no. 28104).

9. Chromatin IP kit (Upstate Biotechnologies: Cat no. 17-295) or EZ kit (Upstate Biotechnologies: cat no. 17-371)

2.2. ChIP Coupled with SAGE

2.2.1. Linker and Primer Sequences

1. Linker WL1: 5′-[biotin]GCGGTGACCCGGGAGATCT-GAATTC-3′ (PAGE-purified).

2. Linker WL2: 5′-GAATTCAGATC-3′ (PAGE-purified).

3. SAGE Linker 1A: 5′-TTTGGATTTGCTGGTGCAGTACAACTAGGCTTAAT-ATCCGACATG-3′(PAGE-purified).

4. SAGE Linker 1B: 5′-TCGGATATTAAGCCTAGTTGTACT-GCACCAGCAAA-TCC[amino mod.C7]-3′(PAGE-purified).

5. SAGE Linker 2A: 5′-TTTCTGCTCGAATTCAAGCTTCTAACGATGTACGTCC-GACATG-3′(PAGE-purified).

6. SAGE Linker 2B: 5′-TCGGACGTACATCGTTAGAAGCTT-GAATTCGAGC-AG[amino mod.C7]-3′(PAGE-purified).

7. SAGE Primer 1: 5'-[dual biotin]GTGCTCGTGGGATTT-GCTGGTGCAGTACA- 3'(PAGE-purified).

8. SAGE Primer 2: 5'-[dual biotin]GAGCTCGTGCTGCTC-GAATTCAAGCTTCT.

2.2.2. Other Reagents

1. DNA END™ -repair kit (Epicentre Biotechnologies, Cat No. ER0720).

2. 10× END-Repair buffer: 330 mM Tris–acetate, pH 7.8, 660 mM potassium acetate, 100 mM magnesium acetate, 5 mM dithiothreitol.

3. T4 DNA ligase (400 U/μL, New England Biolabs, catalog no. M0202S).

4. 10× T4 DNA ligase buffer: 500 mM Tris–HCl, pH 7.5, 100 mM magnesium chloride, 100 mM dithiothreitol, 10 mM ATP, 250 μg/mL bovine serum albumin.

5. Dynabeads binding buffer: 10 mM Tris–HCl, pH 7.5, 1 M sodium chloride.

6. 1× TAE buffer: 40 mM Tris–acetate, 1 mM EDTA, pH 8.0.

7. Pfu enzyme (Stratagene, cat no. 600135).

8. Nla III (New England Biolabs, cat no. R0125S).

9. Dynabeads™ M280 Strepavidin (Invitrogen, cat. no. 1112-05D).

10. Sph I-digested pZero-1™ (Invitrogen).

11. Electromax™ DH10Bs bacteria (Invitrogen).

2.3. Antibodies for ChIP

The success of ChIP is highly dependent on the antibodies used, which must recognize formalin-fixed epitopes. One way of assessing the likelihood that antibodies will work for ChIP is to perform immunofluorescent staining of cells fixed under the same conditions used for ChIP. In addition, if there is a question of whether the immunoprecipitation is successful the ChIPped chromatin can be boiled in SDS loading buffer and analyzed by western blotting. Some of the antibodies that have been successfully used for ChIP are listed below.

2.3.1. Histone Modifications

1. Histone H3 dimethyl lysine 4 (Abcam: #ab7766).

2. Histone H3 trimethyl lysine 4 (Abcam: #ab8580).

3. Histone H3 trimethyl lysine 4 (Upstate Biotechnologies: #07-473).

4. Histone H3 dimethyl lysine 79 (Upstate Biotechnologies: #05-835).

5. Histone H3 trimethyl lysine 27 (Upstate Biotechnologies: 07-449).

6. Histone H3, polyacetylated (Upstate Biotechnologies: #06-599).

7. Histone H3 acetyl lysine 9 (Upstate Biotechnologies: #06-942).

8. Histone H3 acetyl lysine 14 (Upstate Biotechnologies: #07-353).

9. Histone H3 acetyl lysine 27 (Upstate Biotechnologies: #07-360).

10. Histone H4, polyacetylated (Upstate Biotechnologies: #06-866).

11. Histone H4 acetyl lysine 5 (Upstate Biotechnologies: #07-327).

12. Histone H4 acetyl lysine 8 (Upstate Biotechnologies: #07-328).

13. Histone H4 acetyl lysine 12 (Upstate Biotechnologies: #07-323).

14. Histone H4 acetyl lysine 16 (Upstate Biotechnologies: #07-329).

2.3.2. Antibodies for Chromatin-Associated Proteins

1. Rbbp5 (Bethyl Laboratories, Montgomery, TX: cat no. A300-109A).

2. Menin (Bethyl: A300-105A).

3. Estrogen receptor (ER) Ab10 (Lab Vision-Neomarkers, Fremont, CA, TE111.5D11, #MS-315-PO).

4. Estrogen receptor (ER) Ab3 (Lab Vision-Neomarkers AER308, MS-170-PO).

5. MLL1 antibodies (Bethyl: A300-086A).

3. Methods

This protocol is a minor modification of the Upstate Biotechnology protocol that accompanies their chromatin IP kit.

3.1. ChIP and PCR Detection

3.1.1. Fixation

General Fixation

1. For fibroblasts, use 5×10^5 cells per ChIP experiment. For 293 cells, hematopoietic cells or primary human cells, use 5×10^6 cells per ChIP experiment.

2. For histone ChIP or standard transcription factor ChIP (*see* **Note 1**), fix cells for 10 min with 1% freshly made or frozen paraformaldehyde in media at 37°C. For proteins that are members of multisubunit or nucleosome remodeling complexes (*see* **Note 2**), fix cells using the alternate DMP fixation protocol outlined below.

3. For adherent cells, remove media/paraformaldehyde and rinse cells 1× with PBS. Scrape cells into 5 mL PBS with protease inhibitors. Alternatively the protease inhibitor cocktail from EZ ChIP™ kit can be used. Pellet the cells at 364 × g for 5 min. Continue with **step 5**.

4. For nonadherent cells, fix in a small volume of 1% paraformaldehyde in media (~5 mL). When fixation is complete, dilute cells 10× with 45 mL of RPMI. Spin at 364 × g, 5 min, remove the majority of the RPMI. Transfer the remainder to a new tube (10 mL). Rinse with PBS and continue with **step 5**.

5. The pellet can be flash frozen on dry ice at this point and stored at –80°C or you can continue with the protocol at this point. If continuing at this point, freeze/thaw the cells once to facilitate cell disruption. Fixed pellets can be stored frozen for several months without loss of signal.

Alternate Fixation Protocol with Dimethyl Pimelimidate Dihydrochloride (DMP) (Based on Robyr et al. 2004) *(5)*

1. Remove a bottle of dimethyl pimelimidate dihydrochloride from the freezer and allow it to warm to room temperature before opening (it is highly hygroscopic).

2. Rinse cells gently with PBS and then fix cells either directly on the plate or in a 1.5-mL tube by rocking at room temperature for 1 h (for a 10-cm dish use 5 mL DMP/DMSO/PBS, for a 1.5-mL tube use 400 μL DMP/DMSO/PBS).

3. Add 1% paraformaldehyde (in PBS) directly to the plate/tube for a final concentration of 2/3% paraformaldehyde (i.e., add 10 mL 1% paraformaldehyde to 5 mL of DMP solution or 800 μL to 400 μL solution).

4. Seal the plates with Parafilm™ or rotate in 1.5-mL tubes at room temperature in a fume hood for 5–20 h (empirically determine time for different proteins).

5. Spin down at 364 × g, 5 min and rinse cells with PBS being careful not to lose material on the walls of the tube.

6. Add lysis buffer and begin ChIP protocol. Alternatively, the pellet may be frozen at this point. The samples should be aspirated 3× through a 27G needle. The sonication conditions will also need to be increased empirically (for e.g., Bioruptor™ for 20 min on high with a 0.5-min cycle). Continue with **step 4** in **Subheading 3.1.2**.

3.1.2. Lysis and Sonication

1. Add 100 μL of chromatin lysis buffer (+ protease inhibitors) per 5×10^5 MEF cells (or 5×10^6 or more cells per ChIP for "smaller" cell types) and place in 1.5-mL microfuge tube on ice for 10 min.

2. Syringe passage 3× with a 27-gauge needle; centrifuge briefly between passages if mixture gets foamy. Do the first and second passes and spin briefly at 15,000 × g, then follow with third pass.

3. Sonication conditions must be empirically determined depending upon the specific sonicator and the fixation conditions used. As an example, for a 10 min, 1% paraformaldehyde fixation, a Diagenode™ Bioruptor set at high for 10 min (0.5 min cycle) is usually sufficient for sonication of DNA to 200–700 bp. If using the DMP fixation outlined below, sonication should be increased to two cycles of 10-min each.

4. Spin at 15,000 × g for 20 min at 4°C. Transfer supernatant to a 15-mL tube and dilute 10× with chromatin dilution buffer plus protease inhibitors. Save several 50-µL aliquots of diluted chromatin. These aliquots represent input and comprise about 5% of the total chromatin used per ChIP. These should be flash frozen and stored at –20°C to be processed along with the immunoprecipitated samples.

3.1.3. Immunoprecipitation

1. Add antibodies to tubes (usually 1–5 µL/mL, depending on the antibody). One tube without antibody (or pre-immune serum if available) should be used as a no antibody control. We have not found a preclearing step to be necessary.

2. Rotate at 4°C overnight.

3. Collect immune complexes with 60 µL of a 50:50 slurry of agaroseA (or agaroseG for mouse monoclonal antibodies) and salmon sperm DNA slurry (from kit) by rotating for 1 h at 4°C. The slurry is viscous and should be gently mixed immediately before using and transferred using wide bore pipette tips.

4. Pellet beads by centrifugation. Spin tubes briefly until the centrifuge gets up to speed, or by spinning at 94 × g for 1 min. Longer spins may crush the beads. Wash the beads for 3–5 min on a rotating platform with 1 mL of each of the following kit buffers (labeled wash buffers 1–5) (1) Low salt immune complex buffer; (2) High salt immune complex buffer; (3) LiCl immune complex wash buffer; (4) 1× TE; 5. 1× TE. All washes should be performed at 4°C.

5. Elute immune complexes by adding 100 µL of elution buffer to pelleted beads. Vortex briefly at 15,000 × g to mix and incubate at RT for 15 min with rotation. Spin down the beads; carefully transfer supernatant (eluate) to another tube and repeat elution. Combine eluates.

6. Add 8 µL of 5 M NaCl (from kit) to the combined eluates and reverse crosslinks at 65°C overnight. At this point, thaw the input DNA (50 µL) and add 150 µL of elution buffer and 8 µL of 5 M NaCl. Process along with IPs (also 65°C overnight). The tubes can be flash frozen after reversing the crosslinks if desired.

7. The next day, add 4 µL of 0.5 M EDTA, 8 µL of 1 M Tris–HCl, pH 6.5 and 1 µL of 10 mg/mL Proteinase K to the eluate. Incubate for 1 h at 45°C.

8. Recover DNA using a Qiagen Qiaquick™ PCR kit according to the manufacturer's basic protocol. Alternatively, DNA can also be purified either by phenol:chloroform extractions or with the Upstate EZ™ ChIP kit.

9. Analyze ChIPped chromatin using quantitative PCR or ChIP-SAGE (*see* **Notes 3 and 4**).

3.2. Analysis of ChIP DNA Using the Long-SAGE Protocol

A different approach is required if the gene targets of interest are not known. One approach is the use of ChIP–on-chip on genome-wide arrays. Serial analysis of gene expression (SAGE), a technique for high-throughput analysis of gene expression, has also been used for high-throughput analysis of histone modifications and DNA binding proteins. SAGE is based on the principle that short sequence tags contain sufficient information for the identification of a transcript and the number of tags from a particular transcript reflects the absolute abundance of the transcript in the cell. In the modified SAGE protocol (Long-SAGE) *(6)*, the cDNA synthesized from the mRNA isolated from the cells is digested with Nla III restriction enzyme and ligated to a linker containing a class II restriction enzyme sequence (Mme I). Digestion with Mme I cleaves the DNA 21 bp away from its recognition site and releases a 21-bp tag from the cDNA. The short tags are concatenated to 1–2 kb molecules, which are then cloned and sequenced.

ChIP coupled with SAGE has been used to analyze genome-wide histone modification patterns in yeast and human cells *(7–9)*. Because of the quantitative nature of SAGE, this procedure requires minimal normalization. Moreover, it does not require preselected probes and, therefore, can identify any genomic loci that are modified. The combination of this method with the recently developed high throughput sequencing techniques, such as massive parallel signature sequencing (MPSS), provides a comprehensive, quantitative, and economical method for analyzing genome-wide epigenetic modifications of the human genome.

1. After ChIP (**Subheading 3.1.3**), use a DNA END™ -repair kit to blunt the DNA ends by mixing 0.1–0.3 µg of ChIP DNA, 5 µL of 10× END-Repair™ buffer, 5 µL of 2.5 mM each dNTPs, 5 µL of 10 mM ATP, 1 µL of END-Repair™ Enzyme mix (T4 DNA polymerase and T4 polynucleotide kinase). Adjust to 50 µL of volume and incubate at room temperature for 45 min. The DNA is purified using phenol–chloroform extraction and ethanol precipitation.

2. Ligate the annealed biotinylated WL1 + 2 linker to the repaired DNA ends by mixing 38 µL of the ChIP DNA, 5 µL of 10× T4 DNA ligase buffer, 5 µL of 8 µM of the WL1 + 2 linker, 2 µL of T4 DNA ligase (400 U/µL). Incubate at 14°C for 14 h. Purify the DNA using the QIAquick™ column.

3. Amplify the DNA with linkers using the 5′ biotinylated WL1 as the primer by mixing 34 µL of DNA, 5 µL of 10× Pfu buffer, 5 µL of 1 mM dNTPs, 5 µL of 10 µM of WL1, and 1 µL of Pfu enzyme. First incubate the reaction mixture at 74°C for 10 min to synthesize the complementary strand of the linker region. Then cycle as follows: 94°C, 30 s; 58°C, 30 s; 74°C, 45 s; repeat the cycle 17×. Purify the DNA using the QIAquick™ column.

4. Digest the DNA with 10 U of Nla III at 37°C for 2 h. Purify the DNA with phenol–chloroform extraction and ethanol precipitation.

5. Ligate with the SAGE linkers 1(A + B) and 2(A + B): Resuspend the DNA in 66 µL of 1× T4 DNA ligase buffer and dispense it into two tubes (33-µL each). Add 5 µL of 8 µM SAGE linker 1(A + B) to tube 1 and 5 µL of 8 µM long-SAGE linker 2(A + B) to tube 2. Heat the mixture at 50°C for 2 min and incubate at room temperature for 10 min. Add 2 µL of T4 DNA ligase to each tube and incubate at 16°C for 16 h.

6. Combine the two ligation mixtures and dilute with 160 µL of binding buffer. Add the mixture to 1 mg of Dynabeads™ M280 Strepavidin. Incubate at room temperature for 15 min with occasional mixing. Discard the supernatant and wash beads twice with 200 µL of binding buffer and once with 1× TE.

7. Digest beads-bound DNA with Mme I by adding 244 µL of H$_2$O, 30 µL of 10× New England buffer 4, 3 µL of 5 mM S-adenosylmethionine, 3 µL of 100× BSA, and 20 µL of 2 U/µL Mme I. Incubate at 37°C for 3 h with occasional mixing.

8. Collect the supernatant and purify the DNA using phenol–chloroform extraction and ethanol precipitation.

9. Resuspend the DNA in 9 µL of 1× T4 DNA ligase buffer. Add 1 µL of T4 DNA ligase and incubate at 16°C for 16 h.

10. Amplify the ditags using SAGE primers 1 and 2. Mix 100 µL of 10× Pfu buffer, 100 µL of 1 mM dNTPs, 50 µL of DMSO, 35 µL of 10 µM primer 1, 35 µL of 10 µM primer 2, 650 µL of H$_2$O, 10 µL of the ligation mixture, and 20 µL of 2.5 U/µL of Pfu polymerase. Dispense into aliquots of 50 µL. Cycle as follows: 94°C, 20 s; 55°C, 30 s; 74°C, 40 s; repeat 22×.

11. Purify the PCR products using phenol–chloroform extraction. Digest the DNA with Nla III by mixing 320 µL of DNA, 40 µL of 10× buffer 4, 4 µL of 100× BSA, and 40 µL of Nla III (10 U/µL) and incubating at 37°C for 2 h. Stop the reaction by adding 400 µL of 1×TE + 2 M NaCl.

12. Transfer the reaction mixture to an Eppendorf tube containing 1 mg of Dynabeads™ M280 (strepavidin). Mix at room temperature for 15 min.

13. Transfer the supernatant to a new tube containing 1 mg of Dynabeads™ M280 (strepavidin). Mix at room temperature for 15 min.

14. Repeat **step 13** three times.

15. Transfer the supernatant to a new tube and purify the DNA using phenol–chloroform extraction and ethanol precipitation.

16. Resuspend the DNA in 30 μL of 1× TE. Load the DNA into six lanes of a 12% mini acrylamide gel and resolve the DNA fragments by electrophoresis at 100 V for 1 h.

17. Visualize the DNA bands by ethidium bromide staining and excise the band of approximately 38 bps.

18. Spin the gel slices though a 21-gauge hole at the bottom of an Eppendorf™ tube and extract the DNA from the gel with 500 μL of 1×TE + 100 μL of 7.5 M NH$_4$OAc by incubation at 37°C for 2 h with shaking. Purify the DNA with ethanol precipitation.

19. Resuspend the DNA in 9 μL of 1× ligase buffer. Add 1 μL of T4 DNA ligase and incubate at 16°C for 1 h.

20. Resolve the ligation products on 1.4% per 1× TAE agarose gel. Excise the DNA fragments from 500 to 1,000 bp. The DNA is purified using the QIAEX II™ gel extraction kit.

21. Ligate to a sequencing vector by mixing 7 μL of the concatenated DNA, 1 μL of 20 ng/μL of Sph I-digested pZero-1™, 1 μL of 10× T4 DNA ligase buffer, and 1 μL of T4 DNA ligase. Incubate at 16°C for 16 h. Transform Electromax™ DH10Bs bacteria using the ligation mixture by electroporation. Plate the transformation mixture with ampicillin selection. Prepare DNA from individual colonies and analyze the insert by standard enzymatic sequencing reaction.

22. Alternatively, the concatemers can be directly sequenced by the MPSS-like high throughput sequencing services provided by companies such as 454 Lifesciences (Branford, CT). Each sequencing run can generate around 2×10^7 bp of DNA sequences.

23. The sequences obtained either by the traditional sequencing method or the 454 high throughput technique are analyzed using the SAGE2000 v.4.5 program developed by the Johns Hopkins University to extract the 21 bp sequence tags and to quantify the tags. The sequence tags are then compared with a reference library generated from Nla III cutting sites in the human genomic sequence available at UCSC or NCBI databases.

4. Notes

1. Fixation conditions for ChIP must be determined empirically. The optimal conditions appear to vary depending on whether the protein of interest (a) binds directly to a specific DNA sequence such as transcription factors, (b) binds directly to DNA but in a sequence-independent manner such as histones, or (c) binds to DNA only indirectly via interactions with complexes of proteins such as histone methyltransferases or members of nucleosome remodeling complexes (**Fig. 1**). Generally the fixation conditions should be minimized, especially when dealing with histones as lysine residues are structurally altered by fixation. For histone or histone modifications we have had good results with ChIP when cells are fixed for 10 min with 1% formaldehyde at 37°C. The same conditions work well with transcription factors that are directly bound to DNA as the efficiency for DNA:protein cross-linking is very high (**Fig. 1b**).

2. When doing ChIP with proteins that are subunits of large molecular weight complexes, multiple protein:protein as well as protein:DNA fixation steps may be required (**Fig. 1c**). In this case, the signal can often be increased with a multistep fixation procedure employing both a protein:protein cross-linker, such as DMP and then a long formaldehyde cross-linking step. These conditions can increase signal intensity nearly tenfold; however, the conditions need to be optimized because the background signal also increases.
   Sonication conditions must also be empirically determined. The longer the fixation protocol, the more difficult it will be to sonicate the DNA efficiently. We have found that passage of lysed chromatin through a 27G needle before sonication improves the efficiency of sonication. We recommend analyzing the sonicated DNA on agarose gels. For optimal ChIP experiments, DNA fragments should be between 200 and 1,000 bp with a mean fragment size of approximately 500 bp.

3. Although conventional PCR may be used for detection in ChIP, in practice, this approach only works well when the differences between signal and noise are significant. For subtle changes or for weaker ChIP signals, quantitative PCR offers many advantages including analysis in the linear range of the PCR reaction and for a rigorous analysis of IP efficiency. We routinely use TaqMan™ primer/probe sets or SYBR green™. Primer Express™ software (ABI) is helpful for designing primers or primer/probe sets, but care must be taken to visually inspect primers to make sure the GC content is between 20 and 80% and to make sure that the TaqMan probe does not

start with a G. Both SYBR green™ and Taqman™ reactions generate curves that can be analyzed as discussed below.

There is no uniformly agreed approach for quantification of ChIP results. The most common approach is to quantitate immunoprecipitation efficiency as an IP:Input ratio. The two main ways of doing this include using standard curves with a dilution series of an input sample, or comparing input vs. IP signal directly. The approaches yield similar results. For brevity we discuss the second approach. The amount of genomic DNA coprecipitated with antibody is calculated as a percentage of total input using the following formula $\Delta C_T = C_T(\text{input}) - C_T(\text{chromatin IP})$, % total $= 2^{\Delta CT} \times 5.0\%$ (**Fig. 2**). A 50-µL aliquot taken from each of 1 mL of sonicated, diluted chromatin before antibody incubation serves as the input (see protocol). The signal from the input samples represents 5% of the total chromatin used in each ChIP. C_T values are determined by choosing threshold values in the linear range of each PCR reaction (*see* **Fig. 2** for a sample calculation).

4. In using Q-PCR for ChIP analysis, it is important to recognize that quantified values are not direct measures of absolute protein levels. The strength of the ChIP signal is dependent on multiple factors including the strength of the antibody:epitope interaction, the accessibility of the epitope after fixation, as well as the absolute amount of protein present at the locus.

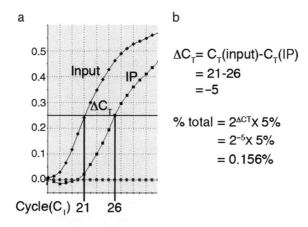

Fig. 2. (**a**) Quantitative PCR curve for input (*black curve*) and chromatin IP (*grey curve*) samples. The threshold value (*horizontal line*) is chosen in a region where the curves are linear. CT is the difference in cycle # at the threshold (i.e., between the input and IP curves there is 5 cycle difference) (**b**) A sample calculation. The difference in cycle number between the input and IP samples is −5 (the higher the cycle number, the lower the amount of starting material). Since each cycle indicates a doubling of material, there is 2^{-5} or about 3/100 the amount of material in the IP sample compared to the input. The input represents 5% of the chromatin used in the ChIP experiment (see protocol); therefore the IP is about 3/100 × 5% or 0.15% of the total chromatin.

A second important factor is that background signal is inherent to ChIP experiments even in the absence of antibody, raising the question of how to distinguish between background and "real" signal. Contamination by cloned DNA representing target sequences when these are also being handled can be a major impediment to successful ChIP. If at all possible, the pre- and post-PCR areas should be separated. Ideally, ChIP experiments should include the following controls:

(a) A cell line lacking the protein of interest to use as an antibody control

(b) A set of gene targets that are not bound or regulated by the protein of interest

(c) A set of positive gene targets that do not change upon experimental manipulation

For example, in **Fig. 3a**, MLL ChIP gives a very strong signal in $Mll^{+/+}$ cells at the *Hoxa9* locus (0.65%). In $Mll^{-/-}$ cells, this signal is reduced to below 0.05%, validating the ChIP assay and establishing this as the background range for this antibody (**Fig. 3a**). At the *Gapdh* locus, which microarray experiments suggest is not regulated by Mll, the signal is below 0.05% in both $Mll^{+/+}$ and $Mll^{-/-}$ cells, indicating that this locus is not bound by Mll.

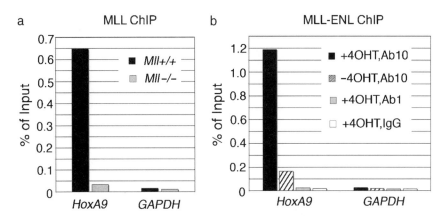

Fig. 3. Comparison of ChIP signal vs. background signal. (**a**) ChIP with antibodies against MLL was performed in MEF cells that were either wild type for *Mll* ($Mll^{+/+}$, *black bars*) or were *Mll* knockout cells ($Mll^{-/-}$, *grey bars*). A strong signal is seen at the *Hoxa9* locus in $Mll^{+/+}$ cells and this signal is reduced to below 0.05% in $Mll^{-/-}$ cells indicating that this is in the background range for this antibody. Binding at *GAPDH* is below this threshold in both cell types indicating that it is negative for Mll binding, at least at the specific region of *GAPDH* examined. (**b**) MLL-ENL-ER, a MLL fusion protein fused to the estrogen receptor, is active only in the presence of 4-OHT (10). Ab10 recognizes the fusion protein and shows a strong binding signal at *Hoxa9* in the presence of 4-OHT (*black bar*). In the absence of 4-OHT, signal is drastically reduced but not completely abolished (*striped bar*). Ab1, (*grey bars*) which does not recognize the fusion protein, gives a similar signal as IgG (*white bars*).

Conditional models are particularly powerful for ChIP experiments (**Figs. 3 and 4**). As an example, when fused to the estrogen receptor (ER), the MLL–ENL fusion protein is only active in the presence of tamoxifen (4-OHT). When ChIP is performed with the antibody Ab10, which recognizes the ER present in MLL–ENL, a strong signal is seen at *Hoxa9* (**Fig. 3b**, black bar) in the presence, but not absence, of 4-OHT (**Fig. 3b**, striped bar, about 0.2%). A small amount of residual binding is seen in the absence of 4-OHT. Two different antibodies that do not recognize the

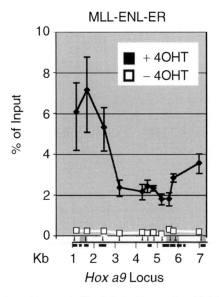

Fig. 4. Using the same experimental conditions as in **Fig. 3**, but with a series of Q-PCR primers (1–7) across the *Hoxa9* locus allows for graphical representation of MLL-ENL-ER binding (reprinted with permission from **ref. 10**).

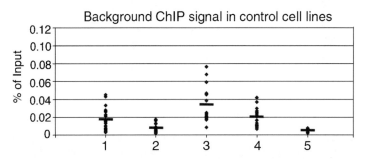

Fig. 5. Background ChIP signals in control cell lines and with control antibodies. *1* MLL ChIP in *Mll*^{−/−} cells, *2* MLL ChIP in *Mll*^{−/−} cells using a Bethyl antibody (cat. no. A300-086), *3* menin ChIP in *menin*^{−/−} cells, *4* rabbit anti-mouse IgG ChIP in *Mll*^{+/+} cells, *5* anti-FLAG ChIP in 293 cells. Each point on the graph represents a separate ChIP experiment quantified for a "positive" gene target (e.g., *HOXA9*) in a control cell line or with a control antibody. Cells were fixed for 10 min in 1% paraformaldehyde. The two MLL antibodies tested in *Mll*^{−/−} cells (1 and 2) produce background signal up to about 0.05%. The menin antibody produces a higher range of background signal (up to 0.08%) in menin^{−/−} cells, but all antibodies are below 0.1%.

fusion protein (Ab1 and general IgG) give a signal again below 0.05% (white and grey bars) and Ab10 in both + and – 4-OHT treated cells gives a signal below 0.05% at *Gapdh*, indicating that the residual binding seen at *Hoxa9* is likely "real."

It is not always possible to include all of these controls. Our general experience is that different antibodies with different fixation conditions generally give a background, nonspecific ChIP signal in the range 0.01–0.08% of input (*see* **Fig. 5**). As a rule of thumb, any signal over 0.1% of input is likely to be significant, while below that is likely in the range of background signal.

Another approach that is particularly informative is to generate a series of primers across the locus to be examined. The graphical representation of the quantitative ChIP data can provide additional information and a higher degree of confidence that small changes in binding seen are significant (*see* **Fig. 4**).

References

1. Orlando, V. (2000). Mapping chromosomal proteins in vivo by formaldehyde-crosslinked-chromatin immunoprecipitation. *Trends Biochem Sci* **25**:99–104.

2. Kirmizis, A. and Farnham, P.J. (2004). Genomic approaches that aid in the identification of transcription factor target genes. *Exp Biol Med* **229**:705–721.

3. Huebert, D.J., Kamal, M., O'Donovan, A., and Bernstein, B.E. (2006). Genome-wide analysis of histone modifications by ChIP on chip. *Methods* **40**:365–369.

4. Shivaswamy, S. and Iyer, V.R. (2007). Genome analysis of chromatin status using tiling microarrays. *Methods* **41**:304–311.

5. Robyr, D., Kurdistani, S.K. and Grunstein, M. (2004). Analysis of genome-wide histone acetylation state and enzyme binding using DNA microarrays. *Methods Enzymol* **376**:289–304.

6. Saha, S., Sparks, A.B., Rago, C., Akmaev, V., Wang, C.J., Vogelstein, B., Kinzler, K.W. and Velculsecu, V.E. (2002). Using the transcriptome to annotate the genome. *Nat Biotechnol* **20**:508–512.

7. Roh, T.Y., Ngau, W.C., Cui, K., Landsman, D. and Zhao, K. (2004). High-resolution genome-wide mapping of histone modifications. *Nat Biotechnol* **22**:1013–1016.

8. Roh, T.Y., Cuddapah, S. and Zhao, K. (2005). Active chromatin domains are defined by acetylation islands revealed by genome-wide mapping. *Genes Dev* **19**:542–552.

9. Roh, T.Y., Cuddapah, S., Cui, K., and Zhao, K. (2006). The genomic landscape of histone modifications in human T cells. *Proc Natl Acad Sci* **103**:15782–15787.

10 Milne A. et al. (2005). Leukemogenic MLL fusion proteins bind across a broad region of the *Hoxa9* locus, promoting transcription and multiple histone modifications. *Cancer Res* **65**:11367–11374.

INDEX